Methods
in
Medical Ethics

Jeremy Sugarman and Daniel P. Sulmasy, O.F.M.,
Editors

GEORGETOWN UNIVERSITY PRESS
WASHINGTON, D.C.

Georgetown University Press, Washington, D.C.
© 2001 by Georgetown University Press. All rights reserved.
Printed in the United States of America

10 9 8 7 6 5 4 3 2 1   2001

This volume is printed on acid-free offset book paper.

Chapter 12, "Experimental Methods," by Marion Danis, Laura Hanson, and Joanne M. Garrett, is not subject to U.S. copyright.
Chapter 13, "Economics and Decision Science," by David A. Asch, © 1996 by the American Public Health Association.

Methods in medical ethics / Jeremy Sugarman, Daniel P. Sulmasy, editors.
    p. cm.
  Includes bibliographical references and index.
  ISBN 0-87840-873-8 (pbk. : alk. paper)
  1. Medical ethics. 2. Medical ethics—Research—Methodology. I. Sugarman, Jeremy. II. Sulmasy, Daniel P., 1956–

R724 .M43 2001
174'.2—dc21   2001023268

For David M. Levine, M.D., M.P.H., Sc.D.,
our fellowship director,
who was always a generous mentor and
genuine mensch. His commitment to our careers
made work on this book possible.

Contents

PART III   RELATIONSHIPS AND APPLICATIONS

Preface

Medical ethics has now become a field of scholarly inquiry that uses a wide variety of methods. These methods derive from the humanities and the social sciences, including anthropology, economics, epidemiology, health services research, history, law, medicine, nursing, philosophy, psychology, sociology, and theology. Although multiple publications examine how problems in medical ethics might be understood within the context of one or more disciplines, we were unable to identify any book that systematically examined all of these disciplines and their multiple methods of inquiry across the entire broad field of medical ethics. Given the multidisciplinary nature of medical ethics, such an examination seems wanting.

Our interest in this area began during our work as fellows in internal medicine at the Johns Hopkins School of Medicine and as graduate students in philosophy at Georgetown University. Our intensive training in both empirical research methods and philosophy made it clear to us that doing quality work in medical ethics requires immersion in one or more of the disciplines that contribute to the field. Moreover, sound training in different disciplines helps make interdisciplinary work productive, relevant, and exciting.

While we had direct experience doing work that involved several disciplines, we were interested in learning more about the ways that other disciplines with which we were less familiar addressed questions in medical ethics. To this end, in the spring of 1994 we conducted a workshop, "Approaching Research Questions in Medical Ethics from Multiple Disciplines," at the annual meeting of the Society of General Internal Medicine in Washington, D.C. We were fortunate to have noted scholars join us in this workshop: Tom Beauchamp, Ph.D. (philosophy); Gregg Bloche, M.D., J.D. (law); Barbara Koenig, Ph.D. (ethnography); Barron Lerner, M.D., Ph.D. (history); Robert Pearlman, M.D. (empirical research); and Edmund Pellegrino, M.D. (clinical ethics). The workshop confirmed our impression that having an accurate grasp of the methods employed in addressing a particular question in medical ethics is essential, not only for engaging in scholarly inquiry, but also for understanding the work that results from it.

Through these and related experiences, we became convinced that a book that examined the many methods of medical ethics would serve as a valuable resource to scholars, teachers, editors, students, and others interested in medical ethics. However, in beginning this project, we struggled with questions about which methods to include. In the end, we settled on approaches that have arguably played a significant role in the contemporary field of medical ethics. Proceeding roughly from normative to descriptive approaches, these are: philosophy; religion and theology; professional codes; law; casuistry; history; qualitative research; ethnography; quantitative surveys; experimental methods; and economics and decision science.

Editing such a book presents multiple challenges of inclusion and exclusion. While we have tried to be comprehensive in our approach, we have also, of necessity, set some boundaries on the scope of this work. First, we do not believe that all medical humanities should be subsumed under the umbrella of methods in medical ethics. These other fields are distinctive. So, for example, we have not included literature or art as methods of medical ethics to be addressed in this book. This is not because we fail to see the possible contributions of literature or the other arts in medical ethics. Quite to the contrary, we think that literature and the arts provide enormously useful tools for teaching, generating discussion, reaching the heart as well as the mind, and putting flesh on the bare bones of research. But unlike research, literature and art do not aim at creating generalized abstract knowledge, explanations, or predictions. Works of literature and art present themselves without explanation. Literature and art can illustrate virtue and vice in health care, or even raise questions for philosophers and theologians to ponder. Literature and art can also remind health care professionals of the immense humanity of their patients, of the privilege that it is to care for them, and of the fact that the encounter in the office or hospital reveals only a fraction of the person. Methods of literary criticism and art history can illuminate the ways that works of literature and art can reflect themes of moral concern in medicine. But these are different fields. It is beyond the scope of this book to describe how a painter, choreographer, or playwright goes about creating such works.

Importantly, one must also be careful to distinguish between narrative approaches to medical ethics and the use of literature or literary criticism in teaching or illustrating medical ethics. Narrative ethics is one among many competing methods of doing philosophical or theological ethics. This approach has challenged some of the major methodological assumptions in these disciplines. Narrative ethics calls for "thicker" descriptions of cases and exposes what may be considered the hidden assumptions of standard methods of philosophical or theological medical ethics. But, used in this way, narrative ethics is not a separate discipline. Recent scholarship argues for a role for narrative theory within medical ethics, primarily in critiquing or supplementing methods in the field, and therefore we have not chosen to dedicate a separate chapter to narrative theory.

In fact, within *each* of the disciplines represented in this book, there are multiple available methodological approaches. This creates challenges in finding the proper balance between comprehensiveness and depth within each chapter. While we have asked the chapter authors to survey the breadth of approaches within their respective disciplines, each author has been necessarily somewhat selective in choosing which approaches to emphasize. In general, the authors have not comprehensively addressed the full range of methodological approaches within their respective disciplines, but have concentrated on the ones with which they are most familiar. So, for example, in chapter 3, DeGrazia and Beauchamp have emphasized principlism and have not engaged in an extensive discussion of narrative, feminist, pragmatist, natural law, or care-based approaches to ethics. In chapter 4, Cahill mentions the literature in medical ethics in other religions, but ecumenically discusses a wide variety of Christian theological approaches. In general, we think our authors have struck the proper balance. We also believe that readers interested in methodological approaches that we could not cover in depth will still benefit significantly from learning to appreciate better the breadth of approaches that we have been able to capture within this one volume.

We begin *Methods in Medical Ethics* with two introductory chapters. In chapter 1, we examine the many methods of scholarship in medical ethics as well as their relationship to one another. We go on to suggest some norms governing the relationship between normative and descriptive ethics. Chapter 2 describes the nature of published empirical research in medical ethics during the decade of the 1980s as a means of demonstrating the diversity of these methods as well as the types of questions that have been addressed.

Particular methods of medical ethics are addressed in chapters 3–13. In order to provide sufficient expertise in each of these methods, we assembled a team of authors based upon their scholarly training and work in medical ethics. We feel quite fortunate that so many talented scholars decided to work with us. In each chapter dealing with a particular method, the author(s) provide an overview, a description of techniques, a critique of the method, and then notes on resources and training in the method.

The concluding chapters are designed to illustrate how these methods can relate to one another and how to assess the quality of scholarship in medical ethics. Specifically, in chapter 14 physician-assisted suicide and euthanasia are used to illustrate the richness of multidisciplinary work in medical ethics regarding a single issue. In chapter 15 the field of medical genetics is an example of how multiple descriptive methods have interrelated in examining the ethical issues in an increasingly important medical field. Finally, in chapter 16 the information gleaned from the preceding chapters is used to offer a proposed approach to being a critical reader of scholarship in medical ethics.

In creating *Methods in Medical Ethics*, we hope that scholars from all disciplines will strive for the kind of methodological excellence described by the contributors to this book, and that all readers of the medical ethics literature will develop an enhanced appreciation of the methods of disciplines other than their own. We also hope that this book will help to facilitate a more productive interdisciplinary discourse across the many methods of medical ethics.

Jeremy Sugarman, Daniel P. Sulmasy
Somewhere in the cyberspace between Durham, N.C., and New York, N.Y.

Acknowledgments

The editors are grateful to Gail Grella, our acquisitions editor at Georgetown University Press, for helping to initiate this project and for providing continuing guidance and support. We are also grateful to Suzanne Ellett for her important work with the contributing authors and in preparing the manuscript.

Contributors

Darrel W. Amundsen, Ph.D.
Department of Modern and Classical
    Languages, Western Washington
    University

David A. Asch, M.D., M.B.A.
Health Services Research, Philadelphia
    Veterans Affairs Medical Center
    and Leonard Davis Institute of
    Health Economics, University of
    Pennsylvania

Tom L. Beauchamp, Ph.D.
Kennedy Institute of Ethics and
    Department of Philosophy, Georgetown
    University

Lisa Sowle Cahill, Ph.D.
Theology Department, Boston College

Marion Danis, M.D.
Department of Clinical Bioethics,
    Warren G. Magnuson Clinical
    Center, National Institutes of
    Health

David DeGrazia, Ph.D.
Department of Philosophy, George
    Washington University

Ruth Faden, Ph.D., M.P.H.
The Bioethics Institute, Johns Hopkins
    University

Joanne M. Garrett, Ph.D.
Division of General Medicine, University
    of North Carolina

Lawrence O. Gostin, J.D., LL.D. (Hon.)
Georgetown University Law Center;
    Johns Hopkins School of Hygiene and
    Public Health

Laura Hanson, M.D., M.P.H.
Division of General Medicine,
    University of North Carolina

Gail E. Henderson, Ph.D.
Department of Social Medicine,
    University of North Carolina School
    of Medicine

James G. Hodge Jr., J.D., LL.M.
Georgetown University Law Center;
    Johns Hopkins School of Hygiene and
    Public Health

Sara Chandros Hull, Ph.D.
Bioethics Research Section, National
    Human Genome Research Institute,
    National Institutes of Health

Albert R. Jonsen, Ph.D.
Medical History and Ethics, University
    of Washington

Nancy E. Kass, Sc.D.
Program in Law, Ethics, and Health,
    Department of Health Policy and
    Management, Johns Hopkins School
    of Public Health; The Bioethics
    Institute, Johns Hopkins University

Barbara A. Koenig, Ph.D.
Stanford University Center for
    Biomedical Ethics

Patricia Loomis Marshall, Ph.D.
Center for Biomedical Ethics, Case
  Western Reserve University

Robert A. Pearlman, M.D., M.P.H.
VA Puget Sound Health Care System and
  the Departments of Medicine, Health
  Services, and Medical History and
  Ethics, University of Washington

Edmund D. Pellegrino, M.D.
Center for Clinical Bioethics, Georgetown
  University

Helene E. Starks, M.P.H.
Department of Medicine, University of
  Washington

Jeremy Sugarman, M.D., M.P.H., M.A.
Center for the Study of Medical Ethics
  and Humanities, Duke University

Daniel P. Sulmasy, O.F.M, M.D., Ph.D.
The John J. Conley Department of
  Ethics, Saint Vincents Hospital, New
  York; The Bioethics Institute, New
  York Medical College

Holly A. Taylor, M.P.H., Ph.D.
Program in Law, Ethics, and Health,
  Johns Hopkins School of Public
  Health; The Bioethics Institute, Johns
  Hopkins University

Judith Weinstein, M.A, M.P.H.
School of Public Health, University of
  Illinois at Chicago

PART I

Overview

The Many Methods of Medical Ethics (Or, Thirteen Ways of Looking at a Blackbird)

Daniel P. Sulmasy and Jeremy Sugarman

The range of scholarship falling under the umbrella of medical ethics is astounding. For instance, the disciplines of anthropology, economics, epidemiology, health services research, history, law, literature, medicine, nursing, philosophy, social psychology, sociology, and theology all have scholars in medical ethics. All of these disciplines and others have made enriching contributions to the field of medical ethics. Some employ unique methods. Others use similar methods, but have different theoretical orientations. However, it is not always clear whether or how work done in many of these disciplines is considered appropriately scholarship in medical ethics. Nor is it always clear how these methods and disciplines relate to each other. In this chapter, we provide a general orientation to the scope of these many methods and offer what we take to be proper interdisciplinary relationships in medical ethics.

TYPES OF ETHICAL INQUIRY

Philosophers hold that there are three basic types of ethical inquiry: normative ethics, metaethics, and descriptive ethics (Frankena 1973).

Normative ethics is the branch of philosophical or theological inquiry that sets out to give answers to the questions, What ought to be done? What ought not to be done? What kinds of persons ought we strive to become? Normative ethics sets out to answer these questions in a systematic, critical fashion, and to justify the answers that are offered. In medical ethics, normative ethics is concerned with arguments about such topics as the morality of physician-assisted suicide or whether it is morally proper to clone human beings.

Metaethics is the branch of philosophical or theological inquiry that investigates the meaning of moral terms, the logic and linguistics of moral reasoning, and the fundamental questions of moral ontology, epistemology, and justification. It is the most abstract type of ethical inquiry, but it is vital to normative investigations. Whether or not it is explicitly acknowledged, all normative inquiry rests upon a fundamental stance regarding metaethical questions. Metaethics asks, What does "right" mean? What does "ought" mean? What is implied by saying "I ought to do X?" Is morality objective or subjective? Are there any moral truths that transcend particular cultures? If so, how does one know what these truths are? Positions regarding all of these questions lurk below the surface of most normative ethical discussions, whether in general normative ethics or in medical ethics. Sometimes it is only possible to understand the grounds upon which people disagree by investigating questions at this level of abstraction. In many cases, however, there is enough general agreement that normative inquiry can proceed without explicitly engaging metaethical questions.

Descriptive ethics does not directly engage questions of what one ought to do or the proper use of ethical terms. Descriptive ethics asks empirical questions such as, How do people think they ought to act in this particular situation of normative concern? What facts are relevant to this normative ethical inquiry? How do people actually behave in this particular circumstance of ethical concern? In medical ethics, the literature is replete with descriptive ethics studies, such as surveys concerning what patients and doctors think about the morality of late-term abortions, about attitudes toward completing advance directives, or about perceptions concerning the risk of being tested for BRCA1/2, breast cancer susceptibility genes.

While all of these types of ethical inquiry are important, normative ethics seems to be at the core of ethical inquiry. This is not to suggest that normative ethics is more intellectual or more worthwhile than other disciplines. Rather, we suggest that the other types of ethical inquiry are only important, meaningful, and useful because of the normative questions that are at stake. One asks, "What does the word 'ought' mean?" because it is very interesting and important to know what one ought to do. As a general rule, one is only interested in knowing what percent of the population thinks something ought to be done in particular circumstances, or how people actually behave in such circumstances, if it is interesting and important to know how one ought to behave in such circumstances. It is relatively uninteresting to ask, "How often should men shine their shoes?" It is much more interesting to know how a physician ought to respond when a patient asks, "Doctor, will you help me die?"

Yet, even if normative ethics is at the core of scholarship in ethics, all these types of research are interesting and important. The methods employed to answer the three types of questions necessarily differ, but each contributes something. They all help to fill in the outlines of ethical inquiry. This can be metaphorically illustrated by the Wallace Stevens poem, "Thirteen Ways of Looking at a Blackbird" (Stevens 1951). Stevens's poem masterfully captures both the complexity and the advantages of looking at anything from a multiplicity of perspectives. Medical ethics is like this poem. Each of the thirteen stanzas of the poem illustrates another view of the blackbird. Each view tells us something about the viewer as well as something about the blackbird. No single view tells us what a blackbird is. But in sum, at the end of the poem, the reader has a better sense of the blackbird. That sense is ineluctably incomplete. But it is ever richer and fuller after thirteen views. As Stevens writes:

> The blackbird whirled in the autumn winds.
> It was a small part of the pantomime.

So it is, we suggest, with medical ethics. Neither the methods employed by philosophy nor theology nor anthropology nor history nor law nor any other methods that contribute to scholarship in medical ethics describe the blackbird called medical ethics in its entirety. But by examining a moral question from the vantage point of several different methods, one gains a richer understanding of that moral question, and a better grasp of an answer. Under ideal circumstances, each method of medical ethics contributes something that is of importance for scholars who employ other, different methods to investigate the same questions. Each method looks at the blackbird from a different angle. And ultimately, in health care, such research is vital not only to scholars, but above all to those practicing the healing professions. After all, medical ethics is, in large part, about what *these people* ought to do. And what these people do obviously has profound implications for persons when they are sick.

ONE FIELD, MANY DISCIPLINES, MANY METHODS

Is medical ethics a discipline in its own right? Recently, Albert Jonsen (1998) suggested that in a "simple sense" it is, but in "the strictest sense" it is not. Some might suggest that medical ethics is now really a single unified discipline in which any scholar can employ any of the methods described in this book that seems proper to the question at hand, jettisoning the disciplinary boundaries and theoretical assumptions that otherwise keep these disciplines from communicating with each other. Witness, for example, the growth of graduate degree programs in "bioethics." Others might suggest that the research "product" would be better if each discipline were to use the methods proper to that discipline to "do" medical ethics without ever bothering to examine how other disciplines examine questions in medical ethics, even if these other disciplines employ the same methods. The result is confusion over what medical ethics research really is, or ought to be.

We would like to bring further conceptual clarity to this discussion by carefully distinguishing between field, discipline, and method. Borrowing from the *Oxford English Dictionary*, we define a *field of inquiry* as a subject matter or set of phenomena or questions addressed by a researcher or researchers. By contrast, we define a *discipline* as a department of learning or knowledge, a community of scholars sharing common assumptions about training, modes of inquiry, the kind of knowledge that is sought, and the boundaries of the subject matter proper to the discipline. Finally, we define a *method* as a systematic procedure, technique, or mode of inquiry employed in examining research questions.

We take the view that medical ethics is a single field of inquiry of great interest to many disciplines, not a discipline in its own right. What medical ethicists share is a common subject matter, not a common disciplinary mode of investigating that subject. Their common subject matter is the normative aspect of health care. This is the medical ethicists' blackbird. It is their field. However, they view it through the eyes of a wide variety of disciplines. These disciplines employ a wide variety of methods, some shared by several disciplines and some unique to a particular discipline. Medical ethics is one field, embracing a variety of disciplines and methods.

Thus, one conducts research in medical ethics as a philosopher, or as a health services researcher, or as a historian. One can certainly be "crosstrained" in one or more of these disciplines. But the quality of scholarship, in our view, will be best when investigators have a disciplinary "home base." This will assure a firm understanding of the assumptions and the limitations of the methods proper to these disciplines, as well as assuring rigor and appropriate peer review of the research.

Yet, we urge an understanding of medical ethics as a genuinely *inter*disciplinary field. While there is constant chatter about interdisciplinary research on university campuses these days, medical ethics is a field of inquiry with enormous potential to make that chatter real. Normative questions, as stated above, are inherently interesting. These questions are of interest to scholars in many disciplines. Sadly, however, what often seems to be missing is genuine interchange between these scholars. For example, the eyes of a lawyer or philosopher often glaze over when someone describes the statistical methods used in a research project about informed consent. Or a health services researcher can be overheard muttering something about "fluff" when a theologian begins to expatiate about the relationship between the concepts of dignity and justice in health care. In this book, we hope to move beyond these stereotypes. We realize that we cannot make a casuist into a decision-scientist in a few pages. However, part of what we hope to make possible for medical ethicists is enough of a rudimentary understanding of the other disciplines in the field to help facilitate a better, genuinely interdisciplinary conversation in medical ethics.

MEDICAL ETHICS AS AN INTERDISCIPLINARY FIELD

If we are correct in our contention that medical ethics is an interdisciplinary field, then it will be incumbent upon us to suggest how the various disciplines and methods should relate to one another. The focus of this discussion will be on the relationship between normative and descriptive methods. Although metaethical questions are important in medical ethics and often lay just beneath the surface of important normative arguments, metaethics is more part of ethics in general than part of the field of medical ethics. We will therefore not discuss metaethics further. We will instead describe the proper role and the limitations of some of the methods commonly employed in normative and descriptive ethics, a topic that has received scant attention in the literature.

We will begin by discussing the fact/value distinction. We believe it is critical to understand this distinction if one is to understand the role and limits of various kinds of medical ethics research. We will then propose a series of guidelines for the proper conduct of genuinely interdisciplinary research among the various empirical and normative disciplines that contribute to medical ethics. In so doing, we hope to spark further conversation, collaboration, and investigation.

THE FACT/VALUE DISTINCTION

There is probably no single principle in ethics that is more important to discuss with respect to the relationship between descriptive and normative studies in medical ethics than the so-called fact/value distinction (Beauchamp 1982). Most (but not all) ethicists subscribe to this distinction, which is also called "the naturalistic fallacy" and the "is/ought distinction." It was originally proposed by David Hume in his *Treatise of Human Nature*, in which he noted that many ethical arguments, particularly in scholastic philosophy, consisted of a series of factual statements using the verb "is," leading to a conclusion using the verb "ought" (Hume 1978). This struck Hume as peculiar. He wondered whether any set of facts ever added up, by itself, entailing any normative conclusion.

Over the ensuing centuries there have been many discussions of this principle. Some who have attacked the fact/value distinction have noted that certain "social facts" do appear to entail normative conclusions. For example, John Searle (1969) points out that the *fact* that I made a promise to do something does seem to imply a normative conclusion, namely that I *ought* to do it. Others have argued that certain facts about the role and purpose of something or someone also seem to entail normative conclusions. Alasdair MacIntyre (1984), for example, points out that the fact that something *is* a knife does entitle one to draw certain conclusions about what an object said to be a knife *ought* to be like. What makes a knife "good" are characteristics such as sharpness, sturdiness, etc. Likewise, he argues that the fact that someone occupies a role as the practitioner of a certain human practice does entitle one to draw conclusions about what makes that individual a good practitioner (e.g., the fact that someone is a soldier implies that if he or she is a "good" soldier, one can expect courage, loyalty, dependability, etc.). Similarly, one might say that the fact that someone is a physician entitles one to draw certain conclusions about what makes that person a "good" physician (e.g., competence, compassion, respectfulness, etc.).

One counterargument to both Searle and MacIntyre might be that these "human purposes" and "social facts" are already implicitly moral. These sorts of facts are different from brute facts about the world that seem to entail no normative conclusions. On this view, social facts and human purposes would not truly violate the fact/value distinction because these sorts of facts already contain implicit moral premises. In reply, it could be argued that there really is a "purpose" to being a physician. If one could better understand what it means to be an excellent physician, one would be well on one's way to having a system of medical ethics (see, for example, Pellegrino and Thomasma 1981). While this discussion cannot be concluded here, it is important to note that questions of fact and value enfold all discussions about the relationship between normative and descriptive work in medical ethics (Pellegrino 1995).

ILLICIT INFERENCE IN MEDICAL ETHICS RESEARCH

These arguments aside, even defenders of the possibility of drawing normative conclusions from certain special facts would tend to agree that the fact/value distinction holds over a variety of important sets of facts. This allows one to conclude that there are some sorts of inferences in medical ethics research that are illicit and can be avoided.

Historical Facts Do Not Entail Normative Conclusions

One might call this the historicist version of the naturalistic fallacy. The historicist fallacy in moral argument is somewhat different from the mistakes of "presentism" and "essentialism" in historical research pointed out by Darrel Amundsen in chapter 8. For example, the mere fact that infanticide was practiced in the early Mediterranean world does not entitle one to conclude that all societies should be free to decide for themselves whether to permit this practice. Likewise, the mere fact that payment for health care has never before been organized with financial incentives for physicians to provide fewer services does not entitle one to conclude that such payment structures are immoral. Whether something has or has not been done in the past does not mean that it is moral or immoral.

Majority Opinions and Behaviors Do Not Entail Normative Conclusions

The opinion survey, a commonly used empirical technique in medical ethics, should *never* be construed to give "the answer." For example, 75 percent of young physicians in a poll might approve of sexual relationships between physicians and patients provided the physician-patient relationship, as such, is terminated once it turns sexual. However, this would not imply that the practice ought to be considered morally permissible. Likewise, the fact that many physicians say that they are willing to falsify medical insurance claims in order to obtain medically indicated treatments for their patients does not imply that such practices are morally appropriate (Freeman et al. 1999). The mere fact that almost everyone says that something is proper, or that almost everyone acts in a certain way, does not make it proper to act that way. The appeal to popular opinion can sometimes amount to an example of the informal logical fallacy of the *argumentum ad populum.* (See also chapter 5.)

As described in chapter 11, quantitative surveys are best viewed as tools to examine what clinical or social factors might be associated with particular opinions about moral issues, pointing out, for example, significant cultural divides. For example, African Americans are less likely to want to forgo life-sustaining treatment than are white Americans (Caralis et al. 1993). But it is critical to understand the limitations of such survey research in ethics. Individuals may not share group beliefs and whole cultures can be mistaken in their moral beliefs.

The Mere Fact That Something Is Legal or Illegal Does Not Make It Moral or Immoral

In general, the moral goodness of a just society will be reflected in its laws. But even Thomas Aquinas thought it unwise for a government to pass laws regarding all aspects of the moral life (Aquinas 1972). Such an effort would probably be impossible. And so, questions about the proper relationship between law and morality will be operative even in morally homogeneous societies.

However, in an increasingly multicultural democratic republic like the United States, in which the rule of law is predicated upon majority rule, it sometimes can be forgotten that laws do not give normative answers. As Hodge and Gostin point out in chapter 6, democratic procedures settle the legal aspects of moral questions by referenda or the vote of a majority of elected representatives, or a judicial decision. But not everything that is legal is moral, and not everything that is moral is legal. Laws can be immoral. Segregation in the United States was once legal, but this does not mean that these practices were moral once, and then became immoral after the law changed. Majority rule, even by free election, can commit moral error. Adolf Hitler, for example, was made chancellor of Germany by the vote of freely elected representatives in a democratic republic. In the end, ethics judges laws as morally good or morally bad.

Nor does the fact that one might be sued constitute a moral argument. The threat of a lawsuit does not render a proposed course of action moral or immoral. Legal consequences are consequences to be weighed with the same moral weight that one generally gives to other types of consequences in making moral decisions. For instance, if one is a strict deontologist, basing decisions solely upon doing one's duty, legal consequences will have no bearing on the decision whatsoever. For others, the threshold might vary for taking a moral stand depending upon practical concerns about consequences. For example, under threat of lawsuit, one might not want to make a moral issue out of a patient's refusal to be weighed daily, even though one might beneficently think that from a moral point of view, daily weights are in the patient's best interest. On the other hand, fidelity to patients and professional integrity does sometimes demand that one do what one thinks is morally correct even under threat of lawsuit.

In the end, the law does not give the answer. To illustrate this, there are cases in which one can be sued no matter which course of action one pursues. For example, if a patient clearly expresses her wishes not to be placed on a ventilator and then goes into a coma, and her husband the lawyer then demands that she be intubated when she develops respiratory distress, one could be sued no matter what course one were to pursue. Successfully resuscitating the patient could invite legal action for battery. Failure to attempt resuscitation could invite legal action for negligence. The law does not settle the moral matter. One must rely on moral analysis and do what one determines to be morally right.

The Opinions of Experts Do Not Necessarily Entail Moral Conclusions

As Edmund Pellegrino argues in chapter 5, under certain specified conditions, tradition and opinion can form important parts of sound moral arguments. There is practical value to reliance upon expertise and tradition. But it is sometimes appropriate to be certain that reliance upon this authority is justified. For example, the mere fact that a clinical ethics consultant has recommended a course of action does not mean that this is the morally correct course of action. Expert advice can and should be obtained in morally troubling cases. The opinions of experts should be taken quite seriously. But experts often disagree, and experts can be wrong. "Expertise" among ethicists, for example, is limited by their training, knowledge, practical wisdom, and potential biases. Appeal to expert opinion represents the informal logical fallacy of the *argumentum ad verecundiam*. Expertise, at times, ought to be appropriately challenged.

The Mere Fact That Something Is Biologically True Does Not Entail Automatic Moral Conclusions

For example, the mere fact that human beings do not have wings does not imply that it is immoral for human beings to fly. Likewise, the mere fact that the human fetus initiates brain wave activity at a certain stage of development does not, in itself, imply anything about the morality of abortion at one stage of development or another.

An often misunderstood moral theory relevant to this issue is known as *natural law*. It is a misconstrual of natural law theory to think that it states that morality is to be read off human biology as if one were reading a script. The way in which natural law ethics operates has more to do with a broad understanding about what it means to be a good human being and what constitutes human flourishing (Finnis 1980). Brute biological facts do not imply immediately clear moral truths.

EMPIRICAL STUDIES AND NORMATIVE ETHICS

Properly conducted empirical studies can help elucidate facts. But as discussed in detail above, the fact/value distinction precludes moral inference from brute facts. This might appear to make empirical studies irrelevant. However, such a conclusion would be premature. There are at least eight ways in which empirical studies can be important in medical ethics.

Purely Descriptive Studies

Purely descriptive studies of what human beings believe about morality, how they change with time, and how they behave in situations of moral concern can be of enormous intellectual interest in and of themselves. Anthropological studies of how human societies differ with respect to the treatment of elderly people, for instance, can be fascinating. Differences in sexual morality can be interesting. Differences in the ways in which cultures pay for medical care, whether by government insurance, private for-profit managed care organizations, or the payment of chickens to the local shaman can be very stimulating to learn about. Such studies need have no normative purpose.

Yet descriptive ethics studies are interesting precisely because they illuminate human responses to normative questions. To study how different cultures grow rice would be of interest to an anthropologist, but not necessarily to an ethicist. When anthropologists or other social scientists apply their techniques to the study of normatively interesting questions, they are "doing" descriptive ethics. In many cases, the relationship between normative ethics and descriptive ethics is only that normative ethics has raised the questions of interest for empirical study.

It is of interest to know, for example, why certain persons have the opinions they do about certain disputed normative questions even if the answers one gathers through survey research are acknowledged to have no normative implications. If Southerners, for example, were to be less concerned about the ethics of vaccinating military recruits without their consent, and this were to be found independent of race and religion, this would be an interesting empirical fact. It might lead one to ask further empirical questions or further normative questions. It deals with an interesting normative issue about research ethics, but has no normative implications in itself.

A good deal of empirical research in ethics is of this nature, carefully describing anthropological, sociological, psychological, and epidemiological facts that are of interest. They are of interest because the subject is normative. But the techniques are descriptive and the conclusions have no immediate normative implications. Nevertheless, empirical findings may introduce facts not already being considered in reaching normative conclusions, thereby better informing this work.

Testing Established or New Norms

Another way in which descriptive studies can be related to normative ethics is through studies that describe compliance with existing moral norms. Again, such studies do not answer the normative question. But provided there is widespread acceptance of a moral norm, it is of interest to study actual behavioral adherence to this norm. In studies of this type, there is no question about the norm itself. What is of interest is the extent to which human beings live up to it, or the extent to which it is legally or socially enforced. For example, in the United States today, almost everyone thinks that if patients do not wish to be connected to a ventilator, they should not receive ventilator therapy. Yet, a multicenter study of critically ill patients has shown that in many cases patients' preferences are overlooked and they frequently receive therapy they do not want (SUPPORT 1995).

In other cases, new policies or procedures designed to operationalize certain moral norms are introduced into clinical settings. Descriptive studies can help to decide whether or not the plan for operationalizing the norm has been successful. For example, studies have shown that the Patient Self-Determination Act, designed to facilitate communication about patients' wishes for end-of-life care, has fallen far short of expectations (Silverman et al. 1995). This does not mean that the norm is morally right or morally wrong. It only means that the implementation of the normative rule may need to be rethought if it is to work in real settings.

Descriptions of Facts Relevant to Normative Arguments

Good ethics depends upon good facts. Failure to understand the facts of a situation thoroughly will clearly lead to perils in moral decision making. Further, many normative arguments depend upon factual information, even though these facts themselves do not confer normative status upon the arguments. For example, one might argue that liver transplantation should be withheld from alcoholics, because the chances of relapse of alcoholism are so high that the prognosis will be poor. In fact, it turns out that the survival of alcoholic patients with liver transplants is equivalent to that of patients transplanted for other conditions (Berlakovich et al. 1994). The moral argument against transplants for alcoholics, based on a presumption of poor prognosis, is thus falsified by the facts disclosed in a descriptive study.

Reliance upon the facts in these sorts of arguments does *not* violate the fact/value distinction. The premises in these arguments both are moral *and* factual, not simply factual. Such arguments are not only permissible, but are essential to moral reasoning.

Ethics is concerned with what to do (Aristotle 1985, 35). Ethics is, in this sense, the most practical of all branches of philosophy. Moral premises relate facts to duties and virtues. Moral arguments often take forms such as,

1. Whenever situation X occurs, it is permissible to do Y
2. If Z is true, then I am in situation X.
3. Therefore, if Z is true, it is permissible to do Y.

Proposition 1 is a moral premise. Proposition 2 is empirical. Empirical studies can make important contributions to ethics if they can show whether a proposition in the form of proposition 2 is always true, or under what conditions Z obtains. Knowing this empirical information is critical to determining whether one is bound by the obligation in proposition 3.

For example, proposition 1 might be the moral rule known in medical ethics as "therapeutic privilege" (Beauchamp and Childress 1994). This states that it is morally permissible to (Y) withhold information from patients if (X) disclosing that information would cause the patient very grave harm. The key to applying this moral rule will be to determine under what conditions situation X is true. Someone might argue (as generations of physicians in the United States did up until the 1970s), that whenever patients have cancer, informing them would cause the patients great harm (Oken 1961). Physicians were constructing a moral argument based upon a proposition of the form of proposition 2: If the patient has cancer (Z), this is a situation in which disclosing the facts will cause them great harm (X). This is precisely the sort of situation in which descriptive ethics can play an enormously important role in medical ethics. In the 1970s, empirical studies were undertaken to show that patients with cancer overwhelmingly wanted to be told of their diagnosis and felt that they had the coping skills to handle it (Alfidi 1971). Further studies were then performed to demonstrate that patients, by and large, felt much better when they were informed of their diagnoses, and perhaps even evidenced better cooperation with treatment and better outcomes. Descriptive ethics studies showed that proposition 2 was false when Z was cancer. Therefore, the moral conclusion, proposition 3, could not be inferred. Physicians' practices changed. By the 1980s, 90 percent of American physicians reported that they routinely informed their patients with cancer of their diagnoses (Novack et al. 1979).

Slippery Slope Arguments

Another way in which empirical studies can uncover facts that are relevant to normative arguments is when so-called "slippery slope" arguments are invoked in moral debates. Slippery slope arguments are those that suggest that if a certain moral rule is changed, other, untoward moral consequences will follow.

These sorts of moral arguments have an empirical form. The facts to which they refer, however, are facts about a possible future that has not yet been realized. Therefore, empirical studies cannot answer the question directly about whether or not a slippery slope will occur, but they can contribute to an understanding of the likelihood that the slippery slope will occur in a given set of circumstances. Descriptive studies that can contribute to an understanding of the likelihood of slippery slopes include: (1) historical studies of similar situations, (2) studies of other settings in which the change in moral norms has already taken place, (3) psychological studies of those likely to be affected by the slippery slope concerns, and (4) legal studies of statutes and case law precedents that might be relevant.

For example, some persons worry about the morality of sex selection in prenatal genetic testing (Wertz and Fletcher 1998) and preimplantation genetic diagnosis (American Society of Reproductive Medicine 1999). One argument against giving the information might be that the percentage of geneticists willing to endorse the practice in opinion surveys appears to be growing (Wertz and Fletcher 1998). This raises the question of whether permitting the disclosure of the gender of the fetus or embryo at all will inevitably lead to psychological acceptance and widespread practice of sex selection. Slippery slope arguments are also frequently invoked in arguments about needle-exchange programs for injection drug users as a means of preventing HIV infection. Descriptive studies could help settle the question of whether this practice inevitably leads to an increase in substance abuse. One might look at the historical experience of other nations that have tried this. One might do intensive interviews with those who regularly inject themselves with illegal substances such as cocaine and/or heroin. Or, one might conduct a small pilot study to see if this result does obtain.

All of these sorts of empirical studies contribute indirectly to the slippery slope argument. To repeat, a slippery slope argument cannot be directly supported by any empirical study. The slippery slope argument envisages a likely future so fraught with moral danger that one ought not to engage in the social experiment of finding out whether the predicted slippery slope will come to pass. The argument is that the social experiment would be too risky to take. Such arguments can be bolstered or attacked, however, by indirect examinations of related facts that help to clarify how realistic such fears might be. Descriptive studies in ethics can thus play a key role in assessing the plausibility of slippery slope arguments.

Assessing Likely Consequences

Empirical studies can also suggest the consequences of certain courses of action in a manner that helps moral decision-makers. One need not be a utilitarian to pay attention to consequences in making moral decisions. For example, if the chances of a patient surviving an operation are only 1 in 5,000, the argument that it would be unjust to withhold the treatment seems much less persuasive than if the chances were 1 in 5. Similarly, data showing that cardiopulmonary resuscitation is unlikely to be effective in patients with widespread metastatic cancer may help those who must make decisions about whether it would be appropriate to use this procedure.

The Empirical Testing of Normative Theories

Sometimes the relationship between normative and descriptive ethics can be very tight and very direct. This is particularly the case when normative theory prescribes practices whose components can be empirically tested. An excellent example of this is the normative theory of substituted judgment. Based upon legal theory and moral philosophy's stress on the importance of respect for the autonomy of individuals who are making biomedical choices, the theory of substituted judgment was developed. According to this theory, when patients lose their decision-making capacity, they ought not thereby forfeit all of their autonomy. What the patient thinks and feels might not be directly known, but one might still express respect for the patient's autonomy if one were to make the decision that one thought the patient would have made if he or she had been able to speak with full decision-making capacity. Thus, one asks clinically not "What would you like us to do for your mother?" but rather, "What do you think your mother would have wanted if she had been able to tell us herself?" Decisions made in the spirit of the latter question are made according to the theory of substituted judgment (Buchanan and Brock 1989).

This is all well and good as a theoretical construct, but one notices quickly that there is an empirically testable question embedded in the theory: Just how well can a loved one predict what the patient would have wanted? Is it a charade to think that human beings, even if closely related, can actually choose what the patient would have chosen? Does asking for a substituted judgment amount to paying mere lip service to the principle of autonomy, or if we were honest with ourselves would we admit that we are choosing according to the "best interests" standard, choosing what we think is in the best interests of the patient?

This sort of provocative question has led to a series of very interesting empirical studies on the validity of substituted judgments (Uhlman, Pearlman, and Cain 1988; Zweibel and Cassel 1989; Seckler et al. 1991; Sulmasy, Haller, and Terry 1994; Sulmasy et al. 1998). In these studies, patients are asked to imagine themselves in a serious clinical situation and to choose the life-sustaining measures they think they would want in that situation. Simultaneously, the patient's surrogate decision-maker is asked what he or she thinks the patient would want. The results are then compared to see how well the surrogate does. Agreement rates have averaged about 70 percent—statistically better than chance alone, but far from perfect. This has led some ethicists to rethink the substituted judgment standard. Others have argued that the moral validity of the standard remains intact, but that what is needed are ways to improve surrogate decision making. Once again, the descriptive facts learned from empirical studies do not answer the normative question. But by calling into question the practicality of a normative ethical rule, descriptive ethics can constructively challenge normative ethics. In Kantian terms, "ought" implies "can" (Rescher 1987). One ought not establish moral duties that are impossible to carry out.

Case Reports

As in other aspects of medical practice, case reports play a role in medical ethics. Careful descriptions of unusual situations can serve as a springboard for substantial normative discussion. Others who might encounter similar situations in the future can benefit from having read and considered the ethical issues in a case encountered by a colleague at another institution. Those who subscribe to the theory of casuistry (moral reasoning by analogies between cases) as their sole method of approaching cases in medical ethics depend heavily upon good case descriptions (Jonsen and Toulmin 1988). Those who appeal to narrative and care-based theories of ethics depend upon "thick" descriptions of the case, including details about interpersonal dynamics and emotions that are often excluded from more traditional case discussions. Since case reports are now generally frowned upon as anecdotal and unscientific in the standard medical literature, in some ways, the case report has experienced something of a revival with the advent of medical ethics. As Jonsen points out eloquently in chapter 7, in ethics there is no escaping the case.

Demonstration Projects

Descriptive ethics studies can be conducted in order to demonstrate the implementation of a normative idea or standard. The empirical project thus can function as a vehicle for the promulgation of a normative idea. This happens frequently in medical ethics. It is particularly common in ethics education. Few people will argue against teaching ethics to medical students or nurses, for example. But it is sometimes important simply to demonstrate that such programs can be successfully implemented (Sulmasy et al. 1994). The content of the program might be shared so that others might benefit by comparing that content with their own program's content, or that others might be inspired to start a program of their own. Pitfalls in the implementation of the program can be discussed for the benefit of others. Such empirical descriptions might also include simple survey data about the acceptability of the course and its perceived value and importance.

Similar descriptive reports can be generated regarding other programs, such as ethics consult services, ombudsperson programs for medical students experiencing ethical conflicts in relation to faculty or residents, or programs on research integrity. All of these can contribute substantially to advancing the field of medical ethics.

Finally, as described by Danis and colleagues in chapter 12, it is possible to conduct controlled trials of such programs. For example, one might test the effectiveness of a new educational program designed to increase awareness about an ethical issue, or to promote a certain behavior that has been deemed morally obligatory or virtuous. Causal inferences about the effectiveness of such programs are most securely made in randomized controlled trials. Even having a concurrent nonrandomized control group is much better than having no control group. Such studies represent an important contribution of empirical research to medical ethics. They provide the best way to assess the efficacy as well as the unintended ill effects of new programs.

NORMATIVE AND DESCRIPTIVE ETHICS: TWO-WAY FEEDBACK

Based on the discussion above, it should be clear that the relationship between normative and descriptive research in medical ethics is one of two-way feedback (Pearlman, Miles, and Arnold 1993). Normative ethics can generate claims that are associated with empirically testable hypotheses, or set normative standards that must be operationalized and can be studied in educational or practice settings. The empirical lessons gained from such studies can, in turn, feed back upon and influence normative theory. Normative arguments may also depend upon facts that can be garnered from empirical inquiry, thus sustaining or refuting the empirical basis for the normative arguments. Descriptive ethics studies can also generate new material for normative study. Anthropological and sociological studies can raise questions about the universalizability of normative claims. Surveys can identify areas of disagreement that are ripe for ethical inquiry. Case studies can give rise to new questions that have never been addressed in normative inquiry, or can supply the entire basis for casuistic, narrative, and care-based work.

The two types of ethical inquiry are thus mutually supportive. Good studies in normative ethics will be grounded in good empirical data. Good descriptive studies will be shaped by ethical theory, providing a framework in which the data will be interpreted. Ethical reflection is enhanced when these two types of investigation are undertaken in an interdisciplinary and cooperative fashion.

CONCLUSION

We have tried, in this chapter, to present a broad overview of a rather extensive field of inquiry—medical ethics. We have distinguished studies in descriptive ethics from studies in normative ethics and metaethics. We have described medical ethics as a single field of inquiry, involving multiple disciplines and multiple methods. We have discussed the importance of the fact/value distinction, and delineated how this distinction helps to understand some illicit inferences in medical ethics research. We have suggested some norms governing the proper relationship between normative ethics and descriptive ethics, and how empirical studies can properly contribute to medical ethics.

Research in medical ethics is exciting, dynamic, and growing. If normative and descriptive work in medical ethics can be pursued in a truly synergistic fashion, we believe there will be extraordinary research opportunities that neither approach could fulfill alone (Singer, Siegler, and Pellegrino 1990). Medical ethics research is among the few academic fields in which truly interdisciplinary study is flourishing. It would be wonderful if the flavor of this interdisciplinary field were enriched further.

REFERENCES

Alfidi, R. J. 1971. "Informed Consent: A Study of Patient Reaction." *Journal of the American Medical Association* 216:1325–39.

American Society of Reproductive Medicine, Ethics Committee. 1999. "Sex Selection and Preimplantation Genetic Diagnosis." *Fertility and Sterility* 72:595–98.

Aquinas, T. 1972. *Summa Theologiae.* I–II, q. 94, a.4, c. Blackfriars Edition. New York: McGraw-Hill.

Aristotle. 1985. *Nichomachean Ethics.* 1103b.28–31. Translated by Terence Irwin. Indianapolis, IN: Hackett.

Beauchamp, T. L. 1982. *Philosophical Ethics: An Introduction to Moral Philosophy.* New York: McGraw-Hill, pp. 336–79.

Beauchamp, T. L., and J. F. Childress. 1994. *Principles of Biomedical Ethics.* 4th ed. New York: Oxford University Press, pp. 150–51.

Berlakovich, G. A., R. Steininger, F. Herbst, M. Barlan, M. Mittlbock, and F. Muhlbacher. 1994. "Efficacy of Liver Transplantation for Alcoholic Cirrhosis with Respect to Recidivism and Compliance." *Transplantation* 58:560–65.

Buchanan, A. E., and D. W. Brock. 1989. *Deciding for Others.* New York: Cambridge University Press.

Caralis, P. V., B. Davis, K. Wright, and E. Marcial. 1993. "The Influence of Ethnicity and Race on Attitudes toward Advance Directives, Life Prolonging Treatments, and Euthanasia." *Journal of Clinical Ethics* 4:155–65.

Finnis, J. 1980. *Natural Law, Natural Rights.* Oxford: Clarendon Press.

Frankena, W. 1973. *Ethics.* 2nd ed. Englewood Cliffs, NJ: Prentice-Hall, pp. 4–5.

Freeman, V. G., S. S. Rathore, K. P. Weinfurt, K. A. Schulman, and D. P. Sulmasy. 1999. "Lying for Patients: Physician Deception of Third Party Payers." *Archives of Internal Medicine* 159:2263–70.

Hume, D. 1978. *A Treatise of Human Nature.* Edited by L. A. Selby-Bigge. 3rd ed. Oxford: Oxford University Press, pp. 468–70.

Jonsen, A. R. 1998. "Bioethics as a Discipline." In *The Birth of Bioethics.* Oxford: Oxford University Press, pp. 325–51.

Jonsen, A. R., and S. Toulmin. 1988. *The Abuse of Casuistry.* Berkeley: University of California Press.

MacIntyre, A. 1984. *After Virtue.* 2nd ed. Notre Dame, IN: University of Notre Dame Press.

Novack, D. H., R. Plumer, and R. L. Smith, H. Ochitil, F. R. Morow, and J. M. Bennett. 1979. "Changes in Physicians' Attitudes toward Telling the Cancer Patient." *Journal of the American Medical Association* 241:897–900.

Oken, D. 1961. "What to Tell Cancer Patients." *Journal of the American Medical Association* 175:1120–28.

Pearlman, R. A., S. H. Miles, and R. M. Arnold. 1993. "Contributions of Empirical Research to Medical Ethics." *Theoretical Medicine* 14:197–210.

Pellegrino, E. D. 1995. "The Limitations of Empirical Research in Ethics." *Journal of Clinical Ethics* 6:161–62.

Pellegrino, E. D., and D. C. Thomasma. 1981. *A Philosophical Basis of Medical Practice: Toward a Philosophy and Ethic of the Healing Professions.* New York: Oxford University Press.

Rescher, N. 1987. "Does Ought Imply Can?" In *Ethical Idealism.* Berkeley: University of California Press, pp. 26–54.

Searle, J. 1969. "Deriving 'Ought' from 'Is'." In *Speech Acts.* Cambridge: Cambridge University Press, pp. 175–98.

Seckler, A. B., D. E. Meier, M. Mulvihill, and B. E. Cammer-Paris. 1991. "Substituted Judgment: How Accurate Are Proxy Decisions?" *Annals of Internal Medicine* 115:92–98.

Silverman, H. J., P. Tuma, M. H. Schaeffer, and B. Singh. 1995. "Implementation of the Patient Self-Determination Act in a Hospital Setting: An Initial Evaluation." *Archives of Internal Medicine* 155:502–10.

Singer, P. A., M. Siegler, and E. D. Pellegrino. 1990. "Research in Clinical Ethics." *Journal of Clinical Ethics* 1:95–99.

Stevens, W. 1951. "Thirteen Ways of Looking at a Blackbird." In *Collected Poems of Wallace Stevens.* New York: Knopf.

Sulmasy, D. P., K. Haller, and P. B. Terry. 1994. "More Talk, Less Paper: Predicting the Accuracy of Substituted Judgments." *American Journal of Medicine* 96:432–38.

Sulmasy, D. P., P. B. Terry, R. R. Faden, and D. M. Levine. 1994. "Long-Term Effects of Ethics Education on the Quality of Care for Patients Who Have Do-Not-Resuscitate Orders." *Journal of General Internal Medicine* 9:622–26.

Sulmasy, D. P., P. B. Terry, C. S. Weisman, D. J. Miller, R. Y. Stallings, M. A. Vettese, and K. B. Haller. 1998. "The Accuracy of Substituted Judgments in Patients with Terminal Diagnoses." *Annals of Internal Medicine* 128:621–29.

The SUPPORT Investigators. 1995. "A Controlled Trial to Improve Care for Seriously Ill Hospitalized Patients: The Study to Understand Prognoses and Preferences for Outcomes and Risks of Treatment (SUPPORT)." *Journal of the American Medical Association* 274:1591–98.

Uhlman, R. F., R. A. Pearlman, and K. C. Cain. 1988. "Physicians' and Spouses' Predictions of Elderly Patients' Resuscitation Preferences." *Journal of Gerontology* 43:M115–21.

Wertz, D. C., and J. C. Fletcher. 1998. "Ethical and Social Issues in Prenatal Sex Selection: A Survey of Geneticists in 37 Nations." *Social Science and Medicine* 46:255–73.

Zweibel, N. R., and C. K. Cassel. 1989. "Treatment Choices at the End of Life: A Comparison of Decisions by Older Patients and Their Physician-Selected Proxies." *Gerontologist* 29:615–21.

2

A Decade of Empirical Research in Medical Ethics

Jeremy Sugarman, Ruth Faden, and
Judith Weinstein

While philosophical, legal, and religious scholarship has traditionally dominated the field of medical ethics, empirical, data-based research with methodological roots in the social sciences has gradually assumed an important role in the field. In this chapter, we set out to describe the inclusion of empirical literature in the field of medical ethics during the first decade in which data on this question are readily available, the 1980s. We provide empirical answers to the following specific empirical questions: What topics in bioethics were empirically studied? What methods were used to study these topics? Who was studied in this research? How did empirical research in medical ethics change?

METHODS

We constructed a database of empirical medical ethics literature by downloading a comprehensive computerized search in BIOETHICSLINE, a database maintained by the National Reference Center for Bioethics (NRCB) that first came on-line in 1979 and is available through the National Library of Medicine. We chose to conduct our search with BIOETHICSLINE because this database is undoubtedly the most comprehensive resource for identifying citations of relevance to medical ethics. Bibliographers for BIOETHICS-LINE use a variety of techniques to capture material that is of relevance to medical ethics, including systematically reviewing journals in which empirical studies in medical ethics are likely to be published (Kahn 1995).

In this analysis, we focus on the empirical research that was published in the first full decade after BIOETHICSLINE came on-line, specifically 1980–89. Since BIO-ETHICSLINE is updated many times each year, making the total number of publications published each year a moving target, we selected as the base for our calculations those postings that would have been present in the database as of June 1992. Selecting this date minimized the likelihood of missing publications due to a delay in cataloging. Although BIOETHICSLINE does not keep such data, it is not unusual for a posting to lag publication date by longer than a year (Kahn 1995). This is consistent with the two-to-three-year lag from publication to entry into the *Bibliography of Bioethics* (Marsh 1987).

The search was designed to be highly sensitive for empirical research in medical ethics.[1] We then reviewed the abstracts, and sometimes the full text, of each of the citations included in the search to determine how many of them actually were reports of empirical studies in bioethics. We defined empirical research in medical ethics as the application of research methods in the social sciences (such as anthropology, epidemiology, psychology, and sociology) to the *direct* examination of issues in medical ethics. Both principal investigators (JS and RF) independently judged each of the citations to determine whether they fit our definition of empirical research in medical ethics. After discussing the coding of the first one hundred citations, both principal investigators rarely disagreed about this characterization. When necessary, we met to discuss any discrepancies in these independent characterizations and to establish consensus on this determination. A coding scheme was developed to characterize these empirical citations according to: (1) the topic under investigation; (2) the methods employed; and (3) the subjects of the research. A uniform coding scheme was required because of changes in terminology that occurred over time, diminishing the usefulness of key words or text words already indexed in computerized databases. For instance, the term "advance directives" was relatively new in the 1980s, although there is a good deal of older literature on advance directives listed under topics such as "living wills." Citations were coded to capture the primary purpose(s) of the report, but not necessarily to include all topics discussed. The coding scheme was pilot tested by having both principal investigators independently code the first 165 empirical postings retrieved. Following a discussion to resolve any inconsistencies, the coding scheme was refined and then used in our review of the entire set of empirical reports. In addition, if a study was performed outside of the United States or if it involved an international comparison, this was indicated. A research assistant with a background in public health (JW) was then trained to help in this review. Relevant citations were entered into a commercially available citation database (Reference Manager, Research Information Systems, Carlsbad, CA) along with topic, method, and research subject key words.[2]

RESULTS

Sample

At our reference point, there were 19,486 total postings that were published between 1980 and 1989 in BIOETHICSLINE. Of these postings, 663, or 3.4 percent, were ultimately determined to be empirical research in medical ethics. Journal articles (n=580) constituted 88 percent of these postings and were published in 251 different journals. Almost 12 percent of the postings were book chapters (n=78) and about 1 percent (n=5) constituted other postings such as newspaper articles or videotapes.

The Growth of Empirical Literature

During the 1980s, the proportion of empirical research to the total postings increased steadily, from 1.5 percent in 1980 to over 5 percent in 1989 (Fig. 2.1). While the proportion of empirical postings published each year in some topic areas such as informed

FIGURE 2.1   *Percentage of Empirical Postings in BIOETHICSLINE by Publication Year*[a]

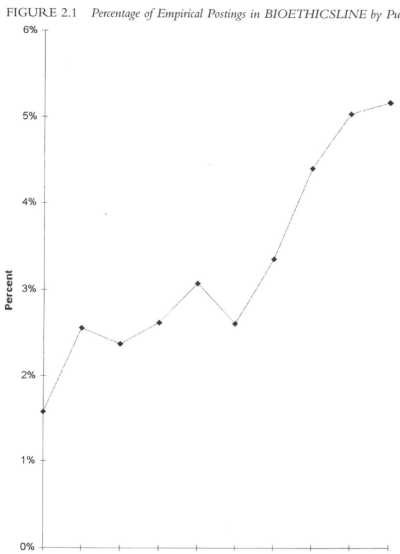

[a]% = no. of empirical research postings/total no. of postings.

consent was fairly consistent, a change in the proportion of publications on other topics, not surprisingly, seems to mirror discussions about that topic in the field. For example, the number of publications related to advance directives increased markedly beginning in 1983, just as the President's Commission for the Study of Ethical Problems in Medicine and Biomedical and Behavioral Research issued its landmark publication, *Deciding to Forego Life-Sustaining Treatment*, and then reached a plateau for the remainder of the decade (President's Commission 1983) (Fig. 2.2).

FIGURE 2.2   *Percentage of Empirical Postings in BIOETHICSLINE for Selected Topics by Publication Year*[a]

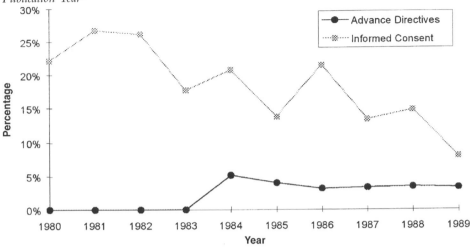

[a]% = no. of empirical research postings on the topic/no. of empirical research postings.

Topics

The prevalence of topics that were studied empirically during the decade is shown in Table 2.1. The range of topics that received empirical attention is quite broad: fifty distinct topics according to our categorization scheme. Nevertheless, certain topics received considerable attention while others were relatively neglected. In fact, four topics together—informed consent, research ethics, mental health, and Do Not Resuscitate orders—accounted for almost 26 percent of the topic assignments.

Research Subjects

The prevalence of types of research subjects in empirical studies of medical ethics are shown in Table 2.2. Of the twenty-six research subject assignments we used, three assignments (patients, physicians, and nurses) accounted for 51 percent of the empirical studies in our sample.

Methods

The methods used in these studies are shown in Table 2.3. For a brief description of each of these methods, see the Methods Glossary (pp. 27–28). Over half (54 percent) of the studies employed cross-sectional surveys. An additional 12 percent of studies used scenarios or vignettes as part of the study. The other fourteen methods that comprised our coding scheme were used less frequently (ranging from meta-analysis, which was never used, to record review, which was used 6 percent of the time).

TABLE 2.1 *Prevalence of Topics in Empirical Studies in Medical Ethics*

Topic[a]	n	Topic	n
Informed Consent	109	Professional Responsibility	20
Research Ethics	69	Patients' Rights	19
Mental Health	58	Advance Directives	18
DNR	55	Nursing Ethics	16
Physician-Patient Relationship	44	Truth-Telling	16
Prenatal Diagnosis	40	Third-party Decision making	14
Codes of Ethics	38	Allocation	14
Confidentiality	34	Transplantation	14
Genetic Screening	34	Intensive Care Units	12
Law	34	Reproductive Technology	12
Ethics Education	32	Compulsory Treatment	11
Genetics	32	Discrimination	9
Newborns	32	Violence	9
Medical Care at the End of Life	31	Medical Nutrition and Hydration	8
Euthanasia	29	Access to Care	6
Abortion	28	Sexual Abuse	3
Clinical Ethics	26	Substance Use	3
Training	26	Insurance	2
Refusal of Treatment	25	Maternal-Fetal Relationship	2
AIDS	24	Rationing	2
Moral Reasoning	24	Surrogacy	2
Competence	22	Gender	1
IRBs	21	Home Care	1
Organ Donation	21	Poverty	1
Death	20	Sex Selection	1

[a] The total number of topic assignments to one of the 50 possibilities listed in the table for all of the 663 empirical postings was 1,124 because some postings were given more than one topic assignment.

Methods that require considerable training or that can be difficult to conduct, such as qualitative research, quantitative observational studies (i.e., studies in which participants are observed and particular behaviors, such as the number of times physicians prompt patients to make their own decisions, are counted), and randomized trials were each used in only 1 percent of the empirical studies in our sample. Seven of the nine studies that employed randomized trial methodology investigated issues in informed consent. In contrast, qualitative research (n=18) was used to examine a variety of topics.

DISCUSSION

Early empirical research in medical ethics addressed a handful of topics. Not surprisingly, these topics were those that seem to have animated substantial discussion during

TABLE 2.2   *Subjects in Empirical Studies in Medical Ethics*

Subject[a]	n
Patients	235
Physicians	192
Nurses	72
Hospitals	66
Students	62
Families	61
Volunteers	60
Newborns	32
Women	32
Elderly	30
Children	18
Ethics Committees	17
Health Care Workers	17
Long-term Care Facilities	13
Adolescents	12
Research Subjects	10
Existing Data	8
Geneticists	8
Veterans	8
Dentists	7
Social Workers	7
Pharmacists	4
Researchers	4
Clergy	3
Corpses	3
Ethicists	2

[a] The total number of subject assignments to one of the 26 possibilities listed in the table for the 663 empirical postings was 983 because some postings were given more than one subject assignment.

the early years of the field, most notably research ethics and informed consent. Relatedly, we observed a marked rise in the proportion of publications about advance directives as major discussions about them were occurring. The reasons why these particular topics were the focus of such attention is a matter of conjecture, yet several factors might be considered relevant. For instance, they simply may reflect the topics in which there was considerable interest and those about which there was considerable public policy debate. After all, questions related to informed consent and research ethics were on the public agenda in the wake of public scandals that led to national commissions prior to similar inquiry into clinical medicine. Second, topics such as research ethics and informed consent were directly relevant to those conducting research, who would be expected to be accustomed to asking empirical

TABLE 2.3   *Prevalence of Empirical Methods Used in Medical Ethics Studies*

Method	n	%
Cross-sectional Survey	360	54
Scenarios/Vignettes	82	12
Records Review	43	6
Quasi-experimental/Time Series	31	5
Longitudinal/Prospective Survey	28	4
Empirical Review	25	4
Qualitative/Descriptive/Ethnographic	18	3
Quantitative Observational Study	14	2
Public Opinion Polls	13	2
Other	11	2
Risk/Utility Assessment/Decision Theory/Modeling	10	2
Case Studies/Case Series	9	1
Randomized	9	1
Secondary Data Analysis	9	1
Methods	2	0
Meta-analysis	0	0
Total[a]	664	100

[a] The total number of method assignments to one of the 16 possibilities listed in the table for the 663 empirical postings was 664 because some postings used more than one method. Rounding brings the total percent to be greater than 100.

questions and having the means with which to answer them. Finally, the topics were uniquely suited to empirical examination.

It is relevant to note that more than half of all the empirical studies in our database used survey research methods. A considerable proportion (12 percent) elaborated on survey methods by using clinical vignettes. However, other powerful research methods, such as ethnography, qualitative research, and randomized trials, were seldom used. It may be that empirical researchers coming from a variety of home disciplines were largely unfamiliar with these methods. Furthermore, as discussed in subsequent chapters in this book, these methods can demand substantial expertise and resources that may not be available to those conducting empirical research in medical ethics.

As will also be discussed in later chapters, whether the research methods are being used appropriately depends on the questions being asked (Kahn and Coutts 1990; Guyatt, Sackett, and Cook 1993; Levine et al. 1994). That is, in order to maximize the validity of the results of empirical studies, researchers must select the proper method according to a carefully refined research question. Consider the following simple hypothetical example: Researchers are interested in determining which of two methods of obtaining informed consent is better, a video presentation about a proposed intervention or a conversation with a nurse. The optimal method to answer this research question likely would be a prospective randomized trial comparing the two methods. Patients in each arm of the trial could be asked about their knowledge and beliefs about the proposed intervention as well as their satisfaction and attitudes toward the informed consent process and their perceptions about the voluntariness of their decisions. These data might then facilitate determining which method was better. In contrast, a simple cross-sectional survey of patients or nurses who had participated in different procedures for soliciting consent might lead to erroneous conclusions because methodological biases inherent in such a cross-sectional design would likely permit factors other than method-of-consent solicitation to mask or enhance differences.

In addition, it is unclear whether empirical research provides the kind of information that is useful in informing deliberations about ethical problems (Arnold and Forrow 1993; Brody 1993). This observation is important as it suggests the need for criteria for selecting issues for empirical investigation that are likely to advance the field.

As discussed in chapter 1, empirical research can and should play an important role in medical ethics. Nevertheless, conducting and including this work in normative deliberations requires an understanding of the strengths and limitations of the methods used, as will be described in subsequent chapters of this book.

Our data indicate that although empirical research in medical ethics experienced a growth phase during the 1980s, it only accounted for about 3 percent of the publications in the field overall. Assuming the trend has continued, this proportion seems likely to increase, although not to the degree, perhaps, that it should given the potential importance of empirical research to the field of medical ethics by prompting discussion and thought about ethical problems in medicine and also by illuminating and sharpening normative questions.

Empirical research today is an accepted and growing component of the literature in medical ethics (Brody 1990; Thomasma 1985). Indeed, some critical questions in medical ethics that are now being addressed in earnest lend themselves to both empirical and normative analysis. For instance, empirical research might be useful in assessing how health care resources should be allocated, in examining the adequacy of current methods of obtaining informed consent, and in delineating the effectiveness of prior review of research by Institutional Review Boards. Thus, the significance of empirical research in medical ethics can only be expected to increase. While no doubt the empirical work in the 2000s will look different from the empirical work of the 1980s, it is important to recognize that empirical research in medical ethics has a history as well as a future.

NOTES

1. The search strategy we used in BIOETHICSLINE was: "(EVALUATION (XXXX) OR EVALUATION STUDIES (XXXX) OR STATISTICS (XXXX) OR SURVEY (XXXX) OR ALL EMPIRIC: (TW))."

2. Several people provided invaluable support for this project. Joy Kahn of the National Reference Center for Bioethics (NRCB) and the chief bibliographer for BIOETHICSLINE helped us design the search strategy used in this study and provided us with generous technical support of the study. The staff at many libraries, especially those at the NRCB, were extremely kind and helpful as we collected articles for analysis. Trevor Myers, M.D., worked efficiently on the early phases of this project, establishing systems to assure accurate review of the articles.

   This project was supported in large part by a grant from the Greenwall Foundation.

REFERENCES

Arnold, R., and L. Forrow. 1993. "Empirical Research in Medical Ethics: An Introduction." *Theoretical Medicine* 14:195–97.

Brody, B. A. 1990. "Quality of Scholarship in Bioethics." *Journal of Medicine and Philosophy* 15:161–78.

———. 1993. "Assessing Empirical Research in Bioethics." *Theoretical Medicine* 14:211–19.

Guyatt, G. H., D. L. Sackett, and D. J. Cook. 1993. "User's Guides to the Medical Literature." *Journal of the American Medical Association* 270:2598–2601.

Kahn, T. J., personal communication, July 1995.

Kahn, T. J., and M. C. Coutts. 1990. "Commentary: Searches of the Medical Ethics Literature." *Journal of Clinical Ethics* 1:198–200.

Levine, M., S. Walker, H. Lee, T. Haines, A. Holbrook, and V. Moyer, for the Evidence-Based Medicine Working Group. 1994. "Users' Guides to the Medical Literature." *Journal of the American Medical Association* 271:1615–19.

Marsh, S. S. 1987. "Bibliography of Bioethics and Index Medicus: Comparison of Coverage, Publication Delay, and Ease of Recall for Journal Articles on Bioethics." *Bulletin of the Medical Library Association* 75:248–52.

President's Commission for the Study of Ethical Problems in Medicine and Biomedical and Behavioral Research. 1983. *Deciding to Forego Life-Sustaining Treatment.* Washington, D.C.: U.S. Government Printing Office.

Thomasma, D. C. 1985. "Empirical Methodology in Medical Ethics." *Journal of the American Geriatrics Society* 33:313–14.

METHODS GLOSSARY

Case studies/case series. Analyzing a case that provides insight, or examining a series of cases about a particular type of problem (e.g., describing a series of cases involving the use of non-heart-beating organ donors).

Cross-sectional survey. Asking questions about knowledge, attitudes, and/or beliefs at a single point in time (e.g., outpatients' knowledge, attitudes, and beliefs about living wills).

Empirical review. Gathering quantitative data from a series of studies in an effort to describe what is known about a particular topic (e.g., reviewing several cross-sectional studies about the use of deception in research).

Longitudinal/prospective survey. Following a group of participants over time (e.g., monitoring the types of ethical issues that a group of nursing students identify in consecutive quarters of their educational program).

Meta-analysis. A statistical technique of combining estimates from several studies to determine the overall best estimate (e.g., combining several studies to estimate the overall likelihood that DNR orders are written for older compared to younger patients).

Methods. A category for those studies that describe the development of new tools for data collection (e.g., new survey instruments) or that evaluate the merits of alternative research tools or techniques (e.g., comparing the use of vignettes to direct observation).

Public opinion polls. Surveys of the attitudes or beliefs of the general public or of a defined subset of the public (e.g., attitudes and beliefs of senior citizens toward physician-assisted suicide).

Qualitative/descriptive/ethnographic. A variety of research methods derived from anthropology to obtain full, thick descriptions of events (e.g., observing the behaviors of different members of a neonatal intensive care unit and family members when treating infants who are likely to die).

Quantitative observational study. Observing interactions, either directly or through some type of recording, and quantifying particular behaviors (e.g., listening to tape recordings of an office visit and counting the number of times the physician makes a clinical decision for a patient and the number of times the patient makes a clinical decision).

Quasi-experimental/time series. Using an event that has occurred to simulate an actual trial (e.g., monitoring the rate of HIV testing of injection drug users in two otherwise similar communities where one community has just adopted a statute requiring mandatory name reporting of those tested while the other has anonymous testing).

Randomized trial. A prospective design in which participants are assigned by chance to receive one of two or more interventions (e.g., determining which of two techniques for obtaining informed consent is better).

Records review. Using medical or other records as a data source (e.g., reviewing hospital records of all patients admitted to determine if palliative care orders are written according to hospital policy).

Risk/utility assessment/decision theory. A variety of methods related to the discipline of decision theory where preferences for interventions or outcomes are quantified and then manipulated mathematically to suggest appropriate courses of action (e.g., developing an algorithm to assist in making intensive care unit admission and discharge decisions by asking patients about their preferences for a variety of health states).

Scenarios/vignettes. Providing case descriptions for respondents, asking them to report what they would do in a particular case (e.g., cases asking physicians whether they would not tell a patient about a medical diagnosis).

Secondary data analysis. Applying statistical methods to existing databases to answer research questions (e.g., reviewing hospital databases to determine whether there are racial differences in the proportion of patients admitted that have advance directives).

PART II

Methods

3

Philosophy

David DeGrazia and Tom L. Beauchamp

What distinctive contributions does philosophy provide to medical ethics? Philosophy's most prominent and influential contribution, on which this chapter focuses, is to provide the critical resources of ethical theory and methodology in ethics.[1] The ambition of *ethical theory* is to provide an adequate normative framework for addressing the problems of moral life. Usually such a framework takes the form of a theory of right action, but it may take the form of a theory of good character (which is sometimes helpful in determining right action). The ambition of *methodology in ethics,* meanwhile, is to provide a procedure or method (1) for producing such a normative framework, (2) for using such a framework once it has been identified, or (3) for navigating the complexities of moral life in the absence of such a framework.

As this book concerns methods in medical ethics, this chapter examines *philosophical* methods in medical ethics. We will explore five leading methods, or models, for doing the work of moral reasoning, with special attention to the problems of medical ethics. Our discussion of particular ethical theories will be relatively compressed, because the application of established ethical theories represents only one of the five methods we explore.

The chapter begins with a section entitled "The Methods of Philosophical Medical Ethics," in which each method or model is described in a subsection and then subjected to one or more important criticisms in a subsection that immediately follows. Following some concluding comments, the chapter ends with a brief section on philosophical training in medical ethics and on leading scholarly resources in the field.

THE METHODS OF PHILOSOPHICAL MEDICAL ETHICS

Moral philosophers have traditionally aspired to normative theories of what is right or wrong that are set out in the most general terms. But it is increasingly questioned whether such general theories can be fruitfully applied in specific cases and contexts. Partly for this reason, it is controversial which philosophical methods best achieve the objectives of "applied ethics" and "practical ethics"—terms that have come into vogue as philosophical ethics has increased its interest in addressing such practical issues as abortion, the use of research subjects, and genetic engineering.

Several methods have been prominent in philosophical medical ethics. Among those influential methods, we will focus on these: (1) tradition and practice as a source of norms in medical ethics; (2) principles, common morality, and specification as the basis of medical ethics; (3) ethical theory as the backbone of "applied ethics"; (4) the use of biomedical cases and their ethical implications; and (5) reflective equilibrium as a technique.

The terrain of method in ethics is considerably broader than the large area that we will sketch here. For reasons of space, we do not discuss, for example, feminist analyses of issues of medical ethics (see, e.g., Holmes and Purdy 1992; Sherwin 1992; and Wolf 1996); considerations of virtue as a form of guidance in medical ethics (see, e.g., Shelp 1985); narrative ethics as a basis for medical ethics (see, e.g., Nelson 1997); and pragmatist approaches to medical ethics (see, e.g., McGee 1999). (Some philosophers might regard one or more of the methods just mentioned as examples of ethical theories that could serve as the backbone of "applied ethics," as in method (3) above, but these approaches are also often regarded as alternatives to the "applied ethics" model.)

Appeals to the Authority of Tradition and Practice Standards

Among the most influential sources of medical and nursing ethics are traditions: the concepts, practices, and norms that have seemingly always guided conduct in these fields. The history and precise character of these traditions have fascinated some philosophers, who find them a logical starting point in reflecting on professional ethics. Great traditions such as Hippocratic ethics deserve respect, but they often fail to provide a comprehensive, unbiased, and adequately justified ethics. The work of the philosopher is to take this history seriously while raising questions about the moral authority of oaths, prayers, codes, published lectures, and general pamphlets and treatises on medical conduct. The idea is to reconstruct traditional norms in a more perspicuous and defensible manner while remaining largely faithful to those norms (see, e.g., Pellegrino 1985; Arras 1988).

It is not always clear whether the statements made in documents that have had great historical influence were primarily descriptive, exhortatory, or self-protective. Some writings describe, for educational purposes, conduct that conformed to prevailing professional standards. Other documents aim at reforming professional conduct by prescribing what *should be* established practice. Still others seem constructed to protect the physician from suspicions of misconduct or from legal liability. Thus, to view prescriptions in codes and similar material at face value, as reflecting prevailing professional opinion in their epoch, may cause serious distortions. Moreover, philosophers want to do more than understand the concepts, practices, and norms that define these traditions; they are not satisfied with historical understanding. The goal is to defend or criticize the concepts, practices, and norms under investigation. Only then has some form of normative ethics entered the analysis.

A defender of the present approach might argue that appreciating the history of medicine is a crucial part of the work of normative ethics. To appreciate the history, according to this argument, helps one to grasp the essential nature (essence) of medicine and of the physician-patient relationship. And from this understanding one can derive or extract an understanding of the ethics of medicine. Edmund Pellegrino, for example, has argued that the nature of illness (which makes a patient uniquely vulnerable), the historically validated fact that medical knowledge is not individually owned, and the physician's public act of taking the Hippocratic Oath together entail that physicians have an obligation to serve patients even when doing so requires some effacement of self-interest (Pellegrino 1987).

Problems with Appeals to Tradition and Practice Standards

The essential problem with attempts to base applied ethics in practice standards and traditional oaths and guidelines is that such resources are not self-justifying. Whether a particular practice standard or oath is justified must be determined by careful ethical reflection, which may conclude that the prevailing norm is inadequate or indefensible from a moral standpoint. Even ethicists and physicians working largely within a traditional framework generally believe that some degree of independent ethical reflection is necessary.

One variant of the traditional approach, however, might seem less susceptible to this line of criticism. As noted above, some traditionalists hold that understanding the history of medical practice helps one to grasp the essential nature of medicine itself, from which one is able to extract a viable medical ethics. Yet the claim that medicine has some essential nature is debatable. Arguably, medicine should be viewed as an evolving set of practices with no intrinsic limits to the possibility for change. Further, even if medicine has a fixed essence or purpose, it is doubtful that ethical norms other than highly abstract statements of general purpose can be straightforwardly derived from facts about this essence.

In any case, it has become clear as a result of historical investigation during the last thirty years that traditional codes and practices of medical and nursing ethics have proved utterly inadequate to address problems arising from modern scientific research, clinical practice, biomedical technology, health policy, and related social developments. The history of medical ethics emanating from the practices of 2,000 years ago is disappointing from the perspective of today's concerns in medical ethics about the rights of patients and subjects and the ways in which society should act to promote the health of its members. Most topics and problems in medical ethics that are of major concern today have been ignored or given but passing notice until the second half of the twentieth century.

The importance of this critique is less to expose the inadequacies of appeals to tradition than to show the need for more. Few philosophers entirely discount appeals to tradition, but few also think that today's medical ethics can be reconstructed from this source alone.

Principles, the Common Morality, and Specification

In part because many observers came to believe that medical tradition was outmoded by modern developments in medicine, representatives of various disciplines sought an explicit recognition of basic ethical principles that would help to identify clinical practices and human experiments that were morally questionable or in need of reform. Since basic moral principles are the province of moral philosophers (at least in secular settings), there was a turn to philosophy to identify and analyze the principles that could serve as a moral framework for medical ethics.

Just as tradition can be a resource, so can common morality—much of which can be summarized in the form of generally accepted principles. Common morality may be understood as the morality shared by morally serious persons throughout the world. It is not a *specific morality* or a *theory*; it is simply morality. It is universal because it contains ethical precepts found wherever morality is found.

In recent years, the favored category to express universality has perhaps been human rights (see, e.g., Dworkin 1977; Thomson 1990; Macklin 1992), but standards of obligation can also be expressed in universal form. These norms constituting shared morality might be called "morality in the narrow sense," because the morality we share is only a small slice of the entire moral life. Morality in the broad sense includes divergent moral norms and positions that spring from particular cultural, philosophical, and religious roots.

Many people, including many philosophers, are skeptical about the idea of a common morality. They think that virtually nothing is shared across cultures and different moral traditions. However, the distinction between broad and narrow morality helps allay these concerns. While the broad sense allows for ample diversity and disagreement, the narrow sense simply captures what we all appreciate about morality. Very general principles that are accepted by all, or virtually all, morally serious persons include *nonmaleficence* (which requires that we not harm others) and *respect for autonomy* (which requires that we respect the decision-making capacities of autonomous persons). Somewhat more specific rules that morally serious persons affirm include the following: "Tell the truth"; "Obtain consent before invading another person's body"; "Do not kill"; "Do not cause pain"; "Do not deprive of liberty"; "Do not steal or otherwise deprive of goods"; and "Prevent harm to others."[2]

It is no objection to these principles and rules that in some circumstances they can be validly overridden by other norms with which they conflict. *All* general norms can be validly overridden in some circumstances in which they compete with other moral claims. For example, one might not tell the truth in order to prevent someone from killing another person; and protecting the liberty or rights of one person may require interfering with the autonomous choice of someone else. When a conflict of two or more principles or rules occurs, the conflict must be addressed to extract the proper content from each. Alternatively, as the context requires, one precept may be found to override the other.

How, then, does one fill the gap between abstract principles and concrete judgments to guide moral decision making sufficiently? The answer is that principles must be *specified* to suit the needs of particular contexts. Specification is the progressive filling in of the abstract content of principles, shedding their indeterminateness and thereby providing action-guiding content (Richardson 1990).[3]

In managing complex or problematic cases involving conflicts, we should begin with the effort to specify norms and eradicate conflicts among them. Many already specified norms will need further specification to handle new circumstances of indeterminateness or conflict. Incremental specification will continue to refine one's commitments, gradually reducing the circumstances of contingent conflict to more manageable dimensions. Increase of substance (normative content) through specification is essential for decision making in clinical and research ethics, as well as for the development of institutional rules and public policy.

The famous case *Tarasoff v. Regents of University of California* (1976) will serve to illustrate specification (as well as the related concept of *balancing*). The practice of psychotherapy has long honored a principle (or rule) of confidentiality, which states that the information divulged in psychotherapy by a patient to the therapist may not be shared with other individuals without the patient's prior consent. This rule is grounded in the need for the patient to trust the therapist as a condition for fully open discussion of the patient's personal difficulties and in respect for the patient's autonomy. But what if a patient divulges the intention to kill an identified third party? Another commonly accepted rule, even if less often explicitly stated, is that one should take reasonable steps to prevent or warn of major harm to another individual if one is uniquely situated to do so and can do so relatively easily. The strength of this obligation may increase if one occupies a professional role such as that of psychiatrist, psychologist, or social worker. Clearly we have a conflict, because maintaining confidentiality is inconsistent with the second rule; taking steps to warn the prospective victim would violate the rule of confidentiality.

How should one manage this conflict? Consistent with the legal judgment that was actually rendered in the case, many therapists and ethicists hold that a serious threat of consequential bodily injury to an identified third party warrants an exception to the rule of confidentiality. Efforts to balance the relevant considerations suggest that the importance of helping the endangered person is weightier than that of confidentiality in such cases. So long as balancing is understood as involving a judgment adequately supported by justifying reasons—and not as a purely intuitive act—the metaphor of balancing fits well with the idea of specification. The reason justifying the resolution can, in effect, be incorporated into a specification of one of the principles or already specified rules (assuming they are regarded as nonabsolute).

In the present case the original rule can be specified as follows: The information divulged in psychotherapy by a patient to the therapist may not be shared with other individuals without the patient's prior consent, unless the patient expresses an intention to cause severe harm to an identified third party. This specification eliminates the dilemma that originally existed because of a conflict between two rules.

But how are particular specifications to be *justified*, since more than one specification is always possible? In the case just described, another possible way to remove conflict would be to preserve confidentiality as an absolute rule and revise the other norm as follows: "One should take reasonable steps to prevent major harm to another individual . . . unless one's professional duties prohibit the only available means for doing so." How can the resolution in terms of making a disclosure to a third party be shown to be more defensible than this *competing* specification?

A particular specification, or any revision in moral belief, is held to be justified if it maximizes the coherence of the overall set of beliefs that are accepted upon reflection.[4] This is, admittedly, a very abstract thesis, and employment of the criteria that together constitute "coherence" in the relevant (rather broad) sense is a subtle and unresolved affair. While we believe at least some of these criteria of coherence—such as logical consistency, argumentative support, and intuitive plausibility—are implicitly accepted by nearly anyone who engages in serious moral reflection and discourse, we cannot further explore the criteria of coherence here. We note, however, that the present principles-based technique or model often employs the technique of "reflective equilibrium," which is described below.

Concerns about Principles and the Common Morality

Several concerns about principles drawn from the common morality have been raised by contemporary writers in medical ethics. Clouser and Gert (1990), for example, maintain that general "principles" function more like chapter headings in a book than as directive rules or normative theories.⁵ Principles, they argue, highlight important moral themes by providing a general label for them, but do not function as practical action guides or furnish a method for medical ethics. Receiving no helpful or controlling guidance from the principle, a moral agent confronting a problem is free, these authors contend, to deal with it in his or her own way and may give the principle whatever weight he or she wishes when it conflicts with another principle.

These deficiencies are alleged to be especially pronounced in the area of justice. We know that justice is concerned with distribution and that we should be concerned about it, but invoking "justice" amounts to little more than a checklist of moral concerns. Since this lack of normative content deeply underdetermines solutions to problems of justice and has no power to guide actions or to establish policies, the agent is free to decide what is just and unjust, as he or she sees fit. Other moral considerations besides the principle(s) of justice, such as intuitions and theories about the equality of persons, must be called upon for real normative guidance. Clouser and Gert think the same problem afflicts all general principles, which alert us to issues, but, lacking an adequate unifying theory, offer no real guidance on their own.

Do principles really lack specific, directive substance? The charge is most plausible in the case of *unspecified* principles. As stated previously, any principle—and any rule, for that matter—will have this problem if the norm is underspecified for the task at hand. A basic principle is necessarily general, covering a broad range of circumstances; in this regard, principles contrast with specific propositions. As the territory governed by any norm (principle, rule, paradigm case judgment, etc.) is narrowed, the conditions become more specific—for example, shifting gradually from "all persons" to "all competent patients"—and along the way it becomes less and less likely that the norm can even qualify as a principle. (For example, while the principle of respect for autonomy applies to autonomous actions generally, the narrower norm of respecting informed refusals by competent patients is more likely to be considered a rule than a principle.)

If general principles can be specified and rendered more useful for particular contexts, why continue to think in terms of general principles at all? One practical reason is that principles must be the sort of thing that can be learned by everyone—not just philosophers, but health professionals, ethics committee members, and laypersons. If morally serious persons thought only in terms of specified principles, the latter's specificity and proliferation would make them very difficult to remember, master, and internalize for practical use.

Ethical Theory as the Basis of Applied Ethics

When the notion of "applied ethics" gained a foothold in philosophy, it was widely presumed that general moral principles or ethical theories were to be *applied* to particular moral problems or cases. This vision suggests that ethical theory develops general principles, rules, and the like, whereas applied ethics treats particular contexts by applying these general norms—either directly to particular cases or through the intermediary of more specific norms.⁶ Applied work does not, it seems, generate any novel ethical content. Applied ethics requires only a detailed knowledge of the areas to which the ethical theory is being applied (medicine, nursing, public health, research, public policy, etc.) and perhaps some skill in drawing out a theory's implications.

This model, which is sometimes called "deductivism" or "top-down application" of general norms, is inspired by justification in disciplines such as mathematics, in which claims can often be shown to follow logically (deductively) from credible premises. In ethics, the parallel idea is that general principles or rules, together with the relevant facts of a situation (in the fields to which the theory is being applied), support an inference to correct or justified moral judgments. In short, the method of reasoning at work is the application of a norm to a clear case falling under the norm.

One version of this approach would feature two or more basic moral principles arranged in a strict hierarchical ordering, so that conflicts between principles are always resolved in the same way. We are not aware of any significant example of a complete ethical theory that has been successfully constructed along these lines.[7]

A more prominent version of the deductivist approach features a single overarching or supreme principle that is presented as foundational for the entire moral domain. The most widely discussed theory of this kind is utilitarianism, which defends the "principle of utility" as supreme. This principle holds that the right action or policy is that which maximizes the balance of good (beneficial) consequences over bad (harmful) consequences. By contrast, deontological theories assert (in different ways, depending on the particular theory) that the right action or policy is to be identified by reference to one or more moral principles that cannot be equated with, or fully derived from, the principle of utility.[8] During the 1970s and much of the 1980s, utilitarian and deontological approaches exerted enormous influence on the literature and discourse of medical ethics, and their characteristic patterns of reasoning are still common today. Therefore a closer look at these theories is warranted.

Utilitarian Theories[9]

The *principle of utility* demands production of the maximal balance of good consequences over bad consequences. But what characteristics determine the value of particular consequences? The answer offered by a particular version of utilitarianism represents that version's *value theory.* These value theories (or theories of the good) point to (1) happiness, (2) the satisfaction of desires and aims, and (3) the attainment of such conditions or states of affairs as autonomy, understanding, various kinds of functioning, achievement, and deep personal relationships. Whatever its value theory, any utilitarian theory decides which actions are right entirely by reference to the *consequences* of the actions, rather than by reference to any intrinsic moral features the actions may have, such as truthfulness or fidelity. Finally, in the utilitarian approach all parties affected by an action must receive *impartial consideration.*

A dispute has arisen among utilitarians over whether the principle of utility is to be applied to *particular acts* in particular circumstances or to *rules of conduct* that determine which acts are right and wrong. An act utilitarian simply justifies actions directly by appeal to the principle of utility. In contrast, for the rule utilitarian, actions are justified by appeal to rules such as "Don't deceive" and "Don't break promises." These rules are themselves justified by appeal to the principle of utility.

Kantian Theories[10]

Deontological theories are now increasingly called Kantian because of their origins in the theory of Immanuel Kant. In this theory, morality provides a rational framework of universal principles and rules that constrain and guide everyone. Kant's supreme principle, called "the categorical imperative," is expressed in several ways in his writings. His first formulation may be roughly paraphrased in this way: "Always act in such a way that you can will that everyone act in the same manner in similar situations," (Kant 1959, 37–42). Kant's view is that wrongful practices, such as lying, theft, cheating, and failure to help someone in distress when you can easily do so, involve a kind of contradiction. Consider cheating on exams. If everyone behaved as the cheater did, exams would not serve their essential function of testing mastery of relevant material, in which case there would effectively be no such thing as an exam. But cheating presupposes the background institution of taking exams, so the cheater cannot consistently will that everyone act as she does.

A second formulation of Kant's categorical imperative, which is more frequently invoked in medical ethics, may be paraphrased in this way: "Treat every person as an end and never solely as a means" (Kant 1959, 47). This principle requires us to treat persons as having their own autonomously established goals. Deceiving prospective subjects in order to get them to consent to participate in nontherapeutic research is one example of a violation of this principle.

Problems with Ethical Theory as a Basis for Applied Ethics

Ethical theories themselves hold a diminished stature in the field of medical ethics, compared with their influence in the 1970s and 1980s. The reasons for the demotion of utilitarian and single-principle deontological theories concern the disadvantages of any approach that attempts to cover or provide a foundation for the entire domain of morality with either one supreme principle or one general viewpoint. Three disadvantages are worthy of note.

First, there is a problem of authority. Despite myriad attempts by philosophers in recent centuries to justify the claim that some principle is morally authoritative—that is, correctly regarded as the supreme moral principle—no such effort at justification has persuaded a majority of philosophers or other thoughtful people that either the principle or the moral system is more authoritative than the common morality that supplies its roots. Thus, to attempt to illuminate problems in medical ethics with a single-principle theory has struck many as misguided as well as presumptuous or dogmatic.

Second, even if an individual working in this field is convinced that some such theory is correct (authoritative), he or she needs to deal responsibly with the fact that many other morally serious individuals do not share this theory and grant it little or no authority. Thus, problems of how to communicate and negotiate in the midst of disagreement do not favor appeals to rigid theories or inflexible principles, which can generate a gridlock of conflicting principled positions, rendering moral discussion hostile and alienating. In our experience—and we believe generally in the experience of teachers of medical ethics—even where people disagree at the level of basic theory, they commonly agree at the level of the principles of medical ethics. These principles, then, may be a more congenial and fruitful starting point for discussion than ethical theories.

Third, there is the problem that a highly general principle functioning as the centerpiece of an entire theory is indeterminate in many contexts in which one might try to apply it. That is, the content of the principle itself does not always identify a unique course of action as right. Thus, single-principle theories are significantly incomplete, frequently depending on independent moral considerations with the help of which the theories can serve as effective guides to action.

Casuistry (Case-Based Reasoning)

In contemporary medical ethics, clinicians and ethicists often concentrate their attention not on principles or theories as the basis of their methods of reasoning, but instead on practical decision making in particular cases and on the implications of those cases for other cases (Jonsen 1995).[11] We can make reliable moral judgments about agents and actions, some philosophers say, only when we have an intimate understanding of particular situations and an appreciation of the record of similar situations.

This approach, commonly called *casuistry,* proceeds by identifying the particular features of and problems present in the case. An analogy to the authority operative in case law is sometimes noted. When the decision of a majority of judges becomes authoritative in a case, their judgments are positioned to become authoritative for other courts hearing cases with similar facts. This is the doctrine of precedent. Defenders of case-based reasoning see moral authority similarly: Social ethics develops from a social consensus formed around cases, which can then be extended to new cases without loss of the accumulated moral wisdom. As a history of similar cases and similar judgments mounts, a society becomes more confident in its moral judgments, and the stable elements crystallize in the form of tentative generalizations about how to handle similar cases. For example, if the case at hand involves a problem of medical confidentiality, analogous cases would be considered in which breaches of confidentiality were deemed justified or unjustified in order to see whether such a breach is justified in the present case. So understood, casuistry partly overlaps with the method of appealing to tradition: Certain cases serve as the focal points of an evolving tradition of ethical reflection and practice.

The leading cases (so-called "paradigm cases") become enduring and authoritative sources for reflection and decision making. Cases such as the Tuskegee syphilis study (in which a group of African American men were intentionally not treated for syphilis in order to follow the course of the disease) are invoked in order to illustrate unjustified biomedical experimentation. Decisions reached about moral wrongs in this case serve as a form of authority for decisions in new cases. These cases profoundly influence our standards of fairness, negligence, paternalism, and the like. Just as case law (legal rules) develops incrementally from legal decisions in cases, so the moral law (moral rules) develops incrementally. From this perspective, principles are less important for moral reasoning than cases. Indeed, principles may even be expendable.

Casuists sometimes write as if cases lead to moral paradigms, analogies, or judgments entirely by their facts alone, but this picture is inaccurate. No matter how many salient facts are assembled, some *value* premises will be needed in order to reach a moral conclusion. The properties that we observe to be of moral importance in cases are picked out by the values that we have already accepted as being morally important. In short, the paradigm cases are value-laden.

The best way to understand paradigm cases is as a combination of (1) *facts* that can be generalized to other cases—for example, "The patient refused the recommended treatment"—and (2) *settled values*—for example, "Competent patients have a right to refuse treatment." The central values are generalizable and must be preserved from one case to the next. For a casuist to reason morally, one or more settled values must connect the cases (hence the necessity of "maxims," or moral generalizations).

Problems with Casuistry

Casuistry is confronted by several challenges. First, it is less independent of principle-based reasoning than its proponents often suggest. Casuists claim that moral certainty is to be found in particular cases. But grasping the ethical significance of a case may not be distinguishable from grasping a moral generalization (principle or rule) under which the case falls. When we perceive that a man's slapping a child without cause is wrong, we also perceive the wrongness of some kind of action, such as harming the innocent or hurting children; after all, something about the action must make it wrong. Thus, there is no basis for claiming that judgments about particular cases are more certain than judgments about more general norms governing the cases; indeed, it is doubtful that the two kinds of judgment can be entirely separated.

Moreover, casuistry sometimes faces difficulties in justifying judgments in particular cases. For example, it is now widely accepted that a competent patient may refuse medical treatment, and courts and commentators have largely agreed that competent patients may also refuse food and water—presumably because the latter sort of case is relevantly similar to refusals of medical treatment. But what supports the claim of relevant similarity here? The casuist is likely to vest authority in community judgment or consensus within the evolving practices and traditions of American medicine. But it is not self-evident that one should accept the ethical judgments woven into these practices and traditions.

Finally, by focusing so heavily on cases, casuistry risks (1) being unable to make progress with especially controversial issues, since consensus on particular cases is elusive, and (2) overlooking very general and fundamental issues, the resolution of which may be relevant to specific cases. As an example of problem (1), casuistry seems of little or no help in illuminating fundamental questions regarding the moral status of animals. Since consensus about the moral status of animals is lacking, any case involving animals to which a casuist might appeal will either elicit incompatible moral judgments from those who consider the case, or elicit agreement to vague or relatively trivial judgements (e.g., "It is wrong to cause animals to suffer unnecessarily"). For an example of (2), consider a casuist who attempts to judge whether some medical treatment should be covered by the government by examining relevantly similar funding decisions. This approach may easily miss broader questions of social justice and access to health care—the resolution of which might vindicate major reform of our health care system, implying different answers to specific funding questions than the answers at which the casuist would arrive.

Reflective Equilibrium (a Form of Coherence Theory)

Many philosophers now defend the view that the relationship between general moral norms and particular moral judgments is bilateral (neither a unilateral "application" of general norms nor a unilateral abstraction from particular case judgments). John Rawls's (1971) celebrated account of "reflective equilibrium" has been the most influential model.

In developing and refining a system of ethics, he argues, it is appropriate to start with the broadest possible set of *considered judgments* (see below) about a subject and to erect a provisional set of principles that reflects them. Reflective equilibrium views investigation in ethics (and theory construction) as a reflective testing of moral principles, theoretical postulates, and other relevant moral beliefs to render them as coherent as possible. Starting with paradigms of what is morally right or wrong, one searches for principles that are consistent with these paradigms as well as one another. Such principles and considered judgments are taken, as Rawls puts it, "provisionally as fixed points," but also as "liable to revision."

Considered judgments is a technical term referring to judgments in which moral beliefs and capacities are most likely to be presented without a distorting bias. Examples are judgments about the wrongness of racial discrimination, religious intolerance, and sexual oppression. By contrast, judgments in which one's confidence level is low and judgments that may reflect self-interest or other forms of bias do not qualify as considered judgments. The goal is to match, prune, and adjust considered judgments and principles so that they form a coherent moral outlook.

This model demands the best approximation to full coherence under the assumption of a never-ending search for consistency and unanticipated situations. From this perspective, just as hypotheses in science are tested, modified, or rejected through experience and experimental thinking, principles and other moral norms are tested, revised (sometimes specified), or rejected. This outlook is very different from deductivism, because the method of reflective equilibrium holds that ethical theories are never complete, always stand to be informed by practical contexts, and must be tested for adequacy by their practical implications.

Problems with the Model of Reflective Equilibrium

The central problem with the reflective-equilibrium model is that the flexibility associated with its bilateral approach is a double-edged sword: While avoiding some of the difficulties associated with (top-down) application of ethical theories and with the case-focused method of casuistry, reflective equilibrium also gives relatively little specific guidance about how to engage in moral reasoning. Several philosophers have endeavored to characterize reasoning within this model in a nontrivial manner (see, e.g, Rawls 1971; Daniels 1979, 1996; Holmgren 1989; Nielsen 1991, chs. 9–11; and DeGrazia 1996, ch. 2). But, theoretically, the model needs further development; and, practically, it is unclear how helpful this model will be to nonphilosophers seeking guidance in moral deliberation.

CONCLUDING COMMENTS

This chapter has presented an overview of major philosophical methods in medical ethics. It began with a characterization of five major methods, or models, for conducting the work of moral reasoning, with special emphasis on the problems that arise in medical ethics. It is one thing to know what a method is, another to have a sense of its adequacy. Therefore, each subsection describing a method was followed by a subsection identifying one or more leading criticisms of that method.

We now conclude the body of this chapter with a few remarks about the limits of philosophy in medical ethics as well as some comments indicating common ground amid the diversity of philosophical contributions to medical ethics.

One limit to what philosophy can accomplish in medical ethics is implicit throughout the above discussions of the methods and major criticisms that they face: Despite the merit of much work in ethical theory and methodology in ethics, no approach has proved so convincing and resilient in responding to criticisms as to convince all or even a majority of philosophers and ethicists to adopt it as the preferred method. This means that everyone interested in methodological issues of medical ethics must think critically about the strengths and weaknesses of the leading approaches.

A second important limit of philosophy is a direct consequence of its nonempirical nature. Philosophy involves a critical perspective from which to evaluate theses, arguments, and viewpoints as well as (in ethics) actions, motives, practices, and institutions. But because it is not an empirical science, philosophy must depend on empirical disciplines in a joint effort of critically evaluating any specific domain of human practice, whether it be medicine, law, international relations, or some other. Therefore, while philosophy can contribute a great deal to medical ethics in the way of ethical theory and, more broadly, methodology in ethics (and make other contributions—see note 1), philosophy can provide reliable moral guidance only to the extent that its empirical assumptions are accurate.

The basic point is commonsensical. If, for example, one argues that physician-assisted suicide is justified—based on the assumption that currently legal means of pain control are ineffective for many patients—one's argument depends on the clinical data that are relevant to assessing the adequacy of legal methods of pain control. Philosophy itself cannot address such a factual issue. Thus, in general, critical moral reasoning in any practical context requires proper empirical data.

Interestingly, philosophy's nonempirical nature motivates what may be the only significant point of methodological consensus among the wide variety of methods in ethics. One is hard-pressed to find methodological claims embraced by all of the major approaches. One might suppose that all of the approaches agree that a theory is rightly tested by the intuitive plausibility of its moral implications (by their "resonance" with our lived moral experience), yet the theory-driven approach of deductivism is not committed to this criterion. Alternatively, one might presume that all of the approaches agree that the evaluation of actions is central to moral reasoning, yet proponents of virtue ethics (or at least some variants of this approach) would dissent. At the same time, all approaches must accept this requirement: The factual assumptions underlying moral reasoning must be reasonably supported by empirical evidence and observation.

On a concluding note, there is probably more agreement about how to write strong papers in philosophical medical ethics than there is on questions of method. Because the present paper has focused on the latter, we will enumerate a few criteria on which there is probably consensus regarding excellence in writing. It is agreed that strong papers in philosophical medical ethics have the following features: (1) clarity of expression and organization (so that, for example, papers are not unnecessarily difficult to read); (2) rigorous argumentation, making it clear to the reader that conclusions are strongly supported by the arguments presented in their defense; (3) a firm command of leading work that has already been published on the topic; (4) novelty, so that the author is not simply duplicating work already published; and (5) an important topic.

NOTES ON RESOURCES AND TRAINING

What sorts of training are available to those who aspire to work in ethical theory or other philosophical areas of medical ethics? Is such training necessary or merely desirable? The answers to these questions turn importantly on an individual's specific goals.

In order to make significant scholarly contributions to philosophical medical ethics, or to teach effectively in that area, there is no substitute for graduate training in philosophy. One possible strategy is to seek admission to a strong philosophy graduate program while planning to take several courses in medical ethics (prioritizing strength in philosophy). Another possible strategy is to apply only to philosophy graduate programs that have a medical ethics track or concentration (making medical ethics more central to one's studies). Both strategies reflect viable paths to philosophical work in medical ethics.

For those seeking basic competence (as opposed to expertise) in specific philosophical areas of medical ethics, less intensive courses of study are available. One or more courses in ethical theory—preferably, but not necessarily, at the graduate level—would be appropriate training for competence in that area. Ideally, such courses would be taken as part of a more extensive graduate training—in a master's program in medical ethics, for example—but they could also prove invaluable to the professional who is auditing courses in her spare time.

In addition to courses at colleges and universities, other opportunities for education in philosophical medical ethics include intensive "short courses" taken over several days, workshops, conferences, and, of course, self-education through reading. Such educational experiences can enrich one's reasoning and discourse about philosophical issues in medical ethics. They can also allow one to learn more from scholarly writings.

There are several leading scholarly resources to which one may turn for information about or work in philosophical contributions to medical ethics. First, one may search journals for articles of particular interest. Leading journals from the standpoint of philosophical medical ethics include *Philosophy and Public Affairs, Bioethics, Public Affairs Quarterly, The Journal of Medicine and Philosophy, The Kennedy Institute of Ethics Journal,* and *Ethics.* Sometimes one can find valuable articles in strong philosophy journals that do not focus on medical ethics or ethical theory. One systematic approach to searching for helpful journal articles is to consult *The Philosopher's Index* (Lineback 1969), which appears quarterly and lists published articles (and books) both by author and by subject. Two encyclopedias offer valuable short articles and bibliographies: *The Encyclopedia of Bioethics,* in its second edition (Reich 1995), and the *Routledge Encyclopedia of Philosophy* (Craig 1998). Some comprehensive textbooks can also be a useful general resource, providing both detailed discussions and leads for further research. Finally, valuable resources, including a unique bioethics database, are located at the National Reference Center for Bioethics Literature ("the Bioethics Library") at Georgetown University in Washington, D.C. Those who are unable to visit the library may call toll-free at 1-800-MED-ETHX.

NOTES

1. Philosophy can and does make other contributions to medical ethics, although we cannot canvass all of them here. Examples include the contributions of action theory to a theory of informed consent and of personal identity theory to views about the definition of death and the authority of advance directives.

2. Appeals to the common morality as the source of universal norms are not intended to suggest that moral reasoning should always lead to conclusions that are commonly accepted, let alone universally accepted. Common moral experience provides the starting point of moral discourse, but critical reflection on specific ethical issues may ultimately vindicate moral judgments that are not widely shared (for example, regarding our obligations to the developing world, or regarding the moral status of animals).

3. For early discussions of this method in bioethics, see DeGrazia 1992; Beauchamp 1994a, 1994b; and Beauchamp and Childress 1994. For discussions of what is now sometimes called "specified principlism," see, e.g., Davis 1995, esp. 95–102; and Levi 1996, esp. 13–19, 24–26.

4. For recent efforts to analyze the idea of justification by coherence, see Daniels 1996 and DeGrazia 1996, ch. 2.

5. Their views are further developed in later writings. See Green, Gert, and Clouser 1993; Clouser and Gert 1994; Clouser 1995; and Gert, Culver, and Clouser 1997, ch. 4.

6. Several different types of ethical theory have been employed in addressing practical problems, including the following: (1) utilitarianism, (2) Kantianism, (3) rights theory, (4) contract theory, (5) virtue ethics, (6) communitarianism, and (7) pragmatism. Many proponents of these theories would argue, however, that specific policy and practical guidelines cannot be simply derived from these ethical theories, and that some additional moral reasoning is always necessary.

7. Rawls (1971) has developed a theory of justice, but not a full ethical theory, that features such a hierarchy of principles.

8. The most classic deontological theory featuring a supreme principle is that of Kant (1959). For contemporary representatives of this approach, see Donagan 1977, a book stressing respect for persons, and Gewirth 1978, which stresses individual rights.

9. For utility-centered theory, see Mill 1979; Frey 1980; Hare 1981; Griffin 1986; Kagan 1989; Brandt 1992; Singer 1993.

10. For prominent contemporary representatives of Kantian ethics, see Herman 1993 and Korsgaard 1996.

11. For a landmark work in the history of the type of reasoning described here, see Jonsen and Toulmin 1988. For additional features of the method, see Jonsen 1996, 37–49, and 1991.

REFERENCES

Arras, J. D. 1988. "AIDS and the Duty to Treat." *Hastings Center Report* 18(2) (Special Supplement):10–18.

Beauchamp, T. L. 1994a. "The Four Principles Approach to Medical Ethics." In *Principles of Health Care Ethics*, ed. R. Gillon. London: John Wiley & Sons, pp. 3–12.

———. 1994b. "Principles and Other Emerging Paradigms for Bioethics." *Indiana Law Journal* 69:1–17.

Beauchamp, T. L., and J. F. Childress. 1994. *Principles of Biomedical Ethics.* 4th ed. New York: Oxford University Press.

Brandt, R. B. 1992. *Morality, Utilitarianism, and Rights.* Cambridge: Cambridge University Press.

Clouser, D. K. 1995. "Common Morality as an Alternative to Principlism." *The Kennedy Institute of Ethics Journal* 5:219–36.

Clouser, D. K., and B. Gert. 1990. "A Critique of Principlism." *The Journal of Medicine and Philosophy* 15:219–36.

———. 1994. "Morality vs. Principlism." In *Principles of Health Care Ethics,* eds. R. Gillon and A. Lloyd. London: John Wiley & Sons, pp. 251–66.

Craig, E., ed. 1998. *Routledge Encyclopedia of Philosophy.* 10 vols. London: Routledge.

Daniels, N. 1979. "Wide Reflective Equilibrium and Theory Acceptance in Ethics." *Journal of Philosophy* 76:256–82.

———. 1996. "Wide Reflective Equilibrium in Practice." In *Philosophical Perspectives on Bioethics,* eds. L. W. Sumner and J. Boyle. Toronto: University of Toronto Press, pp. 96–114.

Davis, R. B. 1995. "The Principlism Debate: A Critical Overview." *The Journal of Medicine and Philosophy* 20:85–105.

DeGrazia, D. 1992. "Moving Forward in Bioethical Theory: Theories, Cases, and Specified Principlism." *The Journal of Medicine and Philosophy* 17:511–39.

———. 1996. *Taking Animals Seriously.* Cambridge: Cambridge University Press.

Donagan, A. 1977. *The Theory of Morality.* Chicago: University of Chicago Press.

Dworkin, R. 1977. *Taking Rights Seriously.* Cambridge, MA: Harvard University Press.

Frey, R. G. 1980. *Interests and Rights.* Oxford: Clarendon Press.

Gert, B., C. M. Culver, and K. D. Clouser. 1997. *Bioethics: A Return to Fundamentals.* New York: Oxford University Press.

Gewirth, A. 1978. *Reason and Morality.* Chicago: University of Chicago Press.

Green, R. M., B. Gert, and K. D. Clouser. 1993. "The Method of Public Morality versus the Method of Principlism." *The Journal of Medicine and Philosophy* 18:477–90.

Griffin, J. 1986. *Well-Being.* Oxford: Clarendon Press.

Hare, R. M. 1981. *Moral Thinking.* Oxford: Clarendon Press.

Herman, B. 1993. *The Practice of Moral Judgment.* Cambridge, MA: Harvard University Press.

Holmes, H. B., and L. Purdy, eds. 1992. *Feminist Perspectives in Medical Ethics.* Bloomington, IN: Indiana University Press.

Holmgren, M. 1989. "The Wide and Narrow of Reflective Equilibrium." *Canadian Journal of Philosophy* 19:43–60.

Jonsen, A. R. 1991. "Casuistry as Methodology in Clinical Ethics." *Theoretical Medicine* 12:299–302.

————. 1995. "Casuistry: An Alternative or Complement to Principles?" *The Journal of the Kennedy Institute of Ethics* 5:246–47.

————. 1996. "Morally Appreciated Circumstances: A Theoretical Problem for Casuistry." In *Philosophical Perspectives on Bioethics*, eds. L. W. Sumner and J. Boyle. Toronto: University of Toronto Press, pp. 37–49.

Jonsen, A. R., and S. Toulmin. 1988. *The Abuse of Casuistry.* Berkeley: University of California Press.

Kagan, S. 1989. *The Limits of Morality.* Oxford: Clarendon Press.

Kant, I. 1959. *Foundations of the Metaphysics of Morals*, trans. L. W. Beck. Indianapolis, IN: Bobbs-Merrill.

Korsgaard, C. M. 1996. *Creating the Kingdom of Ends.* Cambridge: Cambridge University Press.

Levi, B. H. 1996. "Four Approaches to Doing Ethics." *The Journal of Medicine and Philosophy* 21:7–39.

Lineback, R. H., ed. 1969. *The Philosopher's Index.* 1st ed. Bowling Green, OH: Philosophy Documentation Center.

Macklin, R. 1992. "Universality of the Nuremberg Code." In *The Nazi Doctors and the Nuremberg Code*, eds. G. J. Annas and M. Grodin. New York: Oxford University Press, pp. 240–57.

McGee, G. 1999. *Pragmatic Bioethics.* Nashville, TN: Vanderbilt University Press.

Mill, J. S. 1979. *Utilitarianism*, ed. G. Sher. Indianapolis, IN: Hackett.

Nelson, H. L., ed. 1997. *Stories and Their Limits: Narrative Approaches to Bioethics.* New York: Routlege.

Nielsen, K. 1991. *After the Demise of the Tradition.* Boulder, CO: Westview.

Pellegrino, E. D. 1985. "The Virtuous Physician and the Ethics of Medicine." In *Virtue and Medicine*, ed. Earl E. Shelp. Dordrecht, The Netherlands: D. Reidel, pp. 248–53.

————. 1987. "Altruism, Self-Interest, and Medical Ethics." *Journal of the American Medical Association* 258:1939–40.

Rawls, J. 1971. *A Theory of Justice.* Cambridge, MA: Harvard University Press.

Reich, Warren T., ed. 1995. *Encyclopedia of Bioethics.* 2nd ed. New York: Macmillan.

Richardson, H. S. 1990. "Specifying Norms as a Way to Resolve Concrete Ethical Problems." *Philosophy and Public Affairs* 19:279–310.

Shelp, E., ed. 1985. *Virtue and Medicine.* Dordrecht, The Netherlands: D. Reidel.

Sherwin, S. 1992. *No Longer Patient: Feminist Ethics and Health Care.* Philadelphia: Temple University Press.

Singer, P. 1993. *Practical Ethics.* 2nd ed. Cambridge: Cambridge University Press.

Tarasoff v. Regents of the University of California. 1976. 17 Cal. 3d 425.

Thomson, J. J. 1990. *The Realm of Rights.* Cambridge, MA: Harvard University Press.

Wolf, S., ed. 1996. *Feminism and Bioethics.* New York: Oxford University Press.

4

Religion and Theology

Lisa Sowle Cahill

The methods and aims theology brings to medical ethics now can be examined in light of its role in the evolution of the field of modern medical ethics, where theology interacted with developments in moral philosophy. One important factor that has increasingly defined theological medical ethics in the last decade is the social analysis of research and health care, including their expanding international dimensions. This chapter will focus on Christian theology and medical ethics. However, the literature in other religious traditions is growing (Sullivan 1989), and in Judaism is rich and abundant (Bleich and Rosner 1979; Bleich 1981; Feldman 1986; Green 1986; Novak 1990; Davis 1991; Newman 1992; Gellman 1993). In this chapter, I describe characteristics of theological approaches to medical ethics, discuss the history of theology in medical ethics, and then use a paradigm offered by James Gustafson to describe these types of approaches to this field.

The one characteristic that most unifies theological approaches to medical ethics is the grounding of ethical argument in religious claims, and in the history and theological traditions of a religious community. For example, virtually every theologically grounded method in Jewish or Christian medical ethics originates from the conviction that humanity is a creature in a created and interdependent natural world; that the Creator is good, just, and powerful; that humanity is sinful, as well as responsible for good moral behavior; and that God offers human beings healing or salvation from moral and spiritual wrongdoing. These claims are explicated and refined variously in different religious traditions, although the general outlines remain the same.

The differences in theological method as applied to medical ethics result from differences in the way these fundamental claims about God and creation are understood and applied in religious traditions. One key set of differences has to do with the certainty and stability of theologically based moral norms. Another concerns the similarity between religious views of ethics and nonreligious views. Cloning is an example. Some theologians would look for clear norms about right and wrong that can be derived from theological foundations and applied in a reliable, constant manner, consistent with past tradition. They might take the position that since humanity is finite and only God is the Creator, for humans to take such radical control over reproduction as to create children from only one parent would be tantamount to "playing God," and would always be sinful. The sinfulness of cloning is thought to be directly and clearly entailed by the created nature of humanity and the commands of God. Some who would defend clear, stable, theologically grounded moral norms would also support these norms by appealing to a historical tradition of authoritative interpretation. Prominent examples are the Catholic Church's teaching office (*magisterium*) and the Jewish tradition of law (*halakha*), supplemented by the responsa literature, a collection of questions about the law submitted to individual rabbis. In this general approach, in which moral norms are derived more or less directly from theological and traditional premises, a good medical ethics argument is one that cogently demonstrates the connections between premises and conclusions, and the medical ethicist must have command of the theological and legal traditions that provide these premises. This kind of approach can be creative and innovative in the way in which theological tradition or religious law is interpreted, but the innovations are typically presented as being extrapolations, and not departures, from teachings of the past.

Other theological medical ethicists would take issue with the idea that theology provides many very specific, clear, and reliable norms that can be applied so consistently and comprehensively to new or complex situations. They would agree that beliefs about creation, responsibility, sin, and salvation supply parameters and establish concerns and directions of thought. However, concrete applications must be more adaptive to circumstances and emerging developments. Thus, for example, some theologians portray humans as the "created cocreators" with God, and argue that human freedom and responsibility require more flexibility, and even change, in determining what theological ethics requires in medicine today. Here, cloning and other new reproductive and genetic techniques can and should be justified by theological medical ethics. There is a much looser connection between basic theological beliefs and specific moral outcomes. What counts as a good moral argument is proportionately more difficult to specify, but familiarity with basic religious symbols would have to be accompanied by an imaginative application to new circumstances and possibilities. The persuasiveness of an argument would not be primarily logical or deductive, and it would not consist in conformity to tradition. It would lie more in the ability to stimulate readers to share the vision of the author by shifting their perception of the way theological claims relate to the issue at hand. (For an example of this sort of argument about genetic technology, and a discussion of some alternatives, see Peters 1996).

An even more important point of difference in theological methods is whether agreement on, or acceptance of, theological ethics' norms and commitments is perceived to require membership in a specific religious community. All theological ethicists agree that religious identity results in a set of moral commitments that are important for one's life and one's religious tradition, but where they disagree is in relating a religiously and theologically based morality to the larger world. For example, Orthodox Jewish interpreters of the law are not interested in whether society at large accepts the norms they produce, but rather in how Jews can live in faithfulness to their tradition today (Jakobovitz 1975). Similarly, some Christian thinkers write out of the "story" or "narrative" of their religious community, claiming that it provides a distinctive identity that would not be acceptable or even intelligible to outsiders (Hauerwas 1986a). For these ethicists it is more important to be faithful to their own religious and theological ideals than to have a big impact on public medical ethics and policy. A good argument would consist in a faithful delineation of a particular, communally based religious identity and the ways in which it is pertinent to behavior and practices for believers.

A contrasting approach is found in authors or traditions that accept premises like creation, sin, and redemption as the basis of their ethics, but that nevertheless are convinced that other reasonable people can arrive at the same or similar specific judgments about issues in medical ethics, for more generally available reasons. In such an approach, the method of argument would rely quite heavily on philosophy and on information from the natural and social sciences that could be shared with nonreligious persons seeking solutions to the same problems. One example of this approach is the method of Roman Catholic moral theology. Catholic medical ethicists attempt to enter the policy debates on the assumption that there is a common human nature and a generally acceptable ideal of the good society. These debates provide common ground where they can dispute with others whether it is a good idea or a bad one to permit, prohibit, or limit the use of cloning, other reproductive technologies, abortion, physician-assisted suicide, or germ line therapy. The mainline Protestant denominations share a similar approach, although their theological foundations are more the general moral values found in Scripture than they are the values of human nature and the common good. However, it should be noted that Catholicism sometimes falls into the earlier category of a community-relative bioethics, insofar as disputed issues are often referred to Church authority and settled in a manner that avoids philosophical and scientific counterevidence, and is not generally acceptable to thinkers outside Catholicism. (For a discussion of the relative merits of the community-oriented and the public-oriented forms of theological medical ethics, see Verhey 1996.)

An important point to be appreciated in understanding the ways in which theology functions in medical ethics is that the ethical "methods" of theology are neither separate and insulated from one another, nor are abstract theories detached from the realities and dilemmas of particular historical contexts. It is difficult to identify certain methods strictly with corresponding religious traditions, institutions of higher learning, or even followers and students collected around certain leading thinkers (though the latter is perhaps easier). Both the recognizable unity of "theological" medical ethics, and the striking dissimilarities in approach that we see today, must be understood in light of a confluence of factors that brought theologians into the growing field of medical ethics approximately four decades ago. Certain key thinkers were important in this process. The ways in which each of them envisioned theological medical ethics were heavily influenced by the ways they understood religious identity itself, the ways they interpreted new scientific and social challenges, and the opportunities they had for collaboration with nontheologians, for example, in formulating public policy.

HISTORY OF THEOLOGY IN MEDICAL ETHICS

Historical factors defining the relation of theology to modern medical ethics can be described briefly, if in oversimplified terms. In the 1960s, theologians were influential players in defining questions for the emerging field, reintroducing values and principles that had been neglected, and leading the way from general ideals to practical conclusions. Both the theologians and the philosophers who engaged in the modern discipline of medical ethics, and those health professionals who helped flag the sensitive issues, were motivated by the proliferation of new biomedical technologies, as well as a new consciousness of patients' rights and responsibilities that was beginning to replace traditional medical paternalism, especially in light of some well-publicized research abuses. They also recognized that the ethics of medicine could no longer be contained within an individualist patient-physician model and were aware that moral responsibility in medicine might require creativity and an orientation to future possibilities, at least as much as respect for the norms and prohibitions of the past.

Protestant theologians like Joseph Fletcher, Paul Ramsey, and James Gustafson began to think through such issues, drawing on touchstones like self-sacrificial love, covenant, creation, and image of God. They also relied on information from the social and natural sciences to better understand the changing practical context with which to interpret and apply religious themes. Catholic theologians like Richard McCormick, Charles Curran, and Germain Grisez looked for ways to link longstanding traditions of authoritative teaching and moral law to new developments in biomedicine. This was also true of Jewish thinkers like Immanuel Jakobovitz and Fred Rosner, and the Orthodox ethicist Stanley Harakas (Harakas 1980; 1999). They tried to define the appropriate sphere and scope of innovation and flexibility in coming to terms with emerging practices and possibilities.[1]

Theologians like Ramsey (1970), Gustafson (1975), McCormick (1981), and Karen Lebacqz (1983) served on important policy bodies, such as the National Commission on the Protection of Human Subjects of Biomedical and Behavioral Research (1974) and the President's Commission for the Study of Ethical Problems in Medicine and Biomedical and Behavioral Research (1979). They were major players in the formation of the field— helping to create bioethics institutes such as The Institute of Religion at the Texas Medical Center in Houston (1954); The Institute of Society, Ethics, and the Life Sciences, later to become the Hastings Center (1961); and the Kennedy Institute of Ethics at Georgetown University (1971). The first edition of the *Encyclopedia of Bioethics*, whose very existence and title lent substance to the new field, was filled with entries by theologians and other articles written from religious perspectives (Reich 1978; 1996, 90). Theologians were particularly well equipped to advance medical ethics because religious communities had cultivated long-standing traditions of reflection on life, death, and suffering, and had given more guidance on the specifics of moral conduct than had moral philosophy at that time.[2] (See Walters 1986; Reich 1996.)

However, some would say that the influence of the first theological medical ethicists came at a price (Callahan 1990; Lammers 1996). Making themselves heard in pluralistic debates, often touching on public policy, some theological medical ethicists began to operate like moral philosophers. This became more and more true in the 1980s, as more aspiring medical ethicists, even those pursuing theological degrees, were educated specifically for this new field of endeavor and assumed roles in clinical settings. Moreover, many seemed to pay more attention to crises and dilemmas than they did to their theological or even philosophical foundations. Consequently, specifically as theologians, they became marginalized in a field that came to rely increasingly on the kind of moral principles that plausibly could be claimed to be universal, rational, and "secular" and that sought the kind of decision making and policy resolutions that could be squared with U.S. legal traditions and command public support. The preeminent statement of such principles (autonomy, justice, beneficence, and nonmaleficence) was made by Tom Beauchamp and James F. Childress, the latter himself a theologian who studied with Gustafson at Yale (Beauchamp and Childress 1979).

As a result of the perceived marginalization of distinctively theological voices in medical ethics, theologians today are looking for a way to reassert their religious identity while not giving up moral credibility, even in the public and political realms. This search is not just about a theological identity crisis. It is also about a dissatisfaction with the recent tradition of principled, secular medical ethics that, above all, prizes autonomy (and its structural protection, informed consent), in conformity with the dominant U.S. political and legal ethos, which owes so much to Enlightenment ideals of scientific rationality. Theology's search for a new model of thinking in medical ethics corresponds to a simultaneous philosophical development: postmodernism and its concomitant insight that even abstract and supposedly universal principles always come to be articulated out of particular and historical communities of practice and discernment. Maybe such principles do express something universal about the human condition and moral obligation in science and medicine. But it will no longer do to view them as the simple, straightforward products of rational thinking, without looking much more carefully at how they have been contextually shaped (as recognized by Childress 1994). As relevant to the present chapter, this also means that theological "methods" in medical ethics cannot be understood apart from the conditions and individuals that create and use them. They are not merely intellectual products to be deployed scientifically, but tradition-based and contextual strategies for uniting and concretizing a number of concerns and goals having to do with biomedical trends and practices. Moreover, morality as seen from different communal standpoints may not be wholly translatable into a neutral, "secular" sphere. To some observers, this makes communal moralities, including religious moralities and theological ethics, seem like tribal preferences, inappropriate and even dangerous candidates for public consumption (Engelhardt 1996).

But to others, including many theologians, their very marginality should make religious and theological voices more wary of diluting and compromising their own traditions for the sake of participation in a supposedly public square (Callahan 1990; Campbell 1990; Hauerwas 1986a, 1996; Marty 1992). Theology should be more concerned about faithfulness to its own foundational texts, symbols, traditions, and moral practices than about influencing biomedical practice beyond the religious community. Its view will be particular. Its role in social ethics and medical ethics policy should be primarily prophetic. Only by speaking in an authentically religious voice can theology claim to have a method of medical ethics that reaches practical conclusions that are truly theological.

Meanwhile, several theologians on a spectrum seek a middle path (Smith 1996; Gustafson 1996a, 1996b; Reich with dell'Oro 1996; McCormick 1984; Cahill 1992). The commitment to make religiously grounded ideals effective in a public setting has been particularly strong in Roman Catholicism (Hehir 1992; McCormick 1995). Is there some way to reclaim theological identity while participating strongly in a public community of moral discourse?

The remainder of this chapter will address that question, using a paradigm of Gustafson's to sort theological methods in medical ethics into three categories (Gustafson 1996a, 56–72; 1996b). According to Gustafson's paradigm, theology is either autonomous, continuous with other modes of moral knowledge, or in a dialectical relationship with others. After introducing Gustafson's paradigm, I will consider three of the major players in the early development of theological medical ethics: Paul Ramsey, Richard McCormick, and James Gustafson. Then I will turn to a few more recent medical ethicists who have carried forward the theological interests of these "greats" while adapting and changing their agendas in light of recent developments in philosophy, science, and the public culture of the United States. Those making important contributions in theologically informed medical ethics today are far too numerous to treat comprehensively. Selections will be made with a view toward illustrating some major methodological alternatives and differences according to Gustafson's paradigm. Finally, I will outline what I believe are contributions that theology is making, or can make, to medical ethics at the current point in the evolution of the field.

THREE TYPES OF THEOLOGICAL MEDICAL ETHICS: AUTONOMOUS, CONTINUOUS, AND DIALECTICAL

Gustafson's paradigm reflects the general concerns about the nature and role of theological medical ethics: Has religion allowed itself to be marginalized in favor of a secular discourse in medical ethics that is now seen to be impossible, given the contextual and communal nature of all moral thinking (Verhey 1996; Gustafson 1996b)? Has this result been the compromise of the specifically religious context itself? Some theologians want religion to remain an "autonomous" sphere with its own integrity, for secular thinking amounts simply to another, competing, and ultimately hostile ideology. Still others believe that different disciplines do, in fact, offer reliable ways of understanding human behavior and human goods, so the insights generated by a religious community can be "continuous" with such knowledge. Religion's insights can be interpreted or translated into other realms of knowledge in an intelligible and persuasive way. According to Gustafson's third model, religion and other sources of moral knowledge are mutually interactive. Religion is not a privileged source, though it may be distinctive. Moral discernment depends on a "dialectic" between religion and other resources. They may correct one another.

Gustafson defined this basic paradigm of the autonomy, continuity, and dialectic models of medical ethics and applied it to certain types of religious and theological literature. Different warrants for the autonomy model of theological ethics include a postmodern epistemology that relativizes the claims of any and all religious traditions, a strong doctrine of revelation (through sacred texts, traditions, and practices), and respect for institutional authority that guards revelation and tradition. Under the rubric of this model, Gustafson mentions the halakhic reasoning of Orthodox Judaism; Eastern Orthodoxy's focus on the cosmological significance of Christ; forms of Christianity, Judaism, and Islam that focus on the sacred text; Catholic moral theologies that keep change within the parameters of the tradition; and churches where formal or informal structures of authority enforce compliance with revealed or traditional morality. In all cases, "alteration of the religious ethic by the findings of science, medicine, and other disciplines is resisted." Instead, a distinctive, independent, and faithful morality "directs human conduct in medical matters" (Gustafson 1996b, 86).

In direct contrast to this model, the model of theological "continuity" with secular medical ethics proposes that religious or theological medical ethics is not only "intelligible" beyond the religious community, but perhaps even "persuasive." The themes of religious morality can add "depth and scope" to other views. What is "religious," then, about religiously backed medical ethics might be its source in revelation, its authorization by a sacred text, its place in a larger theological framework, or its special obligatory force for religious believers. The actual rules for behavior that these religious origins or qualifications produce, however, are intelligible, understandable, and, even in principle, convincing outside the belief community (Gustafson 1996b, 87–88), as long as outsiders share the same moral anthropology, or basic view of humans. Gustafson mentions religious ethics informed by Aquinas's natural law or the moral anthropology of Kant. On the continuity model, "moral or ethical visions or doctrines of the human are continuous with views of the human articulated for other purposes. . . . " "Religious morality and ethics" is "in continuity with other ethics" (Gustafson 1996b, 91) and therefore can communicate with and transform them.

For the model that is dialectical and interactive, however, religious and theological ethics can itself be changed by other communities and fields of knowledge (Gustafson 1996b, 91). Gustafson seems to prefer this model; it certainly best describes his own theological ethics (to be addressed below). According to the dialectical alternative model, religious language and symbols and theological language do not have to be "translated" to have "some desirable outcome for the practices of morality in a human community more inclusive than those persons who can be socially identified as traditionally religious." A symbol like "image of God" has "disclosive power." Yet, while its meaning of respect for persons may be justified on other grounds, it is not completely reducible to its nonreligious equivalents either. Hence the dialectical relationship between religious and nonreligious views. Sometimes these may turn out to be mutually compatible or complementary, and sometimes they may clash, at least in some respects. When this happens, one or the other may be revised (Gustafson 1996b, 92–93). Sometimes religious backings, symbols, and moralities must be reformulated because nonreligious sources have qualified the truth claims and undermined the credibility of traditional religious interpretations of the human in relation to the divine, and of morality (Gustafson 1984, 7–8).

It is important in understanding the force of these models that they are intended by Gustafson to be ideal types, and not strict means of classification. The three constructs are considered to have "heuristic value" in illuminating "tendencies" and "divergences" in the literature (Gustafson 1996b, 82). Indeed, I would add that virtually all literature and methods in theological medical ethics fit into a broad "dialectical" category, in that their perspectives are highly indebted to concrete developments and innovations in science and medicine. These developments change the very meaning of the human reality, including embodiment, freedom, relation to nature, and social relationships. The moral meaning of religious beliefs and symbols adapts in response to these. No theological medical ethics is insulated or "autonomous" in the full sense of the word. Due to the contextual and historical nature of religious communities and their theological reflection, neither can any community or discipline develop a morality that is simply "continuous" and fully convergent with other viewpoints.

Theology and Other Voices

Gustafson's paradigm may be most fruitfully employed to understand the primary worries and priorities with which a given variety of theological medical ethics enters the dialectic with other discourses. For some, it is important to protect the biblical heritage defining communal identity and its way of life as discipleship, and so to offer a prophetic critique of culture. For others, it is the wisdom and faithfulness of a tradition structured by authoritative teaching institutions that must be safeguarded. For still others, the primary interest, in light of theology's social responsibility, is to ensure that its morality and ethics are articulated on the basis of the best human knowledge and in terms of the most profound and widely shared human ideals, and to enlarge those ideals where possible.

These priorities can change, not only with the particular ways in which religion and theology are perceived, but also with the social and political situations theological ethics addresses. In the 1960s the duty and prerogative of religious spokespersons (such as Reinhold Niebuhr, Martin Luther King, and Pope John XXIII) to exercise leadership on important social issues were less questioned than today. Theologians moved into the medical ethics arena perhaps more confidently, more acceptably, and more warranted in their expectation that their influence could be significant. Therefore, interpreting, "translating," or finding functional equivalents for their religious ideals seemed to be both socially important and of little danger to their essential religious identity.

In the 1990s growing secularism in the public life of this country was accompanied by the privatization of mainstream religious morality and the growing power of a religious right that quite deliberately criticized and countered "reasonable" and "consensus-oriented" discourse on medical ethics and other social issues. Theologians found considerably less opportunity to voice their ethical views with seriousness in the public forum, and less general receptivity when they did do so. Problems of social ethics were resolved politically, or on the basis of the longstanding American principles of autonomy and privacy, heavily pressured in their exercise by the incentives of the market and by consumer opportunity. In this milieu, theological medical ethics turned once again to the distinctive sources of their religious identities, and offered critiques of autonomy and the market that they rightly may have believed would find little cultural resonance. Some theological medical ethicists, more interested in the "autonomy" of religion from cultural forces, now participate in medical ethics debates with diminished confidence in their public persuasiveness and heightened commitment to their religious faithfulness. Others, still believing it important and possible to exert a transformative influence on social values and trends, try to locate points of contact or "continuity" between their own religiously inspired perspectives on human and social well-being and other religious views.

If we use Gustafson's paradigm to appreciate the priorities of the first theological luminaries of modern medical ethics, we discover that they were all dialectical thinkers who energetically participated in public debate and were influenced by it in the presentation of their theological vision. Yet they, too, differed, like thinkers of today, in the relative priority they gave to religious identity or general moral consensus. Ramsey was passionately interested in proclaiming what he considered to be the biblical foundations of ethics, including medical ethics. McCormick wanted to advance the agenda of the Catholic Church's Second Vatican Council to engage with the modern world and to energize moral theology through lively exchanges about a more or less "continuous" interpretation of the person and the common good. Gustafson came to see many expressions of Christian morality as historically relative and therefore as products of culture as well as its critic. While theology can remind medical ethics of limits and dangers that it is tempted to forget, science and history can teach religion and theology that they, too, can embody distortions of human and divine realities. For Gustafson, the divine "ordering of life" cannot be known in any simple way from the bible or tradition. It requires knowing about the concrete conditions of life, particular relationships of humans and of nature, and "the patterns and processes of life in which we are participants" (Gustafson 1984, 319). This requires information from the natural and human sciences, and implies that past interpretations of revelation and tradition may need to be revised or even rejected.

Paul Ramsey

Among those who were influential in the first decades of the field, Methodist theologian Paul Ramsey best exemplifies the concerns of the autonomy model of medical ethics. In his first book, *Basic Christian Ethics* (Ramsey 1951), Ramsey states his purpose as "to stand within the way the Bible views morality" (Ramsey 1951, xi). This way should not be equated with ordinary moral standards: Christian love is obedient, sacrificial, non-preferential love for whatever "neighbor" stands in need of aid (Ramsey 1951, 39–40). Nevertheless, Ramsey was no apolitical Christian idealist. He summed up the relation between Christian love and existing institutions as "the constant criticism and reshaping" of the latter and the "bending" of social policies (Ramsey 1951, 349–50).

In later writings, Ramsey modified this position somewhat by adopting a "mixed" form of a love-based ethic, relying on reason as well as revelation to define the terms of ethics (Ramsey 1967, 29, 122). The theological rationale for this move is Ramsey's eventual conviction that Christ died for "all men," thus including all persons in the covenant established by God in Christ. The ability to recognize and be claimed by altruistic love has become part of "our common humanity" (Ramsey 1967, 43). With this interpretation of his religious base, Ramsey is able to protect the "autonomy" of Christian ethics, at least in theory, while warranting the avid participation in practical medical and policy ethics that characterized his life and work. It also marks a receptivity on Ramsey's part to influences from discourses that are not self-consciously religious.

Two decades after *Basic Christian Ethics*, Ramsey published his key statement of Christian medical ethics, *The Patient as Person*, addressed to "the widest possible audience" (Ramsey 1970, xi). The governing theological categories in this book are "covenant" and "covenant fidelity." The acceptance of covenant responsibilities defines the true fulfillment of even the natural relationships between persons, and can be stated in terms such as justice, faithfulness, care, "canons of loyalty," the sanctity of life, and love or charity (Ramsey 1970, xii–xiii). The Christian ethicist should see that medical ethics is critically informed by these principles and virtues. In *The Patient as Person*, Ramsey addresses the issues of informed consent to experimentation, brain death, care for the dying, organ donation, and the allocation of scarce resources. He translates Christian values into medical ethics primarily in terms of absolute respect for the inviolability of the individual person. No consideration of the common good should be permitted to mitigate the priority of care for the individual patient. And even if a patient is not harmed, he or she may be wronged if caregivers or researchers fail to put his or her individual welfare first and foremost, as protected by personal consent (Ramsey 1970, 39). Thus all experimentation on children, however seemingly benign, is ruled out. Ramsey explicitly rejects the Roman Catholic argument that organ donation can be justified in relation to the donor's own moral identity and holiness; the only possible Christian justification for such an act is charitable sacrifice for another (Ramsey

1970, 176). In writing about the allocation of kidney dialysis, one of the first crises in re-source scarcity brought about by modern technology, Ramsey proposes that only a lottery system, and not any estimation of social worth, is the right way to respect the equal dignity of everyone (Ramsey 1970, 256).

All of the above topics, and others addressed in further writings, were taken up by Ramsey with a quite explicit view to influencing public policy debates and patterns of clinical and research medicine that were urgent at the time. He employs Christian norms, derived from general biblical themes, to advocate the positions he favors. However, it is also quite clear that his understanding of covenant fidelity is focused on the individual and is designed to protect individuals from a technological rationality that measures morality exclusively in terms of good results. His theological medical ethics thus is informed by the moral and social ethos of his time and place, even as it calls that ethos to account by standards of morality that subject individual rights to scientific and social goals. At the same time, his theological perspective is operative in his refusal to define the duty to care equally for all patients in the vocabulary of individual rights (Smith 1993). Ramsey's stress falls much more heavily on duty and obedience: the duty, in obedience to God's saving act in Jesus Christ, to assume the burden of care for the vulnerable. His focus is not on the entitlements of individuals, but on the covenantal obligations of caregivers.

Richard McCormick

Like Paul Ramsey, Richard McCormick sees theological medical ethics as a reflection on a particular religious tradition, and, within that tradition, as being concerned "with what we, as believers in Jesus Christ, ought to be and do (or not do)" (McCormick 1984, 3). However, unlike Ramsey, McCormick was trained theologically in a tradition that not only has a strong central teaching authority, but also claims to base its specific moral conclusions on the "natural law." In other words, morality consists in living up to the goods and ideals apparent in ordinary human experiences and purposes, and Christian morality is the same, at the concrete or substantive level, as the morality of other reasonable persons. This is so not only because the saving actions of Christ apply to all, but also because the goodness of human nature survives sin sufficiently to permit discernment of basic morality and of the requirements of human well-being and the common good.

For example, McCormick elaborates on six themes of medical ethics that can be defended in religious terms but are not exclusive to religious people: the value of life as a basic, but not absolute, good; the inclusion of the unborn in the good of human life; the definition of the highest good of human life not as physical life itself, but as moral and religious experiences; the essential sociality of persons; the unity of the "spheres" of life-giving and lovemaking; and the normative value of heterosexual, permanent marriage (McCormick 1984, 51–57). These values can be backed by experiential and philosophical warrants. The way experience and philosophy are read by McCormick in interpreting the nature of persons and of society no doubt reflects his religious background. Likewise, experiences and theories that have emerged since Vatican II influence the way he interprets the religious tradition. But McCormick would affirm that the basis for discourse between Christianity and other traditions lies in the essential human capacity to know good and evil and to come to reasonable (if necessarily imperfect and revisable) conclusions about what is good or evil morality in practice. Good morality seeks human well-being, while evil conduct undermines and destroys it.

McCormick not only grants that both religious and philosophical morality can change, he views the dialectical relation to culture that came increasingly to characterize Catholic morality after Vatican II as a positive, beneficent, and necessary development. Unlike those who see the authoritative teaching of the Church as a closed system, McCormick believes that the message of Vatican II is that Catholic moral theology is, or should be, inductive, exploratory, sometimes tentative, and "always in flux." It "takes seriously the findings of human experience and human sciences," purifying and modifying past formulations in light of basic Christian and human concerns (McCormick 1984, 4).

This dynamic understanding of theological ethics and medical ethics is reflected in the way McCormick defines the basis of the natural law. Ethics in health and medicine is not just tied to certain prescriptions and proscriptions derived from static human physical faculties and functions. It is based on "the total good of the person," or, to quote Vatican II, "the human person integrally and adequately considered" (McCormick 1984, 15). This definition implies that human freedom, conscience, and relationships, as well as the social interrelatedness of persons, are all essential to defining what human nature and human well-being are. In this way, McCormick interprets the natural law in a manner that is individualized and context sensitive, without losing sight of "objective standards" of what it means to be human and of how morality corresponds to a shared human reality (McCormick 1984, 15, 17; 1989, 1–208).

McCormick has addressed virtually every one of the major issues of medical ethics, carrying forward a tradition that both is based on the natural moral law and mediated by an authoritative institution, and adapting the essential insights of that tradition to contend with new scientific and cultural developments. For example, the distinction between ordinary and extraordinary means of life support has a long history in Roman Catholic ethics and permits withdrawing or foregoing life supports, while forbidding direct euthanasia (Sacred Congregation for the Doctrine of the Faith 1980). McCormick affirms this analysis as making sense of the human condition, valuing patient self-determination, while placing it against the horizon of objective and reasonable best interests and acknowledging the transcendent destiny of the human person (McCormick 1984, 107–23). McCormick also plays this tradition against U.S. court cases; the development of life-prolonging technology; cultural attitudes toward life, death, and medicine; and the drive toward physician-assisted suicide. He takes up the questions of access to adequate health care for all members of society that Paul Ramsey was unable to explore—and that were less publicly visible—before Ramsey's death in 1988.

More than the tradition, McCormick amplifies the spiritual context of care for the dying and also puts decisions to utilize certain types of treatment into the context of the common good and of social institutions. McCormick interprets physician-assisted suicide as a symptom of a society in which mindless, even "violent," technology has become a substitute for "compassion and care" (McCormick 1995, 460–61). If persons were assured of care and pain control, as well as the ability to refuse treatments that violate their quality of life (including artificial nutrition and hydration [McCormick 1995, 461; 1989, 369–87]), they might not define suicide as a necessary option. McCormick also believes the failure to meet the health care needs of the poor reveals a societal attitude of ultimate disrespect for life that is inconsistent with commitment to more humane, albeit more demanding, alternatives to suffering than killing the patient (McCormick 1995, 463).

Over the years, Richard McCormick and Paul Ramsey came into direct conflict on a few issues, though they always remained congenial colleagues and engaged conversation partners. Their disagreements reveal disparities in their basic theological perspectives, differences that also shape the way they formulate their ethical concerns and judgments, including the philosophical principles and categories that seem most adequate to each. For example, Paul Ramsey always maintained that research on those who could give only proxy consent provided for them (children) amounted to "unconsented touching," and could not be justified under any circumstances. His basis was the absoluteness of covenant fidelity, translated as a "deontological" or duty-oriented ethic, in which the object of moral duty is the inviolability of the concrete other or "neighbor." A Christian ethic of obedience to God's commands, most notably advanced in this century by the neo-orthodox theologian Karl Barth, is one way of resisting cultural norms that plead the necessity of advancing short-term good results wherever possible.

McCormick, on the other hand, represents a "teleological" ethic of human goods and purposes, in which the individual good is always seen in relation to the common good. This perspective on morality is typical of Catholic "natural law" and traces its roots back to Aquinas. The common good is not a utilitarian concept in which the good of the many overrides individual rights, but a social ethic comprehending and requiring the participation of all individuals in a larger enterprise from which each benefits. Insofar as the individual is inherently social, contributing to the welfare of others is, in fact, contributory to his or her own well-being as a human person. This is true even of children and incompetent patients. Thus a proxy may give consent to experimentation, provided that there is virtually no risk of harm to the research subject. (For a more extensive discussion of these contrasts, with references, see Cahill 1979.)

James M. Gustafson

Some of the theological foundations of Gustafson's ethics have already been described. He sees the relation between theology and nonreligious forms of discourse as dialectical. From the Reformed tradition in theology, he brings a central commitment to God's sovereignty, particularly the view that ethics and theology should be theocentric, not anthropocentric. In other words, human conduct should not be oriented or judged by the welfare of humans primarily, but by the will of God, and the relation of all things to one another in God. Humans are part of the created universe; they are not its peak or center; and the world does not work so that human beings can, or should, expect all their desires and purposes to be fulfilled.

Among other resources that Gustafson brings to theological ethics, the natural and social sciences are significant. They help shape his view that God's purposes should not be confused with human purposes. They also contribute to his conclusion that the moral life is full of both ambiguity and conflict. The natural sciences, and other experiences of the world, are pathways to a human "sense of the divine." Religious traditions and symbols must be tested against these dialectically related sources. Parallel to the sometimes incompatible needs of creatures in the natural environment, the resolution of a moral dilemma may lie in tragic denial or sacrifice. But human beings can also keep company with one another in the midst of suffering, and sometimes experience God as friend and sustainer. (For a concise and personal presentation of these themes, see Gustafson 1994).

Gustafson's writings in medical ethics generally stay clear of definitive pronouncements on right and wrong conduct. More typically, they introduce and explicate the key theological themes and orientations that should guide Christian engagement with science and medicine (Gustafson 1975); outline models, modes, and parameters within which the engagement should take place (Gustafson 1988, 1996a); or incisively sort out and illustrate the consequences of undertaking the dialectic of theology with certain presuppositions, or in a certain mode, rather than others (Gustafson 1974, 273–86 ["Genetic Engineering and a Normative View of the Human"]). Gustafson can criticize the Christian tradition, for example, by seeing suicide as a "conscientious" decision in some cases of irremediable human suffering and despair (Gustafson 1984, 215). He is one of the first theological medical ethicists to take the global and environmental contexts of medicine and research seriously, for example in surveying the ethics of population and nutrition (Gustafson 1984, 219–50). Certainly, Gustafson exhibits a heightened sensitivity to Western cultural imperialism (political, ethical, or theological); this is a result of his self-avowed "cultural relativism" (which for him is not the same as a thoroughgoing relativism of either God's claim on humans or of ethics). Gustafson distinguishes his position both from traditional Roman Catholicism and from Ramsey's covenantal theology by asserting that God did not so much establish a "moral order" in creation (or redemption) as establish "different patterns of well-being" that could emerge over time (Gustafson 1975, 39). The Christian theologian approaches medical ethics with attitudes not only of respect for life, but also of openness to the new, flavored with appropriate humility and self-criticism, due to the effects of finitude and sinfulness (Gustafson 1975, 54–75). These latter virtues further underwrite the attitude of receptivity with which the theological dialectic with science and medicine is undertaken.

Developments and Complications

The writings of other authors, some of whom have appeared on the theological medical ethics scene more recently, may be assessed in relation to Gustafson's models; many are influenced directly or indirectly by Ramsey, McCormick, and Gustafson.

Autonomy Model

First, let us revisit the autonomy model of theological bioethics. Perhaps the most clear example of such an approach today is Stanley Hauerwas, a student of Gustafson. Hauerwas combines a biblical vocabulary with a strong sense of historical relativity to launch a critique of cultural and theological liberalism that is almost sectarian in tone, compared to the dialectical method of his former mentor. Hauerwas himself would reject the label "sectarian," since his interest in being a public spokesperson on bioethical and political issues (especially war and violence) prevents any sort of isolation from general social concerns. However, Hauerwas does use categories of narrative, story, character, and virtue to define Christian ethics as very much a community-based enterprise that may seem foolish or even senseless to those who judge using worldly or "secular" standards. The theologian approaching medical ethics has the obligation, above all else, to attend to the formation of Christian character within a narrative-based community that is true to its own identity. Christians know that they cannot control science and technology, heal all disease, or end all suffering. What Christians can do is bear Christ's cross by keeping faithful company with those who suffer. In every suffering person, and in suffering itself, the Christian encounters God (Hauerwas 1986a, 1986b, 1990). This is a radical view of Christian theological medical ethics, insofar as Hauerwas, in effect, counsels theologians to stay away from secular philosophy and policy debates, where they can make little impact and where they are likely to be seduced by the temptation to be "relevant."

Somewhat less iconoclastic examples of the view that Christian ethics ought first and foremost to protect its autonomy from alien value systems are Allen Verhey and Gilbert Meilaender. Both are explicitly engaged in influencing medical policy and the cultural discourse about medical ethics at large through writing and professional roles. However, distinctive commitments are also highly important to both. Verhey, an evangelical by background, uses biblical resources more extensively than does Hauerwas and with more attention to exegesis and biblical criticism. Verhey often will interject a biblical reference or refrain into a discussion directed ultimately toward a public or policy outcome on the effective assumption that religious imagery may well evoke some convergence among ethical positions that ultimately will not come into alignment on every point (Verhey 1987). Meilaender, a Lutheran, is also resistant to liberalism and utilitarianism, appealing to a Barthian sense of God's ownership of human life. The Christian vision of the world defines an attitude toward life and death, in which life is understood as a trust from God, and the direct causation of death remains beyond the proper limit of human powers. As did Ramsey, Meilaender often borrows philosophical distinctions developed primarily in Catholic moral theology to define the exact limits of medical interventions; an example is the distinction between direct and indirect intention and action (Meilaender 1982).

Quite a different sort of "autonomist" is the Catholic author Germain Grisez. His theological ethics has much in common with the "continuity" model in that, for Grisez, ethics is based on seven "basic goods" that are shared and knowable by all human beings. These are self-integration; practical reasonableness; justice and friendship; life, including health and the handing on of life; knowledge of truth and appreciation of beauty; work; and play (Grisez 1983, 124; 1993, 567–78). An eighth, marriage, is later added (Grisez 1993, 568). However, Grisez draws conclusions about the practical import of these goods that are not so widely shared. For example, killing in abortion, euthanasia, and war are all wrong (Grisez 1970; Grisez and Boyle 1975; Finnis, Boyle, and Grisez 1987); withdrawal of artificial nutrition and hydration from a comatose patient is wrong (Dennehy and Grisez 1986); and contraception is wrong (Ford et al. 1988). To defend these positions as conclusive and absolute, Grisez appeals to the Christian way of life and to the authoritative teaching of the Roman Catholic Church about what the "natural law" is and demands. Unlike those, such as McCormick, who interpret the natural law in a more "dialectical" mode, Grisez is not open to challenge of certain specific "moral absolutes" in Catholic moral theology, mostly having to do with sexual behavior and the direct killing of "innocent persons" (from conception to death).

Continuity Model

Moving on to the continuity model of ethics, one finds both Catholic and Protestant representatives. First consider the Catholic version. Even a Vatican document like the *Declaration on Euthanasia* (Sacred Congregation for the Doctrine of the Faith 1980), while very committed to preserving authoritative teaching, makes overtures to members of other religions and to the public at large to agree that the good of life is fundamental, and that mercy-killing is not acceptable social policy. This document is somewhat irenic toward those who believe that euthanasia is a form of compassion, or is necessary in the face of human suffering. A similar pro-public stance characterizes statements authored by the U.S. Catholic bishops and directed toward national legal or policy matters, such as health care reform (National Conference of Catholic Bishops 1993; see also Ashley and O'Rourke 1989). Such documents may call on the categories of the modern Catholic tradition of social teaching, focused on the common good and including a "preferential option for the poor," to urge social reforms. They may appeal to a national political tradition and a sense of justice to encourage consensus. While not renouncing official Catholic teaching on such matters as abortion or euthanasia, they may choose in some cases to put the emphasis on social responsibilities for science, research, health, and equitable access to medical care.

Other Catholic authors carry this trajectory further, opening the door, as does McCormick, to revisions of specific teachings about individual "forbidden" behavior. Revisions may be based on interpretations of the human condition as evolving or changing, or on the new moral insights provided by contemporary experience. Proponents typically defend these changes, however, in terms of what they take to be the key or fundamental moral commitments that have always been honored by the tradition itself. For example, John T. Noonan has argued that contraception could be accepted in changing social circumstances on the basis of improved knowledge of the reproductive system and out of continuing respect for the importance of parenthood, its relation to sexual love and commitment, the protection of the unborn, the dignity of women, and the responsibility of parents to nurture children (Noonan 1986). More recently, many Catholic authors have made the case that "quality of life" is a legitimate criterion for deciding to forego certain medical treatments, and that this does not violate the traditional "sanctity-of-life principle" (Walter and Shannon 1990). Others have proposed that the embryo is not fully a person from conception, based on new information about early embryonic development (Shannon and Wolter 1990). These authors exemplify an approach that sees a basic continuity between Christian and other moral insights into practical behavior; they are therefore willing to engage in a dialectic with other sources about morality's specific rules and demands while privileging the basic parameters of the Christian (or even Catholic) moral vision, its definition of moral virtue, and what they consider to be its basic values and principles.

A Protestant example of a dialectically open continuity model of ethics is William F. May, a Methodist like Ramsey and Hauerwas. Like Ramsey, May is interested in covenantal imagery, though he too rarely takes up intensive exegesis of specific biblical texts. He uses covenant to establish a basic orientation of vision and outlook that then informs the way one approaches medical relationships and responsibilities. Like Hauerwas, May believes that the identity of the Christian community should indeed be distinctive and should shape character and virtue in an appropriate way. However, unlike Hauerwas, May draws no strict boundaries between the insights of other communities and Christian morality. In fact, his long-standing use of the covenantal metaphor to understand the physician-patient role and the place of health care and healing within community assumes that the covenant is a type of moral relationship that can be generally recognized and enacted (May 1996, 4, 13–14; see also May 1983, 1991). May is not as focused on concrete distinctions and rules as are many Catholic authors (whether to endorse or reject them). For example, May believes that direct euthanasia or physician-assisted suicide is not the proper covenantal response to suffering patients, who are in need of persevering care and pain relief, not a technological answer to a profound human problem. But May therefore does not propose an absolute norm against mercy-killing as *never* justified. He admits a gray area in decision making and accepts that euthanasia could be acceptable in the rare, exceptional instance (May 1996, 47–48). Like McCormick, May places life-and-death issues in medicine in a larger social picture, in which a health care system that "abandons" the uninsured is part of the push toward legalized euthanasia. Although he grounds the social meaning of covenant responsibilities in religious faith, he also makes his case in philosophical terms: health care is a fundamental good, not the only fundamental good, but a public good nonetheless (May 1996, 99, 103).

Dialectical Model

Since most theological medical ethicists today are dialectical to a greater or lesser degree, and simultaneously are committed anew to maintain intact those tenets of the tradition that they at least perceive to be essential, it is perhaps more difficult than it once was to identify a separate class of those exemplifying the dialectical model. However, there are still some theologians who believe that the dialectical relation of theology and culture cuts both ways—in the sense that religious traditions must sometimes be corrected on basic issues in light of contemporary experience. One such group of thinkers is feminist theologians. Among the many whose work deserves to be mentioned are Barbara Hilkert Andolsen, Sidney Callahan, Dena Davis (who is Jewish), Margaret A. Farley, Christine Gudorf, Beverly Harrison, Karen Lebacqz, and Maura A. Ryan. Among these, I will select just one article, by Margaret Farley, that addresses the defining characteristics of feminist theological medical ethics and that has become something of a "classic" in the genre. In "Feminist Theology and Bioethics," Farley states that feminist theology perceives profound discrimination against women in traditions of religious patriarchy. The major work of feminist theologians to date has been the unmasking of beliefs, symbols, and religious practices that establish and foster this discrimination. What they have found are massive tendencies in religious traditions to justify patterns of relationship in which men dominate women (Farley 1985, 166).

Invoking a feminist perspective that is attentive to relationality, embodiment, and the world of nature, Farley establishes a theological perspective that measures both bible and tradition according to whether, in the words of Rosemary Radford Ruether, they affirm "the full humanity of women" (Farley 1985, 175).

FUTURE DIRECTIONS

Two important trends must be mentioned in concluding an overview of methods in theological medical ethics that has been far too schematic to do justice to the scope and complexity of the authors and works available, or even to cover them all. First, the practice of medicine and the provision of health care in the United States are increasingly scientific rather than humanistic enterprises, and they are even more quickly being directed by marketplace values. Participants in medicine—whether providers or patients—are finding this situation ever less satisfactory at a personal level, and many are raising questions about the kind of society that is sponsoring these shifts. Because they deal in the elemental human experiences of birth, life, death, and suffering, the biomedical arts provide an opening for larger questions of meaning and even of transcendence. Religious themes and imagery can be helpful in articulating these concerns and addressing them in an imaginative, provocative, and perhaps ultimately transformative way. Religious symbolism may be grounded in particular communities and their experiences of God and community, but perhaps it can also mediate a sensibility of transcendence and ultimacy that is achingly latent in the ethical conflicts, tragedies, and triumphs that are unavoidable in biomedicine. The immense current interest in the spiritual dimensions of health care exemplifies this trend (Sulmasy 1997; Guroian 1996; Ashley and O'Rourke 1989, 389–412).

A second, not unrelated, trend is toward investment in the social and even global picture of health care ethics by theologians. In religious perspective, justice in medicine and access to preventive and therapeutic care is seen increasingly in communal terms, not only in terms of autonomy. While philosophical and public policy medical ethics in the United States is still dominated by considerations of autonomy and informed consent, theological medical ethics, even when "translated" into more general, nonreligious categories, tends to prioritize distributive justice and social solidarity over individual rights and liberty. This makes theological medical ethics more resistant to the market forces that so often control what research is funded, where it is conducted and on whom, who has access to the benefits, who profits from new knowledge and its implementation, and how health care is organized within a society as a whole. Biblical foundations can be found for such a perspective, especially in the teaching and example of Jesus about love of neighbor and serving the poor and vulnerable. Warrants can also be found in religious traditions of practice, where care of the sick has often been institutionalized as a work of devotion and self-offering to the divine, and where morality has been communal in nature and definition. In today's world, the "community" in which the neighbor is served and goods shared is increasingly international and global, and theological medical ethics is responding directly to these new global realities (Peters 1998; Keenan 2000).

CONCLUDING COMMENTS

In summary, the methods of theological medical ethics today remain plural, but it is fair to say that, by definition, they orient religious traditions, literatures, symbols, practices, and schools of reflective thought toward a world in which human beings undergo, interpret, and construct some of their most profound experiences. Theology itself is pluralistic on the question of whether its medical ethics should enter that arena with a strong countercultural and religiously distinctive message, or whether it should present its public face as a more familiar visage that invites to mutual communication. Theological medical ethics is agreed, however, that ethics opens onto the transcendence that human persons and communities encounter most fully in the limit experiences of life, suffering, and death, and that compassionate and just solidarity in these experiences defines personal and social virtue in the medical context.

NOTES ON RESOURCES AND TRAINING

As has been indicated by the shape of this chapter, individual theologians have had great influence on shaping the field, and they do not always congregate in identifiable schools of thought that sponsor idiosyncratic programs of education. Theological medical ethics is rather a national (and increasingly international) enterprise, where cross-fertilization occurs through publication, conferences, institutes that gather scholars around special projects or foci, and professional societies whose numerous seminars and groups are devoted to bioethics (American Academy of Religion, Catholic Theological Society of America, College Theology Society, Society of Christian Ethics).

Two axes along which differences in educational opportunities might arise would be Protestant–Catholic–Jewish and academic-clinical. Some of the differences in Protestant versus Catholic approaches to medical ethics will be evident from the main body of this chapter. Perhaps it should also be added that identifiably "Catholic" theological faculties will exist both in universities, some of which include graduate professional schools in health and medicine, and in seminaries. "Protestant" faculties are more likely to exist in smaller religiously affiliated colleges or in seminaries. This is true of Jewish education in medical ethics as well. Seminary faculties, Catholic or Protestant, are, for obvious reasons, dedicated primarily to preparing graduates for work in a particular theological tradition, as are rabbinical colleges. Other Catholic, Protestant, and Jewish theologians teach and engage in scholarly research on interdenominational faculties, and those in church-related institutions often engage in the ecumenical exchange made possible by the institutions and societies mentioned above. Theological education in medical ethics that occurs in universities, as well as in many seminaries and colleges, has an academic, theoretical, scholarly, research-oriented, and properly theological orientation; medical ethics is typically treated as a subspecialty within theological ethics and not as a field of study in its own right. However, universities that incorporate or are in proximity to a medical school, nursing school, or health care facility may have programs in clinical ethics where the focus is more on practical decision making and holistic patient care, in close conversation with medical practitioners and researchers. (Among such universities are Georgetown, Saint Louis University, and Loyola University of Chicago.) In these cases, the approach taken in analysis of decisions and practice, and on pastoral practice, may be flavored by the sponsoring institution (usually Catholic, though with varying accents on the importance of Catholic orthodoxy). It is important not to exaggerate these differences; moreover, many, many more programs in theological ethics that include medical ethics could be mentioned than is possible here.

NOTES

1. For essays on several of the key contributors to theological medical ethics, see Verhey and Lammers, eds. 1993.
2. The Park Ridge Center in Chicago, Illinois, has sponsored a multivolume, international series on "Health and Medicine in the Faith Traditions." The series, *Project Ten*, is edited by Martin E. Marty and Kenneth L. Vaux, and is published by Crossroad (New York).

REFERENCES

Ashley, B. M., and O. P. O'Rourke. 1989. *Health Care Ethics: A Theological Analysis*. 3rd ed. St. Louis, MO: Catholic Health Association.

Beauchamp, T. L., and J. F. Childress. 1979. *Principles of Biomedical Ethics*. New York: Oxford University Press.

Bleich, J. D. 1981. *Judaism and Healing: Halakhic Perspectives*. New York: Ktav.

Bleich, J. D., and F. Rosner, eds. 1979. *Jewish Bioethics*. New York: Sanhedrin Press.

Cahill, L. S. 1979. "Within Shouting Distance: Paul Ramsey and Richard McCormick on Method." *Journal of Medicine and Philosophy* 4:398–417.

———. 1992. "Theology and Bioethics: Should Religious Traditions Have a Public Voice?" *Journal of Medicine and Philosophy* 17:263–72.

Callahan, D. 1990. "Religion and the Secularization of Bioethics." *Hastings Center Report* 20:2–10.

Campbell, C. S. 1990. "Religion and Moral Meaning in Bioethics." *Hastings Center Report* 20:4–10.

Childress, J. F. 1994. "Principles-Oriented Bioethics: An Analysis and Assessment from Within." In *The Foundations of Bioethics,* eds. E. R. DuBose, R. P. Hamel, and L. J. O'Connell. Valley Forge, PA: Trinity Press International, pp. 72–98.

Davis, D. 1991. "Beyond Rabbi Hiyya's Wife: Women's Voices in Jewish Bioethics." *Second Opinion* 16:10–30.

Dennehy, R., and G. Grisez. 1986. *Bioethical Issues*. Cromwell, CT: John Paul II Bioethics Center.

Engelhardt, H. T. 1996. *The Foundations of Bioethics*. New York and Oxford: Oxford University Press.

Farley, M. A. 1985. "Feminist Theology and Bioethics." In *Theology and Bioethics: Exploring the Foundations and Frontiers,* ed. E. E. Shelp. Dordrecht, The Netherlands: Kluwer Academic Publishers, pp. 163–85.

Feldman, D. M. 1986. *Health and Medicine in the Jewish Tradition*. New York: Crossroad.

Finnis, J, J. Boyle, and G. Grisez. 1987. *Nuclear Deterrence, Morality and Realism*. Oxford and New York: Oxford University Press.

Ford, J. C., G. Grisez, J. Boyle, J. Finnis, and W. E. May. 1988. *The Teaching of Humanae vitae: A Defense*. San Francisco: Ignatius Press.

Gellman, M. A. 1993. "On Immanuel Jakobovits: Bringing the Ancient Word to the Modern World." In *Theological Voices in Medical Ethics*, ed. A. Verhey and S. E. Lammers. Grand Rapids, MI: William B. Eerdmans Pub. Co., pp. 178–208.

Green, R. M. 1986. "Contemporary Jewish Bioethics: A Critical Assessment." In *Theology and Bioethics: Exploring the Foundations and Frontiers*, ed. E. E. Shelp. Dordrecht, The Netherlands: Kluwer Academic Publishers, pp. 245–65.

Grisez, G. 1970. *Abortion: The Myths, the Realities, the Arguments*. New York and Cleveland: Corpus Books.

———. 1983. *The Way of the Lord Jesus, Vol. 1*: "Christian Moral Principles." Chicago: Franciscan Herald Press.

———. 1993. *The Way of the Lord Jesus, Vol. 2*: "Living a Christian Life." Quincy, IL: Franciscan Herald Press.

Grisez, G., and J. Boyle. 1975. *Life and Death with Liberty and Justice: A Contribution to the Euthanasia Debate*. Notre Dame, IN: University of Notre Dame Press.

Guroian, V. *Life's Living toward Dying*. 1996. Grand Rapids, MI, and Cambridge, U.K.: William B. Eerdmans Publishing Co.

Gustafson, J. M. 1974. *Theology and Christian Ethics*. Cleveland, OH: The Pilgrim Press.

———. 1975. *The Contributions of Theology to Medical Ethics*. Milwaukee, WI: Marquette University Theology Department.

———. 1984. *Ethics from a Theocentric Perspective, Volume Two: Ethics and Theology*. Chicago: University of Chicago Press.

———. 1988. *Varieties of Moral Discourse: Prophetic, Narrative, Ethical, and Policy*. Grand Rapids, MI: Calvin College and Seminary.

———. 1994. *A Sense of the Divine: The Natural Environment from a Theocentric Perspective*. Cleveland, OH: The Pilgrim Press.

———. 1996a. *Intersections: Science, Theology, and Ethics*. Cleveland, OH: The Pilgrim Press.

———. 1996b. "Styles of Religious Reflection in Medical Ethics." In *Religion and Medical Ethics: Looking Back, Looking Forward*, ed. A. Verhey. Grand Rapids, MI: William B. Eerdmans Publishing Co., pp. 81–95.

Harakas, S. S. 1980. *For the Health of Body and Soul: An Introduction to Eastern Orthodox Bioethics*. Brookline, MA: Holy Cross Orthodox Press.

———. 1999. *Wholeness of Faith and Life: Orthodox Christian Ethics, Part Three: Orthodox Social Ethics*. Brookline, MA: Holy Cross Orthodox Press.

Hauerwas, S. 1986a. *Suffering Presence*. Notre Dame, IN: University of Notre Dame Press.

———. 1986b. "Salvation and Health: Why Medicine Needs the Church." In *Theology and Bioethics: Exploring the Foundations and Frontiers*, ed. E. E. Shelp. Dordrecht, The Netherlands: Kluwer Academic Publishers, pp. 205–24.

———. 1990. *Naming the Silences: God, Medicine and the Problem of Suffering*. Grand Rapids, MI: Wm. B. Eerdmans Publishing Co.

————. 1996. "How Christian Ethics Became Medical Ethics: The Case of Paul Ramsey." In *Religion and Medical Ethics: Looking Back, Looking Forward,* ed. A. Verhey. Grand Rapids, MI: William B. Eerdmans Publishing Co., pp. 61–80.

Hehir, J. B. 1992. "Policy Arguments in a Public Church: Catholic Social Ethics and Bioethics." *Journal of Medicine and Philosophy* 17:347–64.

Jakobovitz, I. 1975. *Jewish Medical Ethics: A Comparative and Historical Study of the Jewish Religious Attitudes to Medicine and Its Practice.* 4th ed. New York: Bloch Publishing.

Keenan, J. F., ed. 2000. *Catholic Ethicists on HIV/AIDS Prevention.* New York: Continuum.

Lammers, S. E. 1996. "The Marginalization of Religious Voices in Bioethics." In *Religion and Medical Ethics: Looking Back, Looking Forward,* ed. A. Verhey. Grand Rapids, MI: William B. Eerdmans Publishing Co., pp. 19–43.

Lammers, S. E., and A. Verhey, eds. 1987. *On Moral Medicine: Theological Perspectives in Medical Ethics.* Grand Rapids, MI: William B. Eerdmans Publishing Co.

Lebacqz, K., ed. 1983. *Genetics, Ethics, and Parenthood.* New York: The Pilgrim Press.

Marty, M. E. 1992. "Religion, Theology, Church, and Bioethics." *Journal of Medicine and Philosophy* 17:273–89.

May, W. F. 1983. *The Physician's Covenant: Images of the Healer in Medical Ethics.* Philadelphia: Westminster/John Knox Press.

————. 1991. *The Patient's Ordeal.* Bloomington, IN: Indiana University Press.

————. 1996. *Testing the Medical Covenant: Active Euthanasia and Health Care Reform.* Grand Rapids, MI: William B. Eerdmans Publishing Co.

McCormick, R. A. 1981. *Notes on Moral Theology: 1965 through 1980.* Washington, D.C.: University Press of America.

————. 1984. *Health and Medicine in the Catholic Tradition: Tradition in Transition.* New York: Crossroad.

————. 1986. "Theology and Bioethics: Christian Foundations." In *Theology and Bioethics: Exploring the Foundations and Frontiers,* ed. E. E. Shelp. Dordrecht, The Netherlands: Kluwer Academic Publishers, pp. 95–113.

————. 1989. *The Critical Calling: Reflections on Moral Dilemmas since Vatican II.* Washington, D.C.: Georgetown University Press.

————. 1995. "Technology, the Consistent Ethic and Assisted Suicide." *Origins* 25:459–64.

Meilaender, G. 1982. "Euthanasia and Christian Vision." *Thought* 57:465–75. Also in *On Moral Medicine: Theological Perspectives in Medical Ethics,* ed. S. E. Lammers and A. Verhey, 1987. Grand Rapids, MI: William B. Eerdmans Publishing Co.

National Conference of Catholic Bishops. 1993. "Resolution on Health Care Reform." *Origins* 23:97, 99–102.

Newman, L. E. 1992. "Jewish Theology and Bioethics." *Journal of Medicine and Philosophy* 17:309–27.

Noonan, J. T. 1986. *Contraception: A History of Its Treatment by the Catholic Theologians and Canonists.* Enlarged Edition. Cambridge, MA, and London: Harvard University Press.

Novak, D. 1990. "Bioethics and the Contemporary Jewish Community." *Hastings Center Report* 20:14–17.

Peters, T. 1996. *For the Love of Children: Genetic Technology and the Future of the Family.* Louisville, KY: Westminster/John Knox Press.

———. 1998. *Genetics: Issues of Social Justice.* Cleveland, OH: The Pilgrim Press.

Ramsey, P. 1951. *Basic Christian Ethics.* New York: Charles Scribner's Sons.

———. 1967. *Deeds and Rules in Christian Ethics.* New York: Charles Scribner's Sons.

———. 1970. *The Patient as Person.* New Haven and London: Yale University Press.

Reich, W. T. 1978. *Encyclopedia of Bioethics.* New York: Macmillan Free Press.

———. 1996. "Bioethics in the United States." In C. Viafora, *Bioethics: A History.* Bethesda, MD: International Scholars Publications, pp. 83–118.

Reich, W. T., with the assistance of R. dell'Oro. 1996. "A New Era for Bioethics: The Search for Meaning in Moral Experience." In *Religion and Medical Ethics: Looking Back, Looking Forward,* ed. A. Verhey. Grand Rapids, MI: William B. Eerdmans Publishing Co., pp. 96–115.

Sacred Congregation for the Doctrine of the Faith (Vatican). 1980. *Declaration on Euthanasia.* Boston: St. Paul Editions.

Shannon, T. A., and A. B. Wolter, O.F.M. 1990. "Reflections on the Moral Status of the Pre-Embryo." *Theological Studies* 51:603–26.

Shelp, E. E., ed. 1986. *Theology and Bioethics: Exploring the Foundations and Frontiers.* Dordrecht, The Netherlands: Kluwer Academic Publishers.

Smith, D. H. 1993. "On Paul Ramsey: A Covenant-Centered Ethic for Medicine." In *Theological Voices in Medical Ethics,* eds. A. Verhey and S. E. Lammers. Grand Rapids, MI: William B. Eerdmans Publishing Co., pp. 7–29.

———. 1996. "Religion and the Roots of the Bioethics Revival." In *Religion and Medical Ethics: Looking Back, Looking Forward,* ed. A. Verhey. Grand Rapids, MI: William B. Eerdmans Publishing Co., pp. 2–18.

Sullivan, L. E., ed. 1989. *Healing and Restoring: Health and Medicine in the World's Religious Traditions.* New York and London: Macmillan.

Sulmasy, D. P. 1997. *The Healer's Calling: A Spirituality for Physicians and Other Health Care Professionals.* New York/Mahwah, NJ: Paulist Press.

Verhey, A. 1987. "The Death of Infant Doe: Jesus and the Neonates." In *On Moral Medicine: Theological Perspectives in Medical Ethics,* ed. S. E. Lammers and A. Verhey. Grand Rapids, MI: William B. Eerdmans Publishing Co., pp. 488–94.

Verhey, A., ed. 1996. *Religion and Medical Ethics: Looking Back, Looking Forward.* Grand Rapids, MI: William B. Eerdmans Publishing Co.

Verhey, A. and S. E. Lammers, eds. 1993. *Theological Voices in Medical Ethics.* Grand Rapids, MI: William B. Eerdmans Publishing Co.

Viafora, C. 1996. *Bioethics: A History.* Bethesda, MD: International Scholars Publications.

Walter, J. J., and T. A. Shannon. 1990. *Quality of Life: The New Medical Dilemma.* New York/Mahwah, NJ: Paulist Press.

Walters, L. 1986. "Religion and the Renaissance of Medical Ethics in the United States." In *Theology and Bioethics: Exploring the Foundations and Frontiers,* ed. E. E. Shelp. Dordrecht, The Netherlands: Kluwer Academic Publishers, pp. 3–16.

5

Professional Codes

Edmund D. Pellegrino

Until very recently, both in Eastern and Western medicine, codes of ethical conduct provided the only source of judgment of good and bad, right and wrong, professional conduct. They were, therefore, the only "method" of ethical argumentation. However, from the beginning of the contemporary era of medical ethics, ethical codes have been challenged by a wide variety of alternate modes of argumentation, as the other chapters in this book attest. Nonetheless, in most of the world, among professionals and laypersons, codes continue to set standards for ethical conduct, to define new ethical issues, and to support one position or another in ethical discourse.

The purpose of this chapter is to examine the use of codes in medical ethics argumentation, to define the sources of their authority, and to delineate their use and abuse in ethical discourse. This chapter will attempt to show that, properly used, professional ethical codes still have an important place in the field, provided their limitations are taken into account.

The chapter consists of five sections: (1) an overview of the ubiquity and historical presence of ethical codes in medicine; (2) the technique or "method" underlying the use of codes in argumentation; (3) a critique of the moral authority of codes, proposed sources of their moral authority, and the use and abuse of codes in ethical argumentation; and (4) advice about training in the use of codes, as well as suggested resources for further study.

THE PERSISTENCE AND UBIQUITY OF CODES

The subject of this chapter is professional codes. It is important at the outset, therefore, to distinguish codes from oaths with which they are frequently confused. Sulmasy has made this distinction quite explicit (Sulmasy 1999). He understands an *oath* to be a formal, solemn, publicly proclaimed commitment to conduct oneself in certain morally specified ways. *Codes*, on the other hand, are simply enumerations, codifications, or collations of a set of moral precepts. One may or may not swear fidelity to a code. When one does swear solemnly to abide by a specific codification of moral precepts, then code and oath coincide but do not lose their separate identities. When I speak of codes in this chapter, I refer to the codification and not necessarily the oath to abide by that codification.

No attempt is made here to summarize the history, variable content, or provenance of the wide variety of ethical codes now extant in the medical and other health professions (Konold 1978; Veatch 1978; Spicer 1995; Etziony 1973; Gorlin 1995). Rather, our focus will be the Hippocratic ethic, that is, the Hippocratic Oath and the other so-called deontological books: *Precepts, Decorum, Law, The Physician,* and *Aphorisms* (Hippocrates 1972, vol. 1; Hippocrates 1981, vol. 2; Hippocrates 1979, vol. 4). The multitudinous medical oaths and codes of the modern era reflect, in significant degree, the prescriptions and proscriptions of these books of the Hippocratic ethic. For this reason, the Hippocratic Oath will be used as a paradigm for this inquiry into the use of codes in ethical argumentation.

Today, the popularity of codes is not limited to medicine. One of the most active areas is in business and corporate ethics. In the early 1980s, businesses in the United States sought to combat the distrust growing in the American public since the late nineteenth century by institutionalizing ethics (Sims 1994). For example, in 1990, of the Fortune 500 companies that responded to a survey, 94 percent had ethics codes, 32 percent had ethics committees, and 15 percent had full-time ethicists (Petry 1993). Many of the same issues addressed in this chapter with regard to medical codes, their use in argumentation, and their moral authority can be found in the expanding literature relative to business codes.

Despite the strength of present criticisms and the doubts about their moral authority, professional codes continue to proliferate. The second edition of the *Encyclopedia of Bioethics* takes 243 pages simply to reproduce the texts of codes related to the health professions (Spicer 1995). Veatch lists forty-one health professions with codes (Veatch 1978). Gorlin presents fifty-one codes in business, health, and law (Gorlin 1995). The Hippocratic Oath is simply an orally verbalized code. Recitation of the Hippocratic Oath, or some variation of it, is regaining popularity in American medical schools after a lapse some years ago (Orr 1997). Clearly, there is a latent attraction to codes as a mark of serious professionalism, even though the degree to which they are observed or felt to be binding is in considerable doubt.

In medicine, professional codes go back at least to the ancient Code of Hammurabi (1792–1750 B.C.E.), which, itself, was probably derived from earlier Sumerian sources dating to 3000 B.C.E. (*Encyclopedia Britannica* 1979; Hamarneh 1993). Since then, every era and all the major cultures—Ancient Greek and Roman, Medieval and Modern Western, as well as Chinese and Indian civilizations—have produced codifications of right and wrong professional behavior (Levey 1977; Temkin 1991; Bar-Sela and Hof 1962; Baker, Porter, and Porter 1993, 1994; Etziony 1973; Muthu 1930). In the West, the dominant "code" of oldest provenance is the Hippocratic Oath and elements drawn from the deontologic books of the Hippocratic corpus. The Oath and its ethic, revised to conform to theological presuppositions, were given added moral authority during late antiquity and the Middle Ages by the major monotheistic religions (Temkin 1991; Amundsen 1996).

All these codes and their variations describe in some detail what was expected in the way of moral conduct, as well as personal decorum of those who professed to be physicians. Taken together, their prescriptions and proscriptions constitute the Hippocratic ethos and ethic, or, more simply, the Hippocratic tradition. They survive, with suitable modification, in the multiplicity of codifications adapted for virtually all the health professions.

To be sure, the Hippocratic ethic has undergone changes in language, interpretation, and emphasis over the centuries (Baker 1993). It was never fully embraced by all physicians in any era. It was frequently violated by individual physicians, or modified or reshaped to suit contemporary mores—just as it is being reshaped today. Some historians have taken those uncertainties of provenance and interpretation as reasons to deny or doubt that the Hippocratic code was ever a universal, unchanging set of moral principles (Baker 1993; Nutton 1995).

Those ambiguities are significant, but they must not obscure several other impressive facts about medical codes. First of all, they have persisted for 2,500 years in Western and Eastern medicine. Despite changes and variations in interpretation, a central core of professional obligations remains intact. There is still substantial agreement across historical eras and cultures on many of these core precepts (Pellegrino 1999). The Hippocratic ethos and its variants have carried, and still carry, significant moral authority for many people.

CODES AS AN ARGUMENT FROM AUTHORITY

Strictly speaking, the use of professional codes in moral discourse and argumentation does not fit precisely under the rubric of "methodology" as that term is used to define other modes of argumentation represented in this book. Codes are not modes of analysis, like the application of *prima facie* principles or the use of paradigm cases, as in casuistry. Nor are they elements of a robust moral philosophy external to medicine, such as Kantian deontology, Millsian utilitarianism, Thomistic natural law, or Aristotelian virtue theory.

Rather, the Hippocratic code and its historical congeners are assertions of moral precepts presented as self-evident in themselves and without formal justification. They are taken to be *prima facie* self-justifying obligations. Nowhere in the long history of codes has there been a concerted effort to justify them through ethical argumentation. Only in the modern era of medical ethics have they or their moral authority been placed under critical and formal scrutiny.

Nonetheless, codes are the reference point of a "method" when they are used in argumentation. Their "method" is the rhetorical method of the argument from authority. In classical logic as well as in scientific reasoning, arguments from authority have often been judged to be the weakest sort of argument. Yet arguments from authority are used universally—in court cases, in everyday discourse, in scholarly papers, and even in scientific investigations. Moreover, argument from authority has been recognized in classical rhetoric as a valid form of argumentation under certain specified conditions that define its valid use (Aubyn 1985; Perelman 1982; Weston 1992; Scriven 1976; Mackin 1969).

In classical logic, the argument from authority was known as *argumentum ad verecundiam*; that is, an argument accepted out of deference for the prestige, stature, or presumed expertise of a person, institution, or office holder. This argument gained a bad reputation because of its frequent misuse and because it was used in the wrong place (e.g., in matters where demonstrable truth was possible) or when the authority cited lacked genuine expertise in the field under examination (e.g., when Nobel laureates in physics or chemistry expatiate on theological or moral matters or on clinical medicine). The strength and validity of any argument from authority vary directly with the strength of the proof of that authority's qualification to command respect.

Thus, in theology, for those who believe in God, argument from authority, as with the Ten Commandments, is the strongest possible argument. It is absolute and thereby overrides every other argument. Believers may differ in their interpretation of precisely what these divine commands require, but not with their authority as binding obligations. For nonbelievers, on the other hand, the decalogue is, at best, a social construction and subject to challenge and doubt.

A related mode of argument is the *argumentum ad populum,* which appeals to general opinion, to categories of persons who hold a certain view, or to a cultural or ethnic tradition. This argument has understandable appeal in democratic societies. Like the argument from authority, great dissonance can result from differences in interpretation of what is popular opinion. *Argumentation ad populum* is classically understood to be a weaker argument than argument from authority—to be used sparingly and only when demonstrable proof, valid expertise, or other arguments are not available (Weston 1992).

The moral authority of a professional act cannot be based, therefore, on the fact that it is sanctioned by a majority of physicians, the law, or the general public. This is to give moral status to social or public opinion, which is per se not a source of moral justification. This is to depend on social construction as moral justification. Pathological communities and societies, for example, have subverted medical ethics for political or social ideology. This is the danger in all forms of social constructions of morals. While more sophisticated than a simple argument by public opinion, social construction suffers the same limitations. Such arguments surface whenever the possibility of objective moral truth is abandoned. When this occurs, the validity of the moral authority of a professional code can be established only by first establishing the moral validity of the community giving it its consensus.

To be valid and effective, any argument from authority must establish the qualifications of the authority, whether that authority is vested in a person, institution, or tradition (Dauber 1996). The authority must be free of conflicts of interest and use expertise in the right circumstances and the right field of inquiry. Genuine qualification and appropriate context are the two essentials of the valid use of authority in argument.

The use of codes in medical ethics argumentation clearly is dependent, therefore, upon the legitimacy of the moral authority of the code in question. Today, the authenticity of the moral authority of any code is under significant attack. An essential step, therefore, in a consideration of codes as a method of argumentation is to examine the criticisms of the paradigm medical ethical code, the Hippocratic Oath, and then to establish its moral authority as clearly as possible. Only then can we proceed to delineate the proper and improper ways of employing codes to define or settle an ethical issue or question.

CHALLENGES TO THE MORAL AUTHORITY OF CODES

In recent years, as a result of intensive historical and social scrutiny, the moral authenticity of the Hippocratic Oath and ethic is frequently and widely judged to be of dubious or little moral authority. Some critics interpret it as a self-serving creed, created by a self-appointed guild to monopolize the healing arts (Berlant 1975). Others reject it because it is unilaterally proclaimed, whereas it should really be a contract negotiated between individual patients, society, and physicians if it is to have any moral weight (Veatch 1991). Still others see physician- and nurse-patient relationships as matters of character: virtuous persons have no need for codes; those who need them are unlikely to respect them (Lebacqz 1985; Warren 1993). Rules may impede the exercise of virtue, displace accountability from persons to codes, and foster "cookbook" ethics (Sanders 1993).

Still further, some see codes as impediments to teaching ethics since they encourage the simplistic reading of codes as duties to be accepted on authority alone (Kluge 1992). In addition, they are thought to stifle individual expression (Downey and Calman 1994). But these are specious arguments. The use of codes may, in fact, require even greater sophistication in ethics than less (Hussey 1996).

An increasingly widespread criticism is that the inherent anachronism of any unchanging code cannot carry moral authority in our times—when so many changes in gender, power, and societal mores have occurred and medicine has become so commercialized and bureaucratized. In the same vein, the admixture of ethics and etiquette in the Hippocratic ethic bespeaks an elitism, insincerity of motive, and obsession with personal comportment out of joint with the times (Foot 1972; Goodfield 1973; Newton 1978; Sugarman 1994).

The more pragmatic critics point out that, in any case, codes have historically been ineffective in making physicians virtuous. This is clear from the many times ethical imperatives have had to be imposed on the profession—for example, the code of Hammurabi (1792–1750 B.C.E.); in Babylonian times, the *Lex Aquilia*; in Roman times, the *Lex Cornelia*; the German "medical police" (*Encyclopedia Britannica* 1979; Castiglioni 1941; Frank 1976) in the nineteenth century; and the medical licensing authorities in the United States today. Moreover, some critics argue that codes could not be effective without better support systems for "whistleblowers" without which self-regulation of the profession becomes a "mockery" (Tadd 1994).

Nutton has recently summarized many of the common criticisms of the Hippocratic Oath. Putting his emphasis on changes in its language, substance, and negative public response and its ineffectiveness in changing behavior, he casts doubt as well on the current resurgence of interest in the Oath, attributing it to a desire for ceremony as a substitute for religious belief and exclusivity (Nutton 1995).

This is not the place to attempt to evaluate or respond to each of those criticisms. Obviously, anyone who intends to use professional codes must be aware that there is some measure of truth in many of them. One must decide whether a code is simply a social construct without any intrinsic claim to moral authority, whether it has a claim to authority that is only transient and subject to change in response to social preferences, or whether the moral authority of medical codes rests in their being stable reflections of moral obligations rooted in the nature of medicine itself.

SOURCES OF MORAL AUTHORITY

It becomes important, therefore, to examine the possible sources of moral authority of professional codes, again, using the Hippocratic Oath and ethic as the paradigm case. These sources of moral authority may be derived externally—that is, from moral theories outside medicine—or internally, from the nature and ends of medicine itself.

External Sources of Moral Authority

Social Construction

A widely accepted source for the moral authority of codes (and the one inherent in most of the criticisms cited above) is some form of social construction. On this view, the ends of medicine are grounded in societal consensus about the uses and goals that medicine should pursue. Here, codes are instruments designed to attain certain predefined social ends of medicine. The ethics of medicine derives from whatever values, guidelines, beliefs, or principles a society chooses to impose upon its practitioners at a particular time.

The requisite consensus can be derived in several ways. One way is by plebiscite or referendum, where a majority vote of the polity would be decisive. This is, in effect, to equate the major tenets of democratic political philosophy with moral discourse. Another way that the precepts of a code could be determined would be by their fitting into a coherence theory; that is, by the "fit" or "misfit" of its precepts within a context of other beliefs already socially accepted. Still another method of social construction is "reflective equilibrium," whereby judgments about particular theories or precepts are tested systematically for congruence or incompatibility with particular judgments and vice versa. The socially preferred or accepted precepts are those that come closest to "equilibrium" between a theory and particular judgments.

Finally, another form of social construction is the "social contract"—as construed by Hobbes, Locke, and Rousseau. On this view, the relationship of a profession with society is in the form of a mutually constructed contract. Society affords certain privileges to a profession in order to gain, in return, the special services that the profession can provide. Here, the moral authority of a code resides in the bilateral obligations of the contracting parties. As a result, the obligations thus incurred are social constructions whose authority is conferred or taken away by societal concurrence.

The moral authority of a socially constructed code is defined by particular social forces in particular historic settings. It is subject, therefore, to continuing processes of change. Today, such codes must accommodate to the prevalent mores of moral pluralism and to moral skepticism about universal, foundational truths. In this setting, linkages between physicians and nurses in different cultures, nations, or historical periods, therefore, would be fortuitous and nonbinding. The notion of a moral tradition would be suspect. As totalitarian regimes have demonstrated, professional ethics are susceptible to subversion and compromise by nonmoral or immoral societal purposes (Pellegrino 1995).

Deontology

Another external source of moral authority would be Kantian deontology. L'tang argues that professional codes are codifications of Kantian perfect duties; that is, duties that are obligatory because they derive from the categorical imperative (L'tang 1992). According to this view, to be valid, such codes would have to be voluntary and arise in the will of the participants, irrespective of personal inclination. Only by that fact could they become duties and moral imperatives.

The difficulty, as with other applications of the categorical imperative, is the paucity of specific content that is precisely what codes strive to make explicit. Codes catalogue specified guidelines or precepts to guide action. L'tang recognizes this limitation but justifies the Kantian approach by what it can contribute to policy formulation and decision procedures and by its insistence on the participation of rational, autonomous human beings (L'tang 1992).

Utilitarianism

Starr justifies the moral authority of codes on grounds of their socially useful consequences, such as the stability of society and establishing a set of expectations that functions as a reference point for laws and policies (Starr 1982). In addition, professional codes yield social benefits for all by encouraging physician compliance. Thus, codes gain moral status in direct proportion to their benefits to society.

Utility as a source of moral authority encounters the usual problems of any utilitarian theory: defining what precisely is in the public interest, doing the necessary utility calculus, and failing to take intention into some account. Moreover, the way utility itself is to be defined is an essential but difficult preliminary step. After all, those elements of professional codes that might serve public interests best might not lead at all to morally defensible acts. Much depends on whether the society to be benefited is, itself, a morally defensible social organism.

Prima Facie Justification

W. D. Ross's notion of *prima facie* obligations has enjoyed wide popularity as a basis for biomedical ethics (Ross 1988; Beauchamp and Childress 1994). It appeals to many professionals as a justification of professional codes as well. According to this view, some set of rules or precepts could gain universal approbation as reflections of a common morality. These rules become *prima facie* obligations to be respected *ipso facto* unless some overriding justification could be offered for violating them.

The problem with *prima facie* principles as the basis of moral authority is that they require assurances of agreement on a common morality. This is more and more difficult to attain in our pluralistic, multicultural, morally divided societies. Also, there remains the problem of reconciling conflicts between *prima facie* rules when they conflict with each other.

Postmodern Ethics

Postmodernism is a multifaceted philosophical and cultural movement with many ramifications for codes of ethics. For one thing, postmodernists would deny the validity of any foundational moral theory for moral authority and, thus, any stable codification of moral precepts. They would read a professional code of ethics as a text that is susceptible, like any other text, to deconstruction. It would be up to individual doctors or patients to give their own meaning to the text and its moral precepts.

The only possible basis for moral authentication would be praxis (Toulmin 1997). If a code "worked"—e.g., in the sense of achieving some measurable difference in conduct—it would be authenticated. The problem, of course, is that what "works" may not be moral. In any case, one would have to define what "works" means and what is "moral." This gets us back into some other justification for moral authority. Some suggest that the normative dimension can be reintroduced by the fact that everyone is a game-player and moral norms are the rules of the "game" (Nuyen 1998). This is a far cry from the ideal of a code. It reduces ultimately to another form of social construction.

Internal Sources of Moral Authority

Two internal sources of moral authority are the practitioners of the profession in question and the activity peculiar to the profession that they practice. In the first case, practitioners themselves discern something special in their art that imposes moral obligations on those who pursue it. As a result of moral reflection, the practitioners, unilaterally, collectively, voluntarily, and publicly assume those obligations as the content of their code. In the second case, a more formal analysis is made of the peculiar nature of the art in question. From its ends, purposes, and phenomena, a set of duties is derived as imperatives if the defined goals are to be achieved.

Moral Reflections of Practitioners

The Hippocratic Oath was developed in the first of the above ways. A group of physicians in ancient Greece saw their art intuitively as a moral enterprise that required a high degree of moral commitment. By their collective Oath, they recognized that commitment, and thus established themselves as a moral community distinct from the main body of practitioners of their day (Edelstein 1943; Carrick 1985). Publicly, they committed themselves to a specified set of moral precepts by an oath, which carried with it the penalty of reproach for its infraction.

The Hippocratics thus combined the notions of code and oath as noted above; however, such combining does not always occur. The American Medical Association (AMA) "code" for example, is not solemnly sworn to. Commitment to its precepts only is implicit in those who join the AMA. In the remainder of this chapter, when oath and code are conflated, the reference is only to the Hippocratic codes and Oath.

As detailed above, the Oath thus proclaimed by the Hippocratics has been shorn of moral authority by many critics. It violates modern democratic principles since it appears unilateral, nondemocratic, authoritarian, sexist, and elitist. Its precepts, on that account, are judged anachronistic. The Oath should be adapted to current mores or discarded and replaced.

Some of these criticisms—those of sexism, elitism, and guild mentality—are justifiable and not ethically defensible. Interestingly, these are in the preamble, but not in the body, of the oath. The main body of the Oath promises beneficence, confidentiality, competence, and fidelity to promises, while abjuring maleficence, abortion, euthanasia, and sexual congress with patients. These moral precepts should be assessed for their moral validity on their own merits, not because of the way the Oath was derived or proclaimed. Even a self-proclaimed, unilateral moral declaration may contain moral truth.

A unilaterally proclaimed code is certainly susceptible to the criticism of self-interest. But it is not, by that fact alone, invalid. Nor is it condemnable solely on grounds that it runs counter to contemporary political philosophy. A self-proclaimed code has two possible claims to moral authority. One is the fact that if taken as an oath it is a freely made promise and, as such, is binding, like all promises, on those who make the promise in good faith. This was the case with those physicians, few or many, who took the Hippocratic Oath in centuries past, and those who take it today.

The second source of moral authority of a self-proclaimed set of moral precepts is the moral status of the precepts themselves. The unilateral nature of those precepts neither validates nor fortifies their moral probity. Only if the precepts of a professional code, themselves, are morally defensible can they constitute a moral imperative. In addition, even morally valid precepts are inadmissible if they are taken as an oath in bad faith or with an intent to deceive or fend off criticism or claim a prerogative.

It matters not who utters the words or precepts of a professional code. What matters is their defensibility as moral statements. To be sure, it is preferable, and recommended, in a democratic society that professional codes be developed cooperatively and with disclosure to the general public. But moral validity transcends societal acceptance.

A Teleological Account of Moral Authority

I contend that what the Hippocratic physicians grasped intuitively as the moral basis for their Oath was the moral imperative embedded in the nature of their art. They took the end of that art to be relief of pain and suffering, lessening "the violence" of the disease—thus, healing. Moreover, the first moral precept of the Oath (its first codification in ethics) is the promise to use medical knowledge for the good of the patient and to refrain from harm—deemed to be that which distinguished medicine from other arts (Hippocrates 1981, vol. 2). Plato discerns this more explicitly, setting medicine apart from carpentry, or navigation, or money-making by its end and function (Plato *Cratylus; The Republic*). For both Plato and Aristotle, medicine was the paradigm of an art, or *tekné*, practiced within a moral framework.

In its classical Platonic, Aristotelian, and Thomistic sense, the term "teleology" refers to the study of ends. This differs from the modern Benthamite or Millsian teleology with emphasis on consequences or outcomes. Classically, the *telos* of a thing is intrinsic to its nature, to what it is, what it is intended for, and what its purpose is. The essence of an act and its *telos* are connected in such a way that an act is a good act of its kind if it attains its proper end or purpose, its *telos*.

In this way, the end or purpose is linked with the good. To know the end is to know the particular excellence that can enable one to attain it with perfection (Guthrie 1971). In moral terms, this idea of the *telos* incorporates an "ought" dimension. Any trait or disposition that enables an agent to achieve the end is a virtue; that is, it confers a power (*virtus*) to attain that end with perfection.

Aristotle incorporated this notion of *telos* in his definition of final causes and his definition of a definition (Aristotle *Metaphysics; Posterior Analytics*). It was further refined by Thomas Aquinas, who defined both the good and the end as being " . . . that for the sake of which other things are done" (Aquinas 1960). Aquinas is quite specific about teleology as the basis for ethics " . . . so the subject matter of moral philosophy is human action as ordered to an end or even man as he is acting voluntarily for the sake of an end" (Aquinas 1960).

This concept of teleology, classically defined, is not consistent with the current preferences for social constructions of the goals of medicine. Indeed, the use of "goals" as opposed to "ends" in a new treatment of this subject is indicative of the contemporary preference (Hanson and Callahan 1999). *Goals* are human societal constructs and can be changed at will. *Ends*, on the other hand, have an ontological status that is not susceptible to manipulation even for ostensibly good reasons. A teleological ethic runs counter to most of the sources of moral authority described above. Those objections notwithstanding, it is important to compare and contrast a teleological account of the moral basis of codes with contemporary theories.

Let us now apply this notion of *telos* and its accompanying ethic of the good to medicine. Medicine exists because humans become ill and want to heal, ameliorate, cure, or prevent this universal human frailty. These are the ends of medicine, those things that define it for what it is. These are, therefore, the "good" for which medicine strives and for which health professionals act.

Physicians, nurses, and other health professionals are the human agents through whom the essential ends of medicine are achieved. They effect these ends in clinical medicine through the physician-patient or nurse-patient relationship. The *telos*, or end, of the clinical relationship is the same as the generic *telos* of medicine as an art. This generic end is brought about clinically through a more proximate and specific end—namely, making and effecting a technically right and morally good healing decision for, and with, a particular patient (Pellegrino and Thomasma 1988). A "right" decision is one that is scientifically correct; that is, it is congruent with the best scientific evidence. A "good" decision is one that is morally good; that is, it is in the best interests of the patient and protects or preserves the good of the patient. The good of the patient is, in turn, a composite notion of four elements: (1) the medical good; (2) the patient's perception of his or her good; (3) the good of the patient as a human being; and (4) the spiritual good of the patient (Pellegrino and Thomasma 1988).

The "good" of the patient thus defined is the immediate end of the clinical encounter attained through making right and good decisions, and these, in turn, serve the more distant good of the restoration of the patient's health, care, cure, or amelioration of illness or disability. Medicine is judged good or bad depending on whether it facilitates those ends. Those ends are intrinsic to medicine, and those who practice this art are under a moral constraint to bring them about. The ethics of medicine arises, therefore, in the nature of medicine, in the definition of its ends, and in the possession, by the medical agent, of those traits of character that enable and empower the closest approach possible to those ends.

The ancient codes of medicine and their contemporary counterparts are public commitments to strive to attain the ends of medicine. They are implicitly proclaimed in the codes that commit doctors to the patient's good through fulfillment of duties and necessary virtues. Thus, in the Hippocratic ethic, one finds the positive duties of beneficence and nonmaleficence; fidelity to trust; preservation of confidences; and not taking sexual advantage of patients, not practicing abortion or euthanasia, and not engaging in practices beyond one's competence. Professional codes of medicine are explicit declarations of commitment to those duties that are required if the ends of medicine are to be attained. They are moral dictates if the physician is to be a good physician.

A teleological validation of moral authority yields a professional code at variance with current moral theory. Such a code is essentialist, stable at least in its core precepts, and universally binding on all who profess to be healers. It would eliminate from the codes those elements that cannot be justified on grounds of the ends and nature of medicine or the other health professions. It would hold all members of a profession who ascribed to the code morally responsible for its observance.

If a minimum core of moral commitments can be fashioned that focus on the obligations of health professionals as professionals, there is every probability that it would eventuate in a code common to all health professions. Such an effort is underway under auspices of the "Tavistock Group," which is attempting to fashion a guide to ethical decision making for all health professionals (Smith, Hiatt, and Berwick 1999). What is proposed is a set of universal principles that might apply to health care systems throughout the world. Allowance would be made for additional ethical principles peculiar to each of the separate professions. Some differences suited to national, sociopolitical, and economic preferences are contemplated as well.

If such a universal code were to succeed, its moral authority would have to be derived from something more fundamental than the interests or assertions of any one of the health professions. The moral grounding in the primacy of the welfare of those to be served, as suggested in this essay, will be essential. Only in this way will the differences between and among health care systems and health professionals be reconciled. Only in this way can a legitimate and morally defensible criterion be established that will distinguish essential from nonessential or self-defeating differences in ethical guidelines.

In today's milieu of moral discourse, the objections to a teleological essentialist derivation of moral authority are many. I list a few with no attempt at responding to them: First is the total negation of any theory of a stable foundation for moral philosophy. Second is the tendency to confuse classical teleology with theological cosmology; that is, the argument for a design built into nature in the form of unbreakable laws. Third is the antimetaphysical conviction of contemporary philosophy since the Enlightenment. Fourth, there is the postmodern resistance to the possibility of grasping moral truths by the use of reason. Finally, any teleological ethic based in objective reality is susceptible to the accusation of the naturalistic fallacy; namely deriving an "ought" conclusion from an "is" sentiment—an error in moral reasoning pointed out by David Hume and G. S. Moore.

This is not the place for a rebuttal of the arguments against the teleological foundation for the moral authority of codes. The purpose of the preceding section has been to illustrate several ways moral authority can be established. Which one is chosen will condition the form of the dialogue. But without some degree of moral authority, there can be no dialogue or argumentation.

THE USE AND ABUSE OF CODES

As indicated at the beginning of this chapter, the "methodology" underlying the use of codes is the rhetorical methodology of the argument from authority. The use or abuse of codes is determined in terms of the criteria for a valid argument from authority. These criteria in moral argumentation reduce to: (1) the authenticity and validity of the authority cited; (2) the use of that authority in the proper context; and (3) the absence of conflicts of interest.

Of course, a prior requirement is the acceptance of the moral authority of codes. If, as some of the criticisms of codes imply, there is no basis for moral authority of codes, argumentation regarding issues in medical ethics cannot even begin. If moral authority is granted, then the particular source of that authority among those given above will determine its use. The shortcomings of each source of authority must be recognized and responded to.

Even if a robust interpretation of the moral authority of a code is accepted, that authority, like any authority, can be misused so that it becomes self-defeating and ineffective. Indeed, some of the current criticisms of codes speak more of their misuse than to a fundamental moral defect. There are many ways to misuse the authority of codes.

For example, the code may be cited to claim or defend some self-serving professional prerogative, such as restricting the exercise of a legitimate technical expertise by members of other health professions. Similarly, some physicians might claim that the code demands so much of them morally that they are thereby justified in assuming moral primacy in team decisions or disputes. Some doctors read the Hippocratic Oath, for example, as giving them automatic headship of the health care team or the right to dictate what is right or wrong without challenge from their colleagues. Still others take the Oath to be a unilateral license to paternalism that brooks no disagreement.

Another misuse of codes is to interpret them legalistically and without the nuances that the use of any moral statement requires. In civil discourse, we are obligated to explain and defend our moral assertions and to subject them to critical inquiry and examination. A code binds those who commit themselves to it by some public act. But it does not per se bind physicians or others who do not subscribe to it. Unless we establish its moral authority beyond mere recitation, no supposedly moral precept is admissible in legitimate discourse.

Some also misuse the code to argue against the need for teaching medical ethics or for further analysis and study of its history, meanings, and interpretations. It is said that everything can be deduced from the Hippocratic Oath or reduced to the simple phrase "Do no harm." This ignores the fact that beneficence, rather than nonmaleficence, is the first moral principle of the code and of the whole Hippocratic ethic. It also ignores the fact that codes, however defensible their moral precepts may be, are subject to continuing analysis of their moral implications as each new clinical dilemma presents itself.

A few physicians may still quote the preamble of the Hippocratic Oath to justify their preferences for elitism, sexism, or the guild mentality. These elements of the Oath may not even have been part of the original text. In any case, they would not survive ethical scrutiny today. Nor were they ever ethically defensible on principled grounds.

Too much emphasis can be placed on the "etiquette" of the so-called "deontological books" of the Hippocratic corpus, resulting in an overemphasis on details of comportment, dress, manner, and style. One facet of the etiquette approach is to place professional loyalty over loyalty to the welfare of patients. This is especially true in matters of malpractice, physicians' personal conduct, or protection of the impaired physician. To do so is to subvert patients' interests to those of physicians—a clear violation of the central commitment of the Oath to patient welfare.

Finally, it is surely an abuse of codes by the critics of medicine to use them to ridicule the profession and to attempt to prove that they are worthless because they have not made all physicians virtuous or were designed to delude the public. Similarly, it is an abnegation of the sense of the code to use it as proof of all physicians' striving to monopolize all health care. Abuse or violation of the code does not vitiate the code itself.

CONCLUDING COMMENTS

Proper use of the code begins with establishing its moral authority by argument and not by simple assertion. It is important that codes or oaths, like any moral statement, be proper subjects for critical examination, explanation, and justification. Readiness to respond to criticism with plausible and principled arguments is crucial to effective use of codes. Codes do not gain moral authority simply because they are espoused by physicians.

But neither do they lose credibility by that fact. A code binds physicians not only because they have voluntarily and publicly proclaimed allegiance to it, but also because its moral precepts can be individually justified and defended by sound moral argumentation.

Despite the emergence of a variety of other powerful methods of "doing" medical ethics, codes will continue to play a prominent role in the indefinite future. They are simple, direct codifications of moral conduct subscribed to by large numbers of today's professionals who have moral and emotional commitments to them. If codes are to satisfy the rhetorical canons for the proper use of arguments from authority, the moral authority of codes will have to be continually validated. This means that scholarly study of codes remains a requisite for sound discourse in medical ethics.

Inquiry into the provenance, content, sociohistorical settings, and social evolution of the meanings of codes will require the knowledge and skills of sociology, history, and politics. Inquiry into the philosophical origins and moral validity of codes and their critical evaluation against modern ethical theory and practice will require the skills of philosophers. Relating these facets of codes to each other will demand a level of interdisciplinary study as yet difficult to attain. In all of this, the error of presentism—that is, interpreting events of the past in terms of the present—must be avoided. Equally seductive is the misuse and abuse of texts simply to score a victory in argument.

In sum, professional codes offer an interesting, challenging, and important research field. The enormous wealth of work already done in no way abnegates the need for ongoing research, deepening of meanings, and careful weighing of moral authority.

NOTES ON RESOURCES AND TRAINING

Those who plan research in professional codes, and especially the Hippocratic code, may do so from a wide variety of perspectives—historical, sociological, philosophical, ethical, etc. Educational requirements will vary with the perspective chosen. What can be assured is that this is a well-tilled field of scholarship. This does not preclude further study, but it does require preparation in depth if new insights are to be added to what is a large and still growing body of literature.

For those who wish to use professional codes in argumentation, but not become themselves expert in some particular aspect of knowledge of the texts, the rules of argumentation and the sociohistorical evolution of the idea of a profession are minimal requirements.

The literature on professional ethics in general, and medical ethics in particular, is voluminous. The citations in the references for this chapter are a small sample, selected for their relevance to the limited question of the use and abuse of codes in bioethical argumentation. Following is also a list of references that provide a portal of entry to a rich field of study. The list is not intended to be comprehensive. Rather, these are resources that will open up various perspectives on the subject. Each contains an extensive bibliography that can be used to extend the reader's studies further.

1. The article on codes in the *Encyclopedia of Bioethics* by Carol Spicer (1995) is the most comprehensive current collation of the content of professional codes.

2. For the AMA code, see: American Medical Association, Council on Ethical and Judicial Affairs, *Code of Medical Ethics: Current Opinions with Annotations* (Chicago: American Medical Association, 1999).

3. Eliot Freidson's *Profession of Medicine* (New York: Dodd, Mead, 1973), Talcott Parson's "The Sick Role and the Role of the Physician Reconsidered," *Milbank Memorial Fund Quarterly* 257(1975): 53ff., and Renée C. Fox's *The Sociology of Medicine: A Participant Observer's View* (Englewood Cliffs, NJ: Prentice Hall, 1989) are excellent examinations of professions in general from the sociological point of view.

4. For the Hippocratic texts, the literature is enormous. For those with the requisite facility, the Greek text will be preferred. Of these, I would single out the following: Loeb Classical Library, eight volumes in Greek and English, at present, with various translators (Cambridge, MA: Harvard University Press); *Hippocratic Writings*, trans. Frances Adams, in the Great Books of the Western World Series, Vol. 10 (Chicago: Encyclopedia Britannica, Inc., 1952).

5. Edelstein's *Ancient Medicine*, ed. Owsei Temkin and C. Lilian Temkin (Baltimore: Johns Hopkins University Press, 1967) represents the work of one of the most respected commentators on the Hippocratic corpus.

6. Paul Carrick's *Medical Ethics in Antiquity* (1985) is an excellent review of specific ethical issues as treated by ancient authors.

7. Owsei Temkin's *Hippocrates in a World of Pagans and Christians* (1991) is a study of the evolution of the Hippocratic ethos during the Christian Era.

8. Wesley D. Smith's *The Hippocratic Tradition* (Ithaca, N.Y.: Cornell University Press, 1979) is an essential commentary on the ways the Hippocratic tradition has been variously interpreted over the centuries and why. Robert Baker's "The History of Medical Ethics" (1993) is a concise, up-to-date history including later codes—e.g., Percival, Gregory, AMA.

9. Anthony Weston's *A Rule Book for Arguments* (1992) is a concise summation of proper and improper use of arguments in discussion.

10. The subject of codes of ethics appears periodically in almost every medical journal. Especially pertinent would be, for example: *Bulletin of the History of Medicine, Hastings Center Report, Kennedy Institute of Ethics Journal, Journal of Clinical Ethics, Journal of History of Medicine and Allied Sciences, Journal of Medicine and Philosophy,* and *Theoretical Medicine and Bioethics.*

11. Electronic resources include: BIOETHICSLINE (http://bioethics.georgetown.edu/bioline.htm); HISTLINE (http://igm.nlm.nih.gov/); Center for the Study of Ethics in the Professions, Illinois Institute of Technology Codes of Ethics On-line Project (http://csep.iit.edu/codes/); and the Library of Bioethics and Medical Humanities Texts and Documents, Center for Clinical Ethics and Humanities in Health Care, University of Buffalo (http://wings.buffalo.edu/faculty/research/bioethics/).[1]

NOTE

1. The author wishes to express his gratitude to Martina Darragh, Reference Librarian, at the National Reference Center for Bioethics Literature, Georgetown University, for

compiling this list of electronic resources. The National Reference Center may be reached at 1-800-MED-ETHX.

REFERENCES

Amundsen, D. W. 1996. *Medicine, Society, and Faith in the Ancient and Medieval Worlds.* Baltimore, MD: Johns Hopkins University Press.

Aquinas, T. 1960. *The Pocket Aquinas,* ed. Vernon J Burke. New York: Washington Square Books, pp. 185, 190.

Aristotle. 1984. "Metaphysics." In *The Complete Works of Aristotle, The Revised Oxford Translation,* ed. Jonathan Barnes. Princeton, NJ: Princeton University Press, p. 1646.

————. "Posterior Analytics" In *The Complete Works of Aristotle, The Revised Oxford Translation,* ed. Jonathan Barnes. Princeton, NJ: Princeton University Press, pp. 154–55.

Aubyn, Saint G. 1985. *The Art of Argument.* New York: Taplinger.

Baker, R. 1993. "The History of Medical Ethics." In *Companion Encyclopedia of Medical History,* ed. B. Bynum and Roy Porter. Vol. 2. London and New York: Routledge.

Baker, R., D. Porter, and R. Porter, eds. 1993. *The Codification of Medical Morality: Historical and Philosophical Studies of the Formalization of Medical Morality, Vol. 1: The Eighteenth Century.* Dordrecht, The Netherlands: Kluwer Academic Publishers.

————. 1994. *The Codification of Medical Morality: Historical and Philosophical Studies of the Formalization of Medical Morality. Vol. 2: The Nineteenth Century.* Dordrecht, The Netherlands: Kluwer Academic Publishers.

Bar-Sela, A., and H. Hoff. 1962. "Isaac Israeli's Fifty Admonitions to Physicians." *Journal of the History of Medicine and Allied Health Sciences* 17:243–54.

Beauchamp, T. L., and J. F. Childress. 1994. *Principles of Biomedical Ethics.* New York: Oxford University Press.

Berlant, J. 1975. *Profession and Monopoly: A Study of Medicine in the United States and Britain.* Berkeley: University of California Press.

Carrick, P. 1985. *Medical Ethics in Antiquity: Philosophical Perspectives on Abortion and Euthanasia.* Dordrecht, The Netherlands, and Boston: D. Reidel/Kluwer Academic Publishers.

Castiglioni, A. 1941. *A History of Medicine,* trans. and ed. E.B. Krumbhaar. New York: Alfred A. Knopf, pp. 226–27.

Dauber, F. W. 1996. *Critical Thinking: An Introduction to Reasoning.* New York: Barnes and Noble, pp. 37–45.

Downey, R. S., and K. C. Calman. 1994. *Healthy Respect.* 2nd ed. London: Faber and Faber.

Edelstein, L. 1943. "The Hippocratic Oath: Text, Translation, and Interpretation." *Bulletin of the History of Medicine* Supp. I.

Encyclopedia Britannica. 1979. "Code of Hammurabi," 15th ed. Vol. 11. Chicago: Encyclopedia Britannica Inc., p. 823.

Etziony, M. B. 1973. *The Physician's Creed.* Springfield, IL: Charles Thomas.

Foot, P. 1972. "Morality as a System of Hypothetical Imperatives." *Philosophical Review* 81:305–16.

Frank, J. P. 1976. *A System of Complete Medical Police.* Baltimore, MD: Johns Hopkins University Press.

Goodfield, J. 1973. "Reflection on the Hippocratic Oaths." *Hastings Center Studies* 1:79–92.

Gorlin, R. A., ed. 1995. *Codes of Professional Responsibility.* Washington, D.C.: Bureau of National Affairs, Inc.

Guthrie, W. K. C. 1971. *Socrates.* Cambridge: Cambridge University Press, p. 146.

Hamarneh, S. K. 1993. "Practical Ethics in the Health Professions." *Hamdard Medicus* 36:11–24.

Hanson, M., and D. Callahan, eds. 1999. *The Goals of Medicine: The Forgotten Issues in Health Care Reform.* Washington, D.C.: Georgetown University Press.

Hippocrates. 1972. *Hippocrates.* Loeb Classical Library 147, with an English translation by W. H. S. Jones. Vol. 1. Cambridge, MA: Harvard University Press, pp. 291–301, 312–33.

———. 1979. *Hippocrates.* Loeb Classical Library 150, with an English translation by W. H. S. Jones. Vol. 4. Cambridge, MA: Harvard University Press, pp. 97–222.

———. 1981. *Hippocrates.* Loeb Classical Library 148, with an English translation by W. H. S. Jones. Vol. 2. Cambridge, MA: Harvard University Press, pp. 190-217, 262–65, 278–301, 305–13.

Hussey, T. 1996. "Nursing Ethics and Codes of Professional Conduct." *Nursing Ethics* 3:250–58.

Kluge, E. H. 1992. "Codes of Ethics and Other Illusions." *Catholic Medical Association Journal* 146:1234–35.

Konold, D. 1978. "Codes of Medical Ethics: History." In *Encyclopedia of Bioethics,* ed. Warren T. Reich. Vol. 1. New York: MacMillan/The Free Press, pp. 162–71.

L'tang, J. 1992. "A Kantian Approach to Codes of Ethics." *Journal of Business Ethics* 11:741–43.

Lebacqz, K. 1985. *Professional Ethics.* Nashville: Abingdon Press.

Levey, M. 1977. "Medical Deontology in Ninth Century Islam." In *Legacies in Ethics and Medicine,* ed. Chester Burns. New York: Science History Publications, pp. 129–44.

Mackin, J. H. 1969. *Classical Rhetoric for Modern Discourse.* New York: Collier-MacMillan, pp. 125–26.

Muthu, D. C. 1930. "The Antiquity of Hindu Medicine and Civilization." London, n.p. Cited in Will Durant. 1994. *Our Oriental Heritage.* New York: Simon and Schuster, p. 530.

Newton, L. 1978. "A Professional Ethic, a Proposal in Context." In *Matters of Life and Death,* ed. John Thomas. Toronto: Samuel Stevens, p. 264.

Nutton, V. 1995. "What's in an Oath?" *Journal of the Royal College of Physicians of London* 29:518–24, 522–23.

Nuyen, A. T. 1998. "Lyotard's Postmodern Ethics and the Normative Question." *Philosophy Today* 42:411–17.

Orr, R. D., N. Pang, E. D. Pellegrino, and M. Siegler. 1997. "Use of the Hippocratic Oath: A Review of Twentieth-Century Practice and a Content Analysis of Oaths Administered in the U.S. and Canada in 1993." *Journal of Clinical Ethics* (Winter): 377–88.

Pellegrino, E. D. 1995. "Guarding the Integrity of Medical Ethics: Some Lessons from Soviet Russia." *Journal of the American Medical Association* 3:1622–23.

———. 1999. "Traditional Medical Ethics: A Reminder." *American Board of Internal Medicine Forum for the Future Report.* Philadelphia: American Board of Internal Medicine.

Pellegrino, E. D., and D. C. Thomasma. 1988. *For the Patient's Good: The Restoration of Beneficence in Health Care.* New York: Oxford University Press.

Perelman, C. 1982. *The Realm of Rhetoric.* Notre Dame, IN: Notre Dame University Press.

Petry, E. D. 1993. "The Wrong Way to Institutionalize Ethics." *Conference Proceedings, Sheffield Business School* (April 1990): 30. Cited in Richard C. Warren, "Codes of Ethics: Bricks without Straw." *Business Ethics* 2:184–91.

Plato. 1982. "Cratylus." In *The Collected Dialogues of Plato Including the Letters*, ed. Edith Hamilton and Huntington Cairns. Princeton, NJ: Princeton University Press, 389c–e, p. 427.

———. "The Republic." In *The Collected Dialogues of Plato,* ed. Edith Hamilton and Huntington Cairns. Book I, 342c–e, p. 592.

Ross, W. D. 1988. *The Right and the Good.* Indianapolis, IN: Hackett, pp. 18–19.

Sanders, J. T. 1993. "Honor among Thieves: Some Reflections on Professional Codes of Ethics." *Professional Ethics* 2:83–103.

Scriven, M. 1976. *Reasoning.* New York: McGraw-Hill, pp. 227–28.

Sims, R. R. 1994. *Ethics and Organizational Decision Making: A Call for Renewal.* Westport, CT: Quorum Books.

Smith, R., H. Hiatt, and D. Berwick. 1999. "Shared Ethical Principles for Everybody in Health Care: A Working Draft from the Tavistock Group." *British Journal of Medicine* 318 (1999): 248–51 and *Annals of Internal Medicine* 130:143–47.

Spicer, C. M., ed. 1995. "Appendix: Codes, Oaths, and Directives Related to Bioethics." In *Encyclopedia of Bioethics,* ed. Warren T. Reich. 2d ed. Vol. 5. New York: MacMillan/Simon & Schuster, pp. 2599–2842.

Starr, P. 1982. *The Social Transformation of American Medicine.* New York: Basic Books.

Sugarman, J. 1994. "Hawkeye Pierce and the Questionable Relevance of Medical Etiquette to Contemporary Medical Ethics and Practice." *Journal of Clinical Ethics* 5:22–30.

Sulmasy, D. P. 1999. "What Is an Oath?" *Theoretical Medicine and Bioethics* 20(4): 329–46.

Tadd, V. 1994. "Professional Codes: An Exercise in Tokenism?" *Nursing Ethics* 1(1): 15–23.

Temkin, O. 1991. *Hippocrates in a World of Pagans and Christians.* Baltimore, MD: Johns Hopkins University Press.

Toulmin, S. 1997. "The Primacy of Practice: Medicine and Postmodernism." In *Philosophy of Medicine and Bioethics: A Twenty-Year Retrospective,* ed. Ronald A. Carson and Chester Q. Burns. Dordrecht, The Netherlands, and Boston: Kluwer Academic Publishers, pp. 41–54.

Veatch, R. M. 1978. "Codes of Medical Ethics: Ethical Analysis." In *Encyclopedia of Bioethics,* ed. Warren T. Reich. Vol. 1. New York: MacMillan/The Free Press, pp. 172–80.

———. 1991. *The Patient as Partner in the Physician-Patient Relationship.* Bloomington, IN: Indiana University Press.

Warren, R. C. 1993. "Codes of Ethics: Bricks without Straw." *Business Ethics: A European Review* 2(4): 185–91.

Weston, A. 1992. *A Rule Book for Arguments.* Indianapolis, IN: Hackett, pp. 28–35.

6

Legal Methods

James G. Hodge, Jr. and Lawrence O. Gostin

The law plays an important role in the understanding and resolution of problems in medical ethics. In this chapter we explain the relation between the law and philosophical ethics and discuss how the law is used to inform and address ethical issues in medicine in the United States (Zatti 1998). We attempt to do this through an examination of the structure and content of the legal system. Too often scholars examine ethical issues in medicine through a narrow lens that focuses on only one facet of the law, primarily case law, and thus fail to examine the larger structure through which cases are decided (and other laws are passed) in the legal system. We believe it is important to understand the basic structure of the legal system in order to examine how the law relates to medical ethics. As a result, we briefly discuss the structural elements of U.S. law.

In subsequent sections, we analyze and discuss the sorts of legal techniques used to address medical ethics inquiries in legislative, executive, and judicial venues. We critique the appropriateness of legal resolution of issues in medical ethics, including a discussion of the strengths and weaknesses of a legal approach to these issues. Finally, we address the types of legal training that can be helpful in applying a legal method to medical ethics and conclude with a synopsis of the many types of resources that exist to facilitate such applications.

THE RELATIONSHIP BETWEEN ETHICS AND LAW

Medical ethics and the law are distinct and yet interdependent. The study and analysis of ethical problems in medicine arises from a moral tradition that serves as a guide to human conduct (Gaare 1989). The moral sphere may be viewed as a preexistent truth or simply as a product of human intelligence (Capron 1979). Medical ethics may be approached broadly by philosophy through consequentialist (e.g., utilitarianism), Kantian, Rawlsian, principlist, or other theories (Finnis 1983; Beauchamp and Childress 1994, 56–62). From these analyses flow *moral* rights that may justify or criticize human conduct in medical settings.

From the law and the legal system flow *legal* rights and responsibilities that may authorize or prohibit human behavior. A law may be defined broadly as a rule enacted by government. In the United States, this means rules enacted by representative government at the federal, state, and local levels (Black 1979, 795). Laws represent the collection of enforceable rights and duties through which individuals relate to one another and their community. The legal system is the means through which society orders and assigns these rights and responsibilities among the competing and often conflicting interests of its citizens (Capron 1979, 403).

While the creation, enforcement, and interpretation of the law are uniquely governmental in nature, they are not divorced from morality. Morality is related to law in at least two ways: (1) the law may codify or supplement accepted moral conduct; or (2) the law may guide human conduct where morality can or does not (Capron 1979, 400–5). Morality greatly influences the law (Gaare 1989). This is particularly observable, historically speaking, in the relationship between the common morality underlying religion and the law (Ariens and Destro 1996; Capron 1979, 402). Law and morality are similar in that they both prescribe human behavior according to a set of rights and duties (Capron 1979, 403). Moral expressions shape individual and public opinions underlying human behavior. Laws may often reflect ethical consensus. Ethical and legal rights and duties often mimic one another (compare the ethical principle of respect for autonomy and liberty interests under the Due Process clauses of the United States Constitution) (Beauchamp and Childress 1994; United States Constitution, Amendments V, XIV). Even some legal and ethical methodologies are similar. For example, compare legal common law with the casuistical method of case-based reasoning, or administrative rule-making with Richardson's specification of norms (Arras 1994; Richardson 1990).

Second, law may replace or clarify morality where ethical principles fail to sufficiently guide human conduct (Beauchamp and Childress 1994). American society ideally functions under moral precepts without significant legal intervention. Common morality helps individuals resolve their differences under accepted norms for conduct. However, where morality fails to resolve conflicts among individuals, is widely questioned, or otherwise breaks down, the law may be relied on to create and enforce affirmative rules to guide human behavior. As Capron argues, in these instances the legal intrusion into the moral sphere may be seen as a " . . . desertion of morals for law. . . . " (Capron 1979, 402).

At least one example of this relationship is seen in the abortion debate. The Supreme Court's unprecedented 1973 decision, *Roe v. Wade,* affirmed a woman's constitutional privacy right to an abortion amidst contentious ethical, religious, and legal debate (*Roe v. Wade* 1973). Though criticized and challenged in subsequent legislation and cases, the benchmark decision has generally withstood scrutiny and provided stability to the debate (Allen 1992; Poland 1997).

The relationships between legal and ethical rights also evince significant differences that help distinguish these fields. Where ethical rights are grounded purely in a moral tradition, legal rights and corresponding duties exist as part of our social structure pursuant to what Hobbes describes as a "social contract" or Walzer's more recent "sphere of security and welfare" (Pence 1998; Walzer 1983). Thus, according to these theorists, laws do not spring forth from a moral foundation, but are simply expressed by a political majority (through legislation), elected or appointed government officials (through administrative law), or members of the judiciary (through case law). Unlike ethical principles that may, or may not, be equally weighted, laws are prioritized within a constitutional-based legal system (Beauchamp and Childress 1994). Constitutional principles are viewed as supreme to legislation that itself can preempt administrative regulations or case law. Assuming a law is not otherwise infirm under such prioritization (e.g., legislation that, as passed, violates the

United States Constitution), it may require an individual to act or not act in ways that are morally acceptable or reprehensible.

The moral response to a law, whether favorable or not, may shape its future existence, enforcement, or interpretation, but it does not make it less binding within a properly functioning legal system under a positivist view; that is, the view that ". . . the law exists only in virtue of some human act or decision" (Dworkin 1985,131). Morality does not compel law anymore than law dictates morality (Beauchamp and Childress 1994). While medical ethics principles and rights emanate from a moral tradition, laws promulgated or interpreted to resolve issues of medical ethics owe their existence to the functioning of a legal system in civilized society, and thus are distinct.

For example, where a physician learns that an unknowing third person is exposed to a communicable disease that she has diagnosed in her patient, the ethical principle of beneficence suggests the physician has a duty to warn the unknowing person of his or her risk of exposure. The principle of autonomy suggests, however, that the physician's duty to the patient is to keep the patient's medical information confidential. Where satisfying the duty to warn may infringe upon the physician's duty of confidentiality, ethical principles may not always sufficiently guide human conduct. However, the law provides an answer to this ethical dilemma, generally upholding a physician's duty to warn under similar circumstances in the 1976 decision *Tarasoff v. Regents of University of California* (*Tarasoff* 1976). The *Tarasoff* decision was criticized by some from an ethical viewpoint precisely because of its abandonment of the physician's duty of confidentiality. As a result, numerous states converted through legislation the *Tarasoff* common law duty to warn into a statutory privilege to warn, thus allowing doctors the discretion to warn third parties of dangers (Gostin and Hodge 1998, 44–50).

THE AMERICAN LEGAL SYSTEM

The United States Constitution is the starting point for any analysis concerning the distribution and exercise of governmental powers in the American legal system. Though the Constitution is said to impose no affirmative obligation on governments to act, to provide services, or to protect individuals and populations, it does serve three primary functions: it (1) allocates power among the federal government and the states (through principles of federalism), (2) divides power among three branches of government (through principles of separation of powers), and (3) limits government power (though protections of individual liberties) (Gostin 2000; Chemerinsky 1997). The Constitution thus acts as both a fountain and a levee; it originates the flow of governmental power and subsequently curbs that power to protect individual freedoms (Areen et al. 1996).

Federalism

Under federalism, theoretically, the division of governmental powers is distinct and clear (Hodge 1997). The federal government is a government of limited power whose acts must be authorized by the federal Constitution (Hodge 1999, 1, 6). By contrast, states retain the powers they possess as sovereign governments (*Gibbons v. Ogden* 1824). These powers include the power to protect the health, safety, morals, and general welfare of the population (police powers) and the interests of minors, incompetent persons, and other specific individuals (*parens patriae* powers). In practice, however, the powers of the federal and state governments intersect in innumerable areas.

Federalism functions as a sorting device for determining which government, federal or state, may legitimately exercise its powers in a given situation. While federal and state governments may exercise their powers concurrently, when conflicts arise, federal laws and regulations preempt state actions pursuant to the constitutional Supremacy Clause (United States Constitution, Article VI, cl. 2).

Separation of Power

The Constitution separates federal governmental powers into three branches: (1) the legislative branch (which has the power to create laws); (2) the executive branch (which has the power to enforce the laws); and (3) the judicial branch (which has the power to interpret the laws). States have similar schemes of governance pursuant to their own constitutions. A consequence of this separation is the varied types of laws that each branch is constitutionally or legislatively authorized to promulgate. The legislative branch may enact legislation and establish executive agencies and courts. The executive branch and its agencies may issue rules and adjudicate administrative matters pursuant to delegated powers from the legislature. Courts interpret the law through the resolution of cases. Each of these sources of law interplays with issues of medical ethics as explained below.

Protection of Liberties

The Constitution functions to limit government power in order to protect individual liberties. While the Constitution grants extensive powers to governments, it also sets forth individual rights, which government cannot infringe without some level of justification. The Bill of Rights (the first ten amendments to the Constitution), together with other constitutional provisions, create a zone of individual liberty, autonomy, privacy, and economic freedom that exists beyond the reach of the government (United States Constitution, Articles I and IV). Interpretations of these individual rights may heavily influence medical ethics debates. Consider, for example, the Supreme Court's interpretation of the liberty clause of the Fourteenth Amendment in *Cruzan v. Director*, where it upheld a person's right to refuse medical treatment subject to proof via clear and convincing evidence as required by Missouri state law (*Cruzan v. Director* 1990).

The limits of federal, state, and local governmental powers thus are dependent on our constitutional system of government. As mentioned above, the federal government must draw its authority to act from specific, enumerated powers. Congress can only act pursuant to constitutional authorization through legislation that does not interfere with any constitutionally protected interest. While the United States government theoretically has only limited, defined powers, political and judicial expansion of federal powers realistically allows it to achieve the objectives of constitutionally enumerated national powers, including the power to tax, spend, and regulate interstate commerce (*McCulloch v. Maryland* 1819).

State and Local Government

Despite an increasingly powerful federal government, states historically and contemporaneously have had a predominant role in American government. The Tenth Amendment of the federal Constitution reserves to the states all those powers not otherwise given to the federal government nor prohibited to the states by the Constitution. States' reserved powers, or police powers, can be generally defined as the inherent authority of state government (and, through delegation, local governments) to enact laws and promulgate regulations to protect, preserve, and promote the health, safety, morals, and general welfare of the people (Hodge 1999, 10–110). To achieve these communal benefits, the state retains the power to restrict, within federal and state constitutional limits, personal interests in liberty (autonomy, privacy, and association), as well as economic interests (freedom to contract and uses of property). Thus, for example, state police powers authorize the enactment of laws requiring the mandatory vaccination of state citizens despite the infringement of individual liberty interests pursuant to the Fourteenth Amendment to the federal Constitution (or similar state constitutional provisions) (*Jacobson v. Massachusetts* 1905).

To the degree local county, city, and special district governments may act, they do so pursuant to specific delegations of state police powers. Local governments in the constitutional system are recognized as subsidiaries of their state sovereigns (Valente and McCarthy 1992; *Bottone v. Town Westport* 1989). As a result, any powers that local governments have must be delegated from the state. Such delegations, which may be narrow or broad, provide local governments with a limited realm of authority, or "home rule," over matters of concern within their jurisdiction (Valente and McCarthy 1992). Absent constitutionally protected delegations of power to local governments, states may modify, clarify, preempt, or remove home rule powers of local government.

THE LAW AND MEDICAL ETHICS

Under this legal framework, it is possible to analyze the sorts of techniques utilized by the three branches of government at the federal, state, or local levels concerning medical ethics. It is important to note that what counts as effective use of the law to inform and address issues in medical ethics is greatly dependent on each government's degree of authority and the prioritization of the action in the American constitutional system. Thus, there is a structure to the law and the legal system through which issues may be addressed. Effective legal arguments in the field of medical ethics stem from a proper allocation of governmental power and are consistent with constitutionally supportable rights.

States possess the broadest of governmental powers (police powers), and may legitimately respond in numerous ways. Their local governments also may take many approaches consistent with their delegation of state powers. However, either government's ability to address issues in medical ethics is contingent on the lawful exercise of federal governmental power. Where the federal government responds to such issues through legislation, administrative regulations, or case law, those laws may preempt inconsistent state and local laws.

Pursuant to principles of separation of powers, discussed above, laws are of three types: (1) federal and state legislatures draft and enact legislation (to proscribe conduct, establish executive agencies or courts, authorize revenue production or expenditures, or other purposes); (2) federal and state executive agencies promulgate legally binding rules (e.g., executive orders and administrative regulations) pursuant to delegated powers from legislatures; and (3) courts craft law through the resolution of cases. Each of these sources of law (legislation, administrative regulations, and cases) employs different techniques and involves different considerations as applied to issues of medical ethics.

Legislation and Medical Ethics

The legislative process in the United States' bicameral system is characterized by compromise. Drafting and enacting legislation at the federal, state, and local levels invariably involves negotiation to accommodate the competing interests of governmental and private actors on any given topic. Rarely is legislation introduced and passed without substantial revision. Rather, the deliberative legislative process involving multiple committee reviews and hearings, amendments, and votes in both legislative houses significantly alters many bills and resolutions (Bach 1996).

Simply getting an issue before a legislative body, especially the federal Congress, is difficult. The ways in which issues in medical ethics enter the legislative process vary. Appropriate topics for legislation may (1) arise from chronic, recurring conditions that demand legislative resolution (e.g., congressional bills concerning health information privacy); (2) stem from political turnover among political parties (e.g., President Clinton's Health Security Reform Act of 1993); or (3) be triggered by a crisis (e.g., the ban on federally funded research concerning human cloning arising from the cloning of sheep in the United Kingdom in 1996), a catastrophic occurrence (e.g., the Ryan White CARE Act of 1990 arising, at least in part, from the death of a hemophiliac boy who contracted HIV from the transfusion of tainted blood), or other focusing events. Depending on the need for legislation, whether properly gauged or not, the legislative process, particularly at the state and local levels, may be expedited. While such legislation may not ultimately be watered down through the legislative process, it may often represent an ill-timed or inappropriate response to a prevailing issue.

Consider, for example, existing state genetics laws that exceptionalize genetic data as deserving special privacy protections. The intent of these statutes (protecting the privacy interests of individuals in their identifiable genetic data) is laudable, but the legislative response is flawed as states struggle to accurately define "genetic information" or "genetic tests" for the purposes of applying privacy protections. Genetic data are increasingly viewed as part of an individual's medical record. Trying to protect one part of individual medical records to the exclusion of other, equally sensitive data is ethically troubling (Hodge 1997).

Administrative Law and Medical Ethics

Administrative rule-making among federal or state executive agencies is another prominent way in which government addresses ethical issues in medicine. The federal Congress has established numerous administrative agencies (e.g., Environmental Protection Agency, Food and Drug Administration, Nuclear Regulatory Commission), departments (e.g., Department of Health and Human Services, Department of Energy), and ethics commissions (e.g., National Commission for the Protection of Human Subjects of Biomedical and Behavioral Research, National Bioethics Advisory Committee) that address issues in medical ethics. States often establish similar entities (e.g., state departments of health, New York State Task Force on Life and the Law) (Brock 1996). These federal and state agencies may be legislatively delegated the power to address issues within their jurisdiction (Gaare 1989). Congressional delegations of powers (which must be reasonably specific and fairly related to the functions and duties of the agency itself) may authorize these agencies to set forth rules and engage in administrative adjudication (*American Textile Manufacturers Institute v. Donovan* 1981; Areen et al. 1996). The legislature may also authorize these agencies and commissions to perform nonbinding functions, such as make policy recommendations or advise the legislature on bioethics issues (*The Belmont Report* 1978; New York State Task Force on Life and the Law 1998).

Like the legislative process, the administrative rule-making process is subject to significant compromise. However, the regulatory process benefits from a more intense, focused approach to issues through a systematic accumulation of information and analysis by individuals from partisan and nonpartisan backgrounds who are usually experts in the field. The regulatory process is geared toward (1) determining and clarifying an issue, (2) examining it through several lenses (e.g., legal, historical, ethical, medical, economic, risk analysis, and comparative analysis), (3) developing consensus on the specific issue, and (4) promulgating effective rules to guide future actions. For example, the federal Department of Health and Human Services recently promulgated sophisticated health information privacy regulations in the absence of congressional legislation as required pursuant to the Health Insurance Portability and Accountability Act of 1996 (Hodge, Gostin, and Jacobson 1999). When properly issued according to detailed administrative procedures, which include public review and comment, these rules have the force and effect of law. Administrative adjudication is similar to judicial case-based decision making, discussed below.

Case Law and Medical Ethics

Many issues in medical ethics are addressed in the legal sphere through judicial case law (Arras 1994). Historically significant cases, such as *Roe v. Wade* (women's right to an abortion), *Tarasoff v. Regents* (physician's duty to warn), *In re Baby M* (surrogate mothers), and *Cruzan v. Director* (right to withdraw medical treatment), and more recent decisions, such as *Washington v. Glucksberg* and *Vacco v. Quill* (physician-assisted death) and *Bragdon v. Abbott* (disability status of individuals with asymptomatic HIV), are milestones in medical ethics debates (*Roe v. Wade* 1973; *Tarasoff v. Regents* 1976; *In re Baby M* 1988; *Cruzan v. Director* 1990; *Washington v. Glucksberg* 1997; *Vacco v. Quill* 1997; *Bragdon v. Abbott* 1998). Although such cases rarely resolve issues in medical ethics, they demonstrate the interplay of medical ethics and the law. Ethical considerations often help resolve difficult cases. Further, decisions themselves become components of scholarship in medical ethics. Consider *Schloendorff v. Society of New York Hospital*, where the New York court declared in 1914:

Every human being of adult years and sound mind has a right to determine what shall be done with his own body; and a surgeon who performs an operation without his patient's consent commits an assault, for which he is liable in damages (*Schloendorff v. Society of New York Hospital* 1914).

This statement by then-Judge Benjamin Cardozo is widely understood to support the legal right to self-determination, which expresses the modern ethical principle of respect for autonomy.

Although courts constitute an important part of the legal system, their scope and powers are limited. Courts can only review legislation and administrative rules pursuant to constitutional challenges or as otherwise authorized by the legislature (Gaare 1989, 1–2). Administrative adjudications are also generally subject to judicial review (Areen et al. 1996). Furthermore, courts are empowered to resolve disputes under the common law, or case law, at the federal and state levels.

Persons having a stake or claim in a controversy may pursue resolution of the claim through judicial review before a court having the power to hear the case. Even where the controversy is not per se a legal one, so long as a party can characterize the claim in legal terms or in the form of a legal dispute, courts may be obligated to assist the parties in resolving the controversy.

The judicial process is unlike the legislative or administrative regulatory processes in that the court (from the judge to the jury) is *ideally* nonpartisan. As a result, the judicial process is guided by legal principles of justice and equity, and less by political influences. Also unlike these other processes, the judicial process is compelled to produce a decision. Improperly deciding, or failing to decide a case, is not acceptable where parties have the right to appeal judicial decisions, except those of the United States Supreme Court or state supreme courts interpreting state law. As a result, the judicial process is driven by the need for a decision, whether good or bad.

Cases are decided based on the interpretation of constitutional, statutory, and administrative law. The decisions in these cases themselves become law. Where the highest court of the federal or state government is interpreting constitutional law, those decisions trump inconsistent laws of any type. Courts accord great precedential value to case decisions (a.k.a. "stare decisis") (Black 1979, 1261). Future cases must generally accord with prior decisions unless changes in other sources of law (constitutional, statutory, or administrative) or public policy justify abandoning prior judicial theory. While shifts in ethical theory or understanding may illuminate issues of law, courts are bound to the precedential value of prior decisions.

While the overwhelming majority of cases filed are settled before trial, remaining cases are generally decided on the basis of significant fact-finding through pretrial discovery, production of factual evidence through lay and expert witnesses during trial, and factual and legal conclusions by the jury (if applicable) and judge, respectively. Attorneys representing the parties' interests must observe sophisticated rules of procedure and evidence at the federal and state levels throughout the judicial process. They must also master the art of researching the law for the purpose of examining a set of issues and arguing for a legal resolution consistent with their parties' interests. The extent of the attorney's direct role is limited to arguing an application of the law to the facts. Technical, scientific, or medical facts cannot be presumed, but rather must be elicited from knowledgeable experts.

CRITIQUING THE ROLE OF LAW IN MEDICAL ETHICS

The techniques utilized by federal and state governments to address ethical issues in medicine through legislation, administrative law, or case law vary significantly in scope, duration, and degree. Yet they each contribute to resolving these issues through the use of the fundamental power of law as an arbiter of issues or controversies. The law, as discussed above, is uniquely positioned to address and attempt to resolve disputes through the use of enforceable mechanisms. Yet, when is it appropriate to use the law to resolve debates in medical ethics?

Appropriate Questions

Issues in medical ethics are often exceedingly difficult to resolve because of the interplay of so many variables and the ethical need for consensus (Zatti 1998). Medical ethics faces the difficulty of assessing the relative moral values of human behavior under scientific, technological, and medical lenses. Even where consensus can be reached on an issue in the ethics community, individuals may not be able or willing to follow ethical recommendations. Failure to adhere to ethical principles may justify turning to the legal system and its varied mechanisms to enforce or require behavior consistent with the law. While the law cannot make people ethical, it may provide teeth to an issue to encourage an ethically desirable result (Nielsen 1998, 44).

The law also plays an important role by providing a stage for these debates. The legal arena can be ideal for intensive fact-finding and sharing of countering views. Since the public is always involved in legal issues (e.g., as voters, interested individuals, parties to a case), ethical issues in medicine needing additional public input are well suited for resolution in the legal system.

The law may as often stand in the way of ethical consensus as it helps to resolve ethical issues in medicine. In these cases, resolving issues, then, must necessarily focus on legal reform. Tactical maneuvering among the branches of government may be needed to obtain an ethically desirable resolution. Consider, for example, the legislative response to the common law duty to warn pursuant to the *Tarasoff* decision previously described.

Strengths of the Role of Law in Medical Ethics

Constitutional protections of individual liberties prohibit government from acting in certain ways that, for example, unnecessarily infringe on personal autonomy. Many legal rights mimic ethical claims. As a result, the existing legal structure, which has devolved from moral codes and expectations, may be well positioned to resolve current and future debates in medical ethics. The legal approach to resolving issues in medical ethics offers many advantages to individuals and society including the following:

Enforcement

As discussed above, the law provides effective enforcement mechanisms in the forms of penalties, fines, imprisonment, incentives, and injunctions. The law can convert ethical duties into legal duties and assign corresponding degrees of civil and criminal punishments for individual failures to act consistent with these duties.

Stability

The law may stabilize public opinion concerning a difficult issue in medical ethics. The law solidifies issues and garners public acceptance of medical, scientific, or technological advances (Nielsen 1998, 43). Insightful lawmakers may anticipate potentially divisive issues and avoid instability through appropriate legislative, regulatory, or judicial actions before they arise.

Protection of Interests

Legal resolution of certain issues may protect the interests of disadvantaged individuals or groups, often through required adjustments in some forms of unethical behavior in the private sector. While economic principles may support a particular form of conduct in the private sector, such conduct may be unethical. The law can intersect these market-driven behaviors for the benefit of persons or groups who are disadvantaged.

Openness

One of the inherent qualities of a democratic, constitutional legal system is its ability to consider numerous societal perspectives and viewpoints through open, public debate. The law and its development are neither secretive, rigid, nor reserved to the views of a few. This is particularly true concerning the legislative and administrative processes. Those who seek resolution of issues in medical ethics solely through the deliberations of a single group (e.g., the medical profession, institutional review boards, or an expert ethics panel) may lack significant public input on matters that are of legitimate public concern, thus contributing to an "Ivory Tower" perception among the public (Nielsen 1998, 42–43). The expertise needed to resolve difficult debates in medical ethics cannot be expected of members of the general public any more than nonlawyers could be expected to draft effective legislation or try a difficult case. However, the resolution of these issues outside the public domain, or without consideration of public views, may be misguided. Though law as enacted, promulgated, or decided may not represent the favored (or even appropriate) ethical response to an issue, it may at least better represent society's response to an issue as judged through the democratic legal process.

Weaknesses of the Role of Law in Medical Ethics

Though there are significant advantages to utilizing the law to resolve issues in medical ethics, the United States legal system is at times ill-suited to address and resolve these questions. The legal approach suffers from several weaknesses:

Lack of Knowledge

The legal process is not well equipped to resolve certain debates in medical ethics. While lawmakers are generally knowledgeable about the law, they may not be knowledgeable about the fields of medical ethics, science, medicine, technology, and risk assessment. They may not be sensitive to the intricacies of relevant relationships (e.g., between doctors and their patients or medical researchers and their subjects). Lawmakers' lack of expertise and sensitivity are compensated to a degree through intensive fact-finding and testimony underlying the legal process. However, resulting legal responses to these issues may still unintentionally have adverse effects.

Focus

One weakness related to the lawmaker's potential lack of expertise is the focus that the law may take concerning an issue in medical ethics. As Brock notes, "there is a deep conflict between the goals and constraints of the public policy process and the aims of academic scholarly activity," through which issues of medical ethics are debated (Brock 1993). Raising these issues in the public policy realm of the legal arena may shift the focus away from ethical arguments to the legal and policy consequences of a variety of actions or inactions. This shift may skew or completely alter the original ethical debate.

Constitutional Limits

The legal system is constrained by constitutional limits on governmental powers. Individual rights and their interpretation by courts may constrain government's ability to resolve an ethical debate consistent with the consensus of the ethics community. Principles of federalism may not allow some level of government, whether federal or state, to act in accordance with needed legal reforms. The federal government may be prevented from directly regulating in areas of traditional state concern (including medical licensing and public health). State and local governments may be preempted from action pursuant to preemptive federal law. One branch of government may be constrained by the actions of another (e.g., a court must adhere to the intentions of the legislature when interpreting statutory law). These structural limits suggest that some issues in medical ethics may lack an appropriate legal response through the level or branch of government addressed, or perhaps altogether.

Resulting Harms

Even where the legal process is equipped and able to address an issue in medical ethics, a resulting law can do more harm than good (Nielsen 1998, 43). To the extent that laws (1) represent compromises among competing interests, (2) are the products of a politically motivated system, (3) apply on a population-wide basis (in the case of legislation and administrative rule-making) or specific parties (case decisions), (4) are often tailored to apply beyond specific issues requiring legal attention, and (5) must be held to examination within the existing legal system, they can be rather blunt instruments of ethical resolution. Lawmakers, like people in general, are poor in judging risk (Breyer 1993). They avoid extending themselves too far on controversial or difficult issues. Their responses to these issues, in the form of law, may not reflect the ethically desirable reaction, but rather the safest or most conservative one. Where legal action is taken, laws may resort to broadly restricting or prohibiting human behaviors to accomplish individual or societal goods. Such well-intended laws (e.g., the federal ban on human cloning research) can be an obstacle toward accomplishing ethical goods (e.g., the performance of valuable medical research on human embryos).

Permanency

Laws take on a degree of permanency. Comprehensive legislation and highly technical administrative regulations are difficult and expensive to amend or repeal once passed. Case decisions take on precedential value and are not often reversed. As a result, legal responses, whether appropriate or not, may guide human conduct for years. This is particularly problematic in medical ethics where scientific, medical, and technological advancements continually reshape the issues. Traditional, acceptable legal responses to these new issues may jeopardize appropriate ethical responses to them.

Governmental Interference

Ethical issues in medicine often involve highly sensitive and personal matters. Consistent with respect for persons, these matters may be viewed as best left to individual decision making and discretion. Turning to the legal system to resolve these highly sensitive issues necessarily requires government to intrude into private lives and interests. Not only are governmental interferences politically and culturally unpopular in the United States, they themselves present ethical issues, particularly where the law inappropriately resolves ethical debates under purely legal principles, thus stripping individuals of their ability to decide such issues themselves (Wills 1999; Capron 1990).

Interpretation

One of the principle consequences of legal responses to medical ethics issues is the need to incorporate these responses into the legal system. Legislation, administrative regulations, and case decisions all contribute to the legal sphere. Each must be interpreted consistently in a coherent, functional legal system. Because interpreting the law is difficult, particularly in areas that are highly technical, great variance in legal interpretation exists among jurisdictions or between branches of government. As a result, the law may not be evenly or consistently applied across jurisdictions, raising ethical concerns about violations of the principles of justice.

CONCLUDING COMMENTS

The ways in which the law and medical ethics intersect are complex. To further appreciate how the law interrelates with medical ethics requires a sophisticated understanding of the American legal system. Consistent with our constitutional system of government, the role of the law in medical ethics is critically dependent on the structure in which law is created, enforced, and interpreted. Effective use of the law to inform issues in medical ethics thus depends on the validity of the legal argument within the constitutional, federalist, and tripartite structure of government. As a result, using the law to guide, interpret, or resolve ethical issues is difficult and problematic for the layperson, but not impossible. Significant legal scholarship and ready access to legal statutes, administrative regulations, and case decisions facilitate legal research. When supplemented with legal training, an individual can reasonably interpret and appreciate the law and its relation to debates in medical ethics.

NOTES ON RESOURCES AND TRAINING

As we have described, the analysis of legal approaches to issues in medical ethics requires an understanding of the legal system, the techniques through which various laws are enacted, made, or decided, and the ability to interpret legislation, administrative regulations, and cases in the legal infrastructure. These basic requirements may be supplemented through understanding of the philosophy of law and jurisprudence, jurisprudential history, legal procedure, public policy processes, principles of risk assessment, and other fields (e.g., economics, religion). Given the intersection of law and medical ethics, the understanding of moral traditions, codes, and philosophy, specifically related to medicine, is also advisable.

In the United States, fundamental training in the law is the Juris Doctor (J.D.) degree offered by approximately 180 law schools approved by the American Bar Association. The J.D. is a postgraduate degree requiring no less than three years of full-time legal study. Law school courses concentrate on the fundamentals of the legal system (e.g., Constitutional Law, Legal Process, Civil and Criminal Procedure, Comparative Law, and Conflict of Laws), broad legal subject matters (e.g., Torts, Contracts, and Property), and legal skills (e.g., Legal Research and Writing and Appellate Advocacy). Other courses allow students to develop specific expertise in health law and policy and medical ethics. Through rigorous legal studies required to earn the J.D. degree, individuals learn how to successfully analyze, interpret, and argue the law in all its forms.

Post-J.D. degrees, including the Master of Laws (LL.M.) degree and the rarely pursued Doctor of Juridical Science (S.J.D.) degree, allow J.D. candidates to pursue specific legal areas of interest. Much individual development of legal skills occurs, however, through an individual's practice of law in the legal system. Lawyers may practice their skills in many settings, including private law firms, government agencies, courts, legislative bodies, and academic institutions.

There is no substitute for a formal legal education and experience acquired through legal practice. However, law-related courses in colleges and universities and other graduate schools (medical schools, public health schools, health policy programs) may assist nonlawyers to understand the intricacies of the legal system. Other training opportunities include nonacademic conferences, lectures, and an abundance of legal publications (discussed below).

An array of primary and secondary resources exists to facilitate analysis and interpretation of the law as applied to issues in medical ethics. Many of the resources, however, require significant training to be utilized effectively. While each of the nation's ABA-approved law schools (and many government agencies, law firms, and public libraries) house significant bound collections of legislative volumes, administrative regulations, and case reporters, effective use of these primary materials requires legal research skills. This is also true for electronic legal databases, including Westlaw and Lexis/Nexis, and many other web-based legal resources (specifically government-supported and academic legal websites).

Completely understanding the law involves a broad examination of its many parts. A common error in legal research arises where an individual focuses exclusively on one type of law (e.g., legislation) to the exclusion of others (e.g., administrative regulations, case law) in attempting to provide a legal answer to a particular question. Even if it is determined that a piece of federal legislation answers an existing question, it is also necessary to determine how this legislation is interpreted by the courts and promulgated through administrative regulations. Furthermore, it is necessary to examine critically the extent to which the federal law is valid in a federalist system of government. Has Congress exceeded its own powers in enacting the law? Are constitutional guarantees of individual rights infringed by the legislation? These are critical questions that require sophisticated comprehension of the legal system.

Individuals may benefit from the review of many secondary resources. Professional legal publishers produce legal encyclopedias (e.g., *Corpus Juris Secundum, American Jurisprudence*); annotations of law (e.g., *American Law Reports*); procedural guides (e.g., *Federal Rules of Civil Procedure, Federal Rules of Evidence*); legislative chronicles (e.g., *Congressional Record*); administrative news (e.g., *United States Code Congressional & Administrative News, Code of Federal Regulations*); and condensed legal case reviews (e.g., *United States Law Week*). Lawmakers, judges, practitioners, scholars, and students of the law regularly contribute to legal knowledge through the production of legal and policy articles, comments, treatises, and instructional texts. These materials, which include student-operated law reviews, subject-matter treatises, casebooks, and policy reviews, present broad overviews of legal subjects, allowing readers to learn a great deal on specific subjects without having to perform original legal research. Occasionally nonlawyers may publish articles on medical ethics in such venues, although this is not common.

Many additional articles and educational treatments of the law and its relation to medical ethics are published in medical journals (e.g., *Journal of the American Medical Association, New England Journal of Medicine);* health policy journals (e.g., *Journal of Law, Medicine, and Ethics, American Journal of Law and Medicine*); public health journals (e.g., *American Journal of Public Health, Morbidity and Mortality Weekly Reports*); and ethics/philosophy journals (e.g., *Philosophy and Public Affairs, Journal of Medicine and Philosophy, Kennedy Institute of Ethics Journal, Hastings Center Report)* (Fluss 1998). Government and private organization publications and reports can also be a beneficial source of information.

Law-related articles on topics in medical ethics range in quality, context, and scope. It may be difficult for the nonlawyer to critically analyze the legal arguments presented, although the best scholars manage to seamlessly explain the law and its intersection with medical ethics. Fortunately for the layperson, law articles often feature intensely cited passages where references to laws, treatises, articles, and other resources are provided for the reader's edification and subsequent research. To properly assess the validity of a legal article on medical ethics, one must clearly understand the interplay between law and medical ethics.

REFERENCES

Allen, A. L. 1992. "Autonomy's Magic Wand: Abortion and Constitutional Interpretation." *Boston University Law Review* 72:683–98.

American Textile Manufacturers Institute, Inc. v. Donovan, 452 US 490 (1981).

Areen, J., P. A. King, S. Goldberg, L. O. Gostin, and A. M. Capron. 1996. *Law, Science and Medicine.* Westbury, NY: The Foundation Press, Inc.

Ariens, M. S., and R. A. Destro. 1996. *Religious Liberty in a Pluralistic Society.* Durham, NC: Carolina Academic Press.

Arras, J. D. 1994. "Principles and Particularity: The Roles of Cases in Bioethics." *Indiana Law Journal* 69:983–1014.

Bach, S. 1996. *The Legislative Process on the House Floor: An Introduction.* Washington, D.C: Congressional Research Service.

Beauchamp, T. L., and James F. Childress. 1994. *Principles of Biomedical Ethics.* New York: Oxford University Press.

The Belmont Report: Ethical Guidelines for the Protection of Human Subjects of Research. 1978. Washington, D.C.: Department of Health, Education, and Welfare.

Black, H. C. 1979. *Black's Law Dictionary.* St. Paul, MN: West Publishing Co.

Bottone v. Town Westport, 553 A2d 576 (Conn. 1989).

Bragdon v. Abbott, 524 US 624 (1998).

Breyer, S. 1993. *Breaking the Vicious Circle: Toward Effective Risk Regulation.* Cambridge, MA: Harvard University Press.

Brock, D. W. 1993. "Truth or Consequences: The Role of Philosophers in Policy-making." In *Life and Death: Philosophical Essays in Biomedical Ethics.* Cambridge: Cambridge University Press.

———. 1996. "Public Moral Discourse." In *Philosophical Perspectives on Bioethics,* ed. L.W. Sumner and J. Boyle. Toronto: University of Toronto Press.

Capron, A. M. 1979. "Legal Rights and Moral Rights." In *Biomedical Ethics and the Law,* ed. J. M. Humber and R. F. Almeder. New York: Plenum Press.

———. 1990. "The Burden of Decision." *Hastings Center Report* 20(3): 36–41.

Chemerinsky, E. 1997. *Constitutional Law: Principles and Policies.* New York: Aspen Law and Business.

Cruzan v. Director, Missouri Dept. of Health, 497 US 261 (1990).

Dworkin, R. 1985. *A Matter of Principle.* Cambridge, MA: Harvard University Press.

Finnis, J. 1983. *Fundamentals of Ethics.* Washington, D.C.: Georgetown University Press.

Fluss, S. S. 1998. "An International Overview of Developments in Certain Areas, 1984–1994." In *A Legal Framework for Bioethics,* ed. C. M. Mazzoni. Boston: Kluwer Law International.

Gaare, R. D. 1989. "Introduction to the Legal System." In *BioLaw,* ed. James F. Childress, Patricia A. King, Karen H. Rothenberg, Walter J. Wadlington, and Ruth D. Gaare. Bethesda, MD: University Publications of America.

Gibbons v. Ogden, 22 US 1 (1824).

Gostin, L. O. 2000. *Public Health Law: Power, Duty, Restraint.* Berkeley: University of California Press.

Gostin, L. O., and J. G. Hodge, Jr. 1998. "Piercing the Veil of Secrecy in HIV/AIDS and Other Sexually-Transmitted Diseases: Theories of Privacy and Disclosure in Partner Notification." *Duke Journal of Gender Law and Policy* 5:9–88.

Hodge Jr., J. G. 1997. "Implementing Modern Public Health Goals through Government: An Examination of New Federalism and Public Health Law." *Journal of Contemporary Health Law and Policy* 14:93–126.

———. 1998. "The Role of New Federalism and Public Health Law." *Journal of Law and Health* 12:309–57.

———. 1999. "Privacy and Anti-discrimination Issues: Genetics Legislation in the United States." *Journal of Community Genetics* 1:169–74.

Hodge Jr., J. G., Lawrence O. Gostin, and Peter Jacobson. 1999. "Privacy, Quality, and Liability: Legal Issues Concerning Electronic Health Information." *Journal of the American Medical Association* 282:1466–71.

In re Baby M, 537 A2d 1127 (NJ 1988).

Jacobson v. Massachusetts, 197 US 11 (1905).

McCulloch v. Maryland, 17 US (4 Wheat.) 316 (1819).

New York State Task Force on Life and the Law. 1998. *Assisted Reproductive Technologies.* New York: New York State Task Force on Life and the Law.

Nielsen, L. 1998. "From Bioethics to Biolaw." In *A Legal Framework for Bioethics,* ed. C. M. Mazzoni. Boston: Kluwer Law International.

Pence, G. E. 1998. "Ethical Theories and Medical Ethics." In *Classic Works in Medical Ethics,* ed. G. E. Pence. Boston: McGraw Hill.

Poland, S. C. 1997. "Landmark Legal Cases in Bioethics." *Kennedy Institute of Ethics Journal* 7:191–209.

Richardson, H. S. 1990. "Specifying Norms as a Way to Resolve Concrete Ethical Problems." *Philosophy & Public Affairs* 19:279–310

Roe v. Wade, 410 US 113 (1973).

Schloendorff v. Society of New York Hospital, 105 NE 92 (N.Y. 1914).

Tarasoff v. Regents of University of California, 551 P2d 334 (Cal. 1976).

Vacco v. Quill, 521 US 793 (1997).

Valente, W. D., and D. J. McCarthy, Jr. 1992. *Local Government Law.* St. Paul, MN: West Publishing Co.

Walzer, M. 1983. *Spheres of Justice: A Defense of Pluralism and Equality.* New York: Basic Books, Inc.

Washington v. Glucksberg, 521 US 702 (1997).

Wills, G. 1999. *A Necessary Evil: A History of American Distrust of Government.* New York: Simon & Schuster.

Zatti, P. 1998. "Towards a Law for Bioethics." In *A Legal Framework for Bioethics,* ed. C. M. Mazzoni. Boston: Kluwer Law International.

7

Casuistry

Albert R. Jonsen

One of the defining features of modern medical ethics is the presence of persons trained in the disciplines of moral philosophy and moral theology as participants in the conversation with health professionals, scientists, and legal scholars about moral questions in medicine and science. The philosophers and theologians naturally desired to bring to that conversation methods of analysis that are identified with their disciplines. When they entered the conversation, they quickly learned that in medical care the moral questions are stimulated by cases, particular instances in which actual persons are being treated in specific ways in definite circumstances. Scholars might have recalled the words of Aristotle, "Agents are compelled at every step to think out for themselves what the circumstances demand, just as happens in the arts of medicine and navigation . . . Prudence is not concerned with universals only; it must also take cognizance of particulars, because it is concerned with conduct, and conduct has its sphere in particular circumstances" (Aristotle 1976, II, ii, 1104; IV, vii, 1141).

This intense concentration on the particulars of medical cases presented a problem for those trained in moral philosophy who worked on these issues in the early part of modern medical ethics. That discipline had, for many years, cultivated an approach to ethics that turned away from cases and toward theory. One of the seminal books of modern moral philosophy, G. E. Moore's *Principia Ethica*, opened with the assertion that there is "a study different from Ethics and one much less respectable, the study of Casuistry . . . (although Ethics cannot be complete without it)." He goes on, "The defects of Casuistry are not defects of principle; no objection can be taken to its aim and object. It has failed because . . . the casuist had been unable to distinguish, in the cases which he treats, those elements upon which their value depends" (Moore 1903, 4-5). Many of Moore's predecessors in Continental and British moral philosophy had, since the late Renaissance and Enlightenment, reflected on the natural, psychological, and logical foundations of moral reasoning and constructed theories to ground the rationality (or in some instances the irrationality) of morality. After Moore, most moral philosophers in the English tradition turned their attention to the meaning of the peculiar vocabulary of moral discourse: What do words such as "right" and "good" mean, since they do not appear to refer to the objects of empirical perception? Casuistry, a "less respectable branch of moral philosophy" in Moore's words, was hardly noticed. Philosophers neither analyzed cases nor did they reflect, in anything but a cursory way, on the theoretical conditions under which universal principles could be brought to bear on particular circumstances.[1]

In one corner of the scholarly world of ethics, however, a tradition of case analysis had survived. Roman Catholic moral theology had developed casuistry to a high art in the seventeenth century and, although that art had been severely ridiculed and had eventually deteriorated into a tired and rather shabby technique, it had retained an important place. That place was guaranteed by the Roman Catholic practice of private confession of sins to a priest for absolution. Priests were required to judge the seriousness of sins confessed and impose proportionate penance. Thus, the exact circumstances of an action, the relevance of excuses, and the persuasiveness of justifications entered into their judgment. In addition, Roman Catholicism imposed upon its faithful a variety of moral and ritual obligations, and all of these needed to be interpreted in the circumstances of actual life. Thus, casuistry remained an integral part of Roman Catholic (and Anglican) moral theology. It also remained vigorous within Orthodox Judaism, but Talmudic methods of reasoning did not easily translate into the secular discourse of modern medicine in the United States, as did that of Catholic casuistry.

Catholic scholars, familiar with historical casuistry (and often disdainful of the debilitated casuistry of latter-day moral theology), became active participants in the conversation about medical ethics. Recognizing the interest in medical cases as an analogue to their own concern about judgment in particular moral cases, they saw possibilities for a contribution to the methodology of the new medical ethics. In 1988, Albert Jonsen and Stephen Toulmin published a study of historical Catholic casuistry, suggesting that its methods could be rehabilitated and re-invigorated for use in modern ethical discourse (Jonsen and Toulmin 1988). In the same year, Baruch Brody, a philosopher familiar with Talmudic reasoning, also proposed that casuistic reasoning could be drawn into the debates about medical ethics (Brody 1988).[2] A considerable scholarly literature followed these works, and casuistry, once a word of ridicule in common discourse, began to regain its righteous place as a method of moral reasoning in the Aristotelian tradition. It was not, however, without its drawbacks, as many commentators noted. This chapter will describe one form of casuistry and discuss the advantages and disadvantages of casuistry as a method of moral reasoning.

Specifically, this chapter explains the casuistic method by reviewing its three main features: (1) the role of circumstances and topics in the construction of a case; (2) the importance of moral maxims, or principles; and (3) the use of paradigm cases and analogies in argumentation about cases. A review of criticisms of casuistry as a method of moral argument follows and, after some concluding comments, the chapter ends with a note on resources for the study of the casuistic method and on the intellectual stance that facilitates sound casuistic reasoning.

CASUISTIC METHOD

Circumstances and Topics

"Method" means many different things, but in its simplest meaning it designates instructions about how to get from here to there: method is derived from the Greek *meta* and *odos*; literally "on the road." Road travel is facilitated by maps; the travel of the mind through a problem is facilitated by method. Methods differ in different disciplines, depending on the materials that the discipline studies and the sorts of problems to be solved. A method suited to the philosophical analysis of ethics will be very different from a method made to solve an engineering or a mathematical problem. Even a philosophical problem of ethics can be posed in ways that require rather different methods. So, one might ask, "What are the ethical principles that should govern research with human subjects?" One philosopher, facing that question, might have recourse to a well-established ethical theory, such as Kantian deontology, and move from the theoretical presuppositions of that theory to general conclusions. Thus, the philosopher, working out the implications of the categorical imperative, "So act as to treat humanity, whether in thine own person or in that of any other, in every case as an end withal, never as means only," might conclude that no one should be the subject of research unless full and voluntary consent has been given. Another philosopher might have recourse to the theory of rule utilitarianism and come to the same conclusion through a quite different line of argument. Both routes travel from a theory and general principle to a conclusion. Both are properly philosophical methods of argument.

Both routes are well-marked maps. Any astute philosopher who uses these maps is aware that certain paths of the map are perilous because they lead into logical intricacies from which it is difficult to emerge. The philosopher will halt his journey and examine the path in exquisite detail, attempting to work out a logically defensible way of proceeding, and, if that cannot be found, the intellectual journey toward the conclusion must end. This is the typical philosophical manner of thinking about ethics: attention is directed to the moves of the mind, definition of terms, assumptions, implications, entailments, and proofs. The voyage, however, is more than a movement of mind along certain conceptual and logical paths. It also moves through a terrain peopled with individuals of certain age, gender, and status, situated in real settings of time, place, and problem. These are the circumstances of which Aristotle spoke, saying that, "agents are compelled at every step to think out for themselves what the circumstances demand, just as happens in the arts of medicine and navigation."

The question is: How does one "think out . . . what the circumstances demand"? The original Greek of that passage says "to examine what must be done according to the occasion." How should one examine or take into account the contingencies of occasions, the particularities of situations? Classical philosophical reflection about ethics offers little direction. It prefers to contemplate the abstractions of the map rather than plunge into the thickets of actual cases. Casuistry, on the other hand, works in the terrain, taking into account the lay of the land, distance, the vegetation, and the weather. Aristotle likens this sort of reasoning to the way in which doctors and sailors go about their work. In both medicine and navigation there are theories and principles, but the physician treating a sick person is guided by the changing symptoms and the varying response to treatments; the sailor trims his sails as the wind and current shift. So the ethical analyst must know the meaning and relevance of the multifarious circumstances of the case, as well as the principles and theories. Indeed, the principles and theories by themselves do not get a person anywhere; the moral mind and imagination are moved by circumstances.

Classical casuistry did not explicate its methodology in any detail. However, the classical casuists worked in an intellectual tradition in which ethics and rhetoric were closely linked. They had read Aristotle and Cicero and saw that both ethics and rhetoric aimed to persuade persons about choices and courses of action by the presentation of reasons. The explicit methods of classical rhetoric are equivalently the methods of moral casuistry (Tallmon 1993, 1995). The method of the classical rhetorician consisted, in large part, of the elucidation of topics, the exploration of the range of maxims, and the exploitation of analogical reasoning. It was the intention of the authors of *The Abuse of Casuistry* to revise the classical rhetorical and casuistical methodology for use in contemporary moral argumentation.

What is a case? The English word "case" is a homonym: one of its meanings is "a thing that befalls or happens to anyone; an event, occurrence . . . and instance or example of the occurrence." The other meaning is "a thing fitted to enclose something else; a receptacle, holder, box," such as a suitcase or a briefcase (*Oxford English Dictionary* 1989). The first derives from the Latin, *casus*, an event, from *cadere*, to happen; the second derives from the Latin, *capsa*, from *capere*, to hold, which comes into the Romance languages as "cassa." These are very different meanings and derivations, yet for the purpose of explaining "case method," they are very illuminating. The most colloquial use of the first meaning (for example, "well, it was the case that . . . ") is made into technical jargon in medicine and in law (for example, "this is a case of pneumonia," or "this is a case of treason"), meaning this is a particular instance of the general condition called pneumonia or the crime called treason. This jargon use can remind us of the second meaning of case. A complex human event, filled with behaviors, beliefs, motivations, emotions, is "boxed." Its components, which are so tumbled together in life, are sorted out into compartments so that they can be seen more distinctly. In general, a medical text will describe pneumonia in terms of certain changes in respiration and body temperature, certain findings on the chest X-ray and in the sputum, and certain physiological responses to administration of antibiotics. A legal text will describe treason as actions and intentions, by persons with certain characteristics, such as nationality and occupation, in relation to certain rules of law. These are the general descriptions that are intended to fit many cases, each of which has certain features that presumably correspond to the general description, but that present themselves in unique and somewhat different ways. Thus, the doctor might say, "It looks like this patient has pneumonia, but there are atypical features"; the prosecutor may say, "this government scientist communicated with foreign scientists about classified material, but was the communication of such a nature as to violate the law?"

This sorting out, or boxing, is, in part, what the classical rhetoricians called the elucidation of topics. A topic (*topos* in Greek means "place") designates a standard "place in the mind" that stores certain common and invariant lines of reasoning, either about some general feature of existence, such as causality, proportion, or sequence, or about some particular form of existence, such as the human institutions of marriage, education, warfare, administration of justice, and so forth. The classical rhetoricians suggested that, whenever, for instance, one was making an argument about causality, one would have to refer to the contiguity of cause and effect, the temporal priority of one over the other, and the sufficient and necessary relationship of both. This form of argument penetrated all cases in which causality was in question. Readers of murder mysteries will recognize this common topic as the sleuth's reasoning, and those familiar with the law will be reminded of the structure of argument about negligence. The special topics comprise certain elements that seem essential to particular human institutions and activities. Marriage, for example (in its traditional form), will consist of two persons of opposite gender, joined by agreement or contract, in a lasting union involving cohabitation and mutual sexual activity for the procreation and education of children. Arguments about the advisability and value of marriage, and about responsibilities within it, will dwell within this general pattern. Although many variations to this defining pattern are possible, it gives a recognizable structure to a human institution. Similarly, warfare involves aggression between the organized military units of two or more political entities, with the objective of gaining ascendancy in authority. Arguments about the advisability of warfare, its justification, and its manner presuppose these invariant features. The point of the ancient rhetorician-casuists in proposing the relevance of topics is to place the particular circumstances of any instance of either marriage or warfare, or any other human activity, within a general framework that distinguishes that activity from others. This situates or places the argument so that particular assertions can be associated with familiar features, and persons can be helped to appreciate the issues that are at stake. Human actions and performances are the subject matter of ethics, but most human actions and performances take place within recognizable "practices" ; that is, "sets of considerations, manners, uses, observances, customs, standards, canons, maxims, principles, rules, and offices specifying useful procedures or denoting obligations or duties which relate to human actions and utterances" (Oakeshott 1975, 55). Performances, such as eating, are, in the human world, practices that can be described and distinguished: banquets, family meals, snacking, noshing, grazing, etc. Human "grazing" is, despite is highly informal nature, quite different from the grazing of cows: essays can be written about the former in which its ethics and etiquette might be criticized and its environmental effects deplored. Many human performances take place within much more formal cultural institutions in which certain bodies of knowledge and skill are deployed by certain qualified persons for certain purposes in relation to the expectations of certain populations: "faith communities," the banking business, the insurance industry, the police force, etc. Medicine and health care is one such institution in Western culture.

The contemporary medical ethicists, Jonsen, Siegler, and Winslade, suggest that the complex practices of the institution of medicine can be seen to consist of at least four morally relevant features or topics. These are the first "boxes" into which all particular cases of health care can be sorted. The first topic is *Medical Indications*; the physical signs and symptoms that suggest to persons that they seek the aid of health professionals, and that health professionals recognize as reasons to respond to requests, and as starting points for employment of their skills of diagnosis and therapy. The second topic is *Patient Preferences*; the perceptions, assessments, and choices that lead people to seek help, direct its progress, and to obtain its results. The third topic is *Quality of Life*; the physical, intellectual, affective, and social states that persons wish to attain by means of health interventions, and the objective ability of those interventions to contribute to such states. The fourth topic is *Contextual Features*; the social, organizational, administrative, financial, and legal structures within which health interventions take place, and that enhance or limit their efficacy. Any particular instance of the medical relationship takes place within these four topics; every case has these four dimensions.

Take a particular case: a man is brought to an emergency department (ED) bleeding severely. The doctors and nurses recognize that he needs a blood transfusion. He says he is a Jehovah's Witness and refuses the transfusion. What should the doctors and nurses do?

"Bleeding" and "needs a transfusion" are medical indications. "Says he is Jehovah's Witness and refuses the transfusion" are patient preferences. The clinicians know the patient's quality of life will be nil, since he will be dead; the patient believes his quality of life will be in the splendor of salvation, if he dies faithful to God's command. The fact that the patient is the father of several young children, the mission of the hospital and its emergency department, the extant law, the possibility for malpractice claims, the distress of the ED staff, the doctrine of the Jehovah's Witness faith, and the rallying of the local congregation to support its brother are contextual features (Jonsen, Siegler, and Winslade 1998). This is, then, a "case of refusal of medical care." While it is easy to recognize it as such, it is not easy to analyze the particular case at hand. A general philosophical response to the case might be, "The principle of respect for autonomy dictates that the patient's refusal be respected," and the philosopher might go on to provide strong arguments to justify the principle of respect for autonomy. However, those faced with the question, "What shall I do?" (which includes the patient, his family, and fellow believers, as well as the doctors, nurses, administrators, and legal counsel), cannot be satisfied with that response. It is generally accepted, in ethics and in law, that competent patients may refuse medical care, but in this case, can that general principle be implemented?

This question can be answered only when we examine in detail the actual features of this case. We need quite specific information about this patient's medical condition, its causes, his past medical history, and his physical and psychological status at admission. We need to know just how urgent is the need for transfusion and whether there are alternatives. We have to be better informed about his personal beliefs and the tenets of his faith, as well as about the relevant policies and legal provisions that might apply. In other words, each of the four topics must be filled with information specific to this case. When this is done, it might be seen that, given the blood loss, the need for blood transfusion is not urgent or, conversely, that even a transfusion might be useless. We might learn that someone who brings him, rather than he, himself, is expressing this preference or that he expresses it only vaguely in his confusion. We might find that, while we believed that he would be expelled from his congregation if we administered blood against his will, he would be received with love as one who had been wronged. We might be astonished to learn from legal counsel that the hospital policy and the state law acknowledge the right of Jehovah's Witnesses to refuse transfusions, even at risk to life. These features of this particular case are crucially important: they allow us to move toward an ethical resolution. Thus, the first casuistic act is to determine the topics of relevance to the general enterprise within which the case arises; the second act is to sort out the details of the specific case into the appropriate topics.

Maxims and Principles

Up to this point, this chapter has focused on the factual details that constitute the case. Specific cases are, in reality, always a riot of detail, and it is the details that attract attention. Casuistry revels in those details. Yet casuistic reasoning begins by sorting those details in an orderly way. The development of topics is the technique or method for doing such sorting. However, the conjunction of the topics and the factual details reveals not merely an empirical state of affairs. It begins, as well, to disclose the moral dimensions of the case. Recall the definition of "practice" cited above: it refers to "principles, maxims, rules, duties."

Human practices are shaped not only by conventional and customary understandings and ways; they have embedded in them a host of normative features that say not only how persons engaged in that practice behave, but also how they ought to behave. Morality, in itself, is not an institution or practice; it is a particular way of acting within a variety of institutions and practices, and the particular way is dictated by what are generally called moral principles, rules, or values. The classical rhetorician-casuist spoke of "maxims." These were the *maxima sententia,* or "significant opinions" that expressed in pithy ways the standards of behavior that any rational person, who understood the practice, would see as obligatory or prudently wise. Maxims served as the fulcrum of any persuasive argument. They were statements that the hearers would acknowledge at face value, needing no proof in themselves, but giving the color of truth to the conclusions drawn about the case. There are multitudes of moral maxims, invoked in all sorts of cases. Some maxims are framed as common sense advice, such as "honesty is the best policy," or "the truth will out." Other maxims take a more lofty tone, such as "truthfulness is the essential ingredient in trust" or "thou shalt not bear false witness." Moral arguments pivot on these maxims. Thus, someone might say, "The president was wrong to deceive the American people, because he forfeits their trust: after all, truth is the essential ingredient in trust." The argument may then go on to show that trust is the basis for political authority and effectiveness, using other maxims to make that point. Maxims go by very fast in moral discourse, since it is seldom necessary to stop and demonstrate, explain, or justify the maxims invoked. However, maxims themselves might be challenged and then the argument moves to another plane where the relatively unreflective maxims must be transmuted into principles. Principles are stated in a more general fashion, as "universal," and are related to more general theories of moral justification. Contemporary moral philosophy has concentrated intently on the problem of giving theoretical explanations for the origin and certainty of moral principles. So much intellectual effort was expended on this search that the more humble maxims of classical rhetoric-casuistry have been forgotten. Instead of the multitude of maxims that inhabit common moral discourse, modern moral philosophy attempts to identify one or several very general principles that encompass a wide swath of moral issues. Modern medical ethics, for example, commonly refers to four fundamental principles: respect for autonomy, nonmaleficence, beneficence, and justice. The challenge to moral discourse consists in how to relate the very specific details of particular cases to these abstractly defined moral principles. How does the principle of respect for autonomy resolve the case of this Jehovah's Witness believer arriving in this emergency department at this time? It should be clear that, in addition to the principle of autonomy, many other moral maxims are at play in the case: How can this patient be helped and not harmed? Are we somehow bound by a belief that we do not understand and share? Is it right to let a person do himself in because of a belief that is not rationally justifiable? Is it right to allow this person, who is the father of a family, to leave his wife without a husband and his children fatherless? Would it not be better to force a transfusion on him and let him be welcomed back to family and congregation not as a sinner but as one whom we have sinned against? These and other maxims provide the moral ambiance of the case. Still, how do we find the route to travel between these moral maxims and the facts of the case, so that we might arrive at a resolution useful to those who must make a decision?

The metaphor of "balancing and weighing" is favored by many ethicists trying to explain how principles relate to decisions in particular cases. For example, in *Principles of*

Biomedical Ethics, Beauchamp and Childress (1994) reject theories, such as classic utilitarianism, that rely on a single principle by which all cases are resolved. They propose what they call a "composite theory," which "permits each basic principle to have weight without assigning a priority weighting or ranking. Which principle overrides in a case of conflict will depend on the particular context, which always has unique features." They then recall philosopher W. D. Ross's thesis that when two or more obligations conflict, balancing is necessary and "we must examine the situation carefully until we form 'a considered opinion (it is never more)' that one obligation is more incumbent in the circumstances than any other" (Ross 1930, 19–36). Ross invokes the metaphor of "weights moving on a scale" to describe how principles are balanced. Yet, even with this departure from the rigid adherence to a single theory and a univocal principle, we are left with some mystery. What does it mean to say, as Beauchamp and Childress do, "what principle overrides . . . will depend on the particular context, which always has unique features" (1994, 33, 104–11)? How do the unique features of a particular context provide weight to a principle or tip the balance toward one rather than the other?

At the most abstract level, two principles—beneficence and respect for autonomy—strive for attention in the case of the bleeding Jehovah's Witness who refuses blood transfusion. These principles are in apparent conflict. As the factual details of the case emerge, however, these abstract principles begin to take on (or lose) weight. If the details show that the patient had, in fact, reached critically low hemoglobin levels to sustain organic perfusion and life, and also reveal that he is a truly committed believer and is (or was at the moment of admission to the Emergency Department Room) clear and competent in expressing his beliefs, the two competing principles remain in balance. This patient can be benefited by transfusion; but he competently rejects transfusion. However, as more detail about the nature of his beliefs and the doctrines of his church appear, and as possible medical alternatives are considered, weight may begin to shift. Without pursuing the case in detail, the accumulation of details may finally weigh down the principle of autonomy to the point where its importance becomes manifest: it may become clear that the beneficence that sustains organic life by blood transfusion is not, for this patient, a benefit. It will give him not the gift of life, but a burden of guilt, perhaps not even his own but, in his belief, a sin he has occasioned for others. Even his continued fatherly presence may be less a benefit than an example of infidelity to divine commands. The abstract principles of beneficence and autonomy take on their respective weight as the factual details relative to the topics and maxims are filled out and amplified. This is the essential method of casuistic reasoning.

Another case, dealing with policy rather than with clinical decision, may further illustrate this method. In 1974, Congress established The National Commission for Protection of Human Subjects of Biomedical and Behavioral Research. This was the first public body in the United States charged with the task of relating ethics to public policy. As such, it had to bring speculative moral philosophy into the real world of moral commitments and moral conflict. It had to turn abstract principles into practical resolutions. Congress specified the tasks of the commission: it was to study several particular problems, such as research with the human fetus, with children, with the mentally infirm, and with prisoners; it was also charged with developing general ethical principles relevant to research with human subjects. The commission's report, "Research Involving Children" (hereafter, "The Children's Report"), was issued in September 1977, and its recommendations were issued as regulations in the *Federal Register*, March 8, 1983. These were among the most difficult recommendations to issue from the commission. One reason for the difficulty lay in the formulation of the congressional mandate, "to identify the requirements for informed consent . . . by children . . . or their legal representatives."

It has often been noted that the first principle of the *Nuremberg Code*, "voluntary consent . . . is absolutely essential," was shaped in response to the moral abominations of the Nazi concentration camp experiments. The victims of this deadly exploitation were as far from volunteers as humans could be. Persons in captivity were the center of attention. It has also been noted that so primary and absolute a principle unequivocally excludes from research children or others who are mentally incompetent. This exclusion was eliminated by the *Declaration of Helsinki* in 1964, which authorizes the consent of legal guardians for such subjects (Jonsen, Veatch, and Walters 1998). However, at this point a moral paradox appears: since a research procedure and its risks are directed not to the good of the subject but to the good of future knowledge and improved care for future patients, may anyone other than the subject consent to the procedure? May parents, who exercise the power of proxy consent only for acts that promote the welfare of their children, ever consent to their inclusion in a research study?

The commission's "Belmont Report" subscribed to some basic principles that should govern all research with human subjects, namely, respect for persons, beneficence, and justice (National Commission 1979a). It associated these three general principles with the practices of informed consent, risk-benefit assessment, and fair selection processes, respectively. These three practices would incorporate the three principles into the actual conduct of research in the clinical setting. The "Belmont Report" did not suggest how these practices might be "weighed or balanced" should conflict arise between them, nor did it provide clues about whether the practices were ever open to exception or limitation. It did not give detailed recipes about how particular "tough cases" should be resolved. Recognizing, however, that these questions would arise, the commission endorsed the policy of establishing Institutional Review Boards (IRBs) in each research institution. IRBs would be charged with the interpretation and application of the principles and practices in every case in which an investigator wished to use a human person as a research subject. They would have to resolve most of the tough cases.

The basic ethical principles of "Belmont" certainly looked like W. D. Ross's *prima facie* principles. The commissioners, most of whom had never read a word by Professor Ross, were thinking like him, and they eventually found themselves faced with the same problems that he left unsolved in his books: How does one determine actual duty when several principles conflict? "The Children's Report" pushed that problem from the speculative to the practical and required an answer that could be translated into public policy. The commissioners listened to two distinguished ethicists arguing cogently for each side of the paradox. Professor Paul Ramsey of Princeton maintained that a child could never be the subject of any research procedure that did not directly benefit that individual child subject. Jesuit theologian Richard McCormick countered that nontherapeutic research could be permitted when there can be a reasonable presumption that the child would consent. The commissioners were swayed by Father McCormick's thesis but realized that they must go beyond a statement of principle. They must decide on such matters as the degrees of risk that a "reasonable child" would accept, the significance and the likelihood of anticipated benefit to the child, and the importance of the results of the research to other children and to the society itself. Only so would the phrase "reasonable presumption" make any sense. Thus, the recommendations of *The Children's Report* are studded with terms like "minimal risk," "minor increase over minimal," "more than minimal risk," "experiences reasonably commensurate," and "significant benefit." The commissioners realized that these terms required definition. At the same time, they realized that the terms could not be defined without positing from whose point of view, for what end, and under what circumstances minimal risk might be proposed and undertaken. Unbeknown to themselves, the commissioners had been transmogrified into a covey of casuists, debating not the principles of things, but the "who, what, when, where, why, and how much" of particular situations (National Commission 1979b, 41–53).[3] Each one of the many circumstances cannot be defined down to a sharp point: their relevance to the weight of the principles can only be judged in the full context of the case as it presents itself to those who must decide. "Circumstances make the case" advises an old adage familiar to lawyers and doctors and beloved of casuists.

However, even if circumstances exert a powerful pull on the abstract principles, the casuist must appreciate that principles and maxims, abstract though they may be, carry some weight in themselves. Failure to appreciate the weight of principles allows good casuistry to collapse into *situationism*: the ethical doctrine that circumstances alone determine the moral quality of decision and action (Jonsen 1993). Further examination of the metaphor of weighing may advance the appreciation of the role of principles in casuistic reasoning. Weight, in classical physics, is the result of the pull of gravity toward a center. A moral principle is weighty when it falls to the center of consideration within the universe of moral considerations relevant to the problem at issue. Its weight is its importance or significance in deliberation about the issue. That weight derives from several related sources. First, it comes from the way in which a society in a particular cultural tradition cultivates certain ideas and values, enacting and reinforcing them in its intellectual, social, and religious life. Second, it comes from the critical examinations to which such central ideas are subjected by scholars of the society. A third source of weight derives from the aggregation of the factual circumstances to the principles in particular cases.

The first source of moral weight is the intellectual, social, and cultural traditions of a community. Certain moral notions accumulate weight as a tradition rolls through time. Robert Bellah's book, *Habits of the Heart*, records how the idea of "individualism" has permeated American culture. Bellah writes, "American cultural traditions define personality, achievement, and the purpose of human life in ways that leave the individual suspended in glorious, but terrifying, isolation" (Bellah et al. 1985, 6). This is the modern precipitate from a long "historical conversation" that includes "biblical and republican strands." Our current American emphasis on "respect for autonomy" as an ethical principle is the precipitate of that tradition. The tradition of political and moral liberalism, as it becomes mainstream within a culture, has pushed to the margins of our culture other principles that are incompatible or fit, at best, clumsily. For example, religious zealotry demanding that all conform to an orthodoxy is intellectually and politically incompatible with liberalism and respect for autonomy. Thus, not without strife it is pushed to the margins and, not without strife, may be kept there. It has little or no weight in deliberations about moral and social issues within the dominant culture, although it may flourish within minority communities. The failure of Marxist principles, in their totalitarian form, to capture the American mind, even in the depths of the Depression and in the midst of labor turmoil, is another example of the marginalization of a moral principle.

Thus, in our culture, respect for persons is a principle that has considerable weight. It outweighs the marginalized principles mentioned above. It also outweighs other principles that are commonly accepted as worthy but that have "lost weight" by attrition of the social conditions in which they flourished. For example, it would be commonly accepted that "family loyalty" or "respect for elders" were good things but, given significant changes in the sociology and economics of the family in American culture, these good things are much less weighty as ethical notions than they were in earlier times. Clearly, the principle of autonomy outweighs a panoply of other moral notions that may serve major purposes in other cultures but are only minor functions in our own. Punctilious etiquette toward persons of various social classes, rigorous conventions of honor, and elaborate linguistic formulas are important morally in other societies, but not in the United States. Thus, in this sense, it not difficult to find some principles that have more weight than others within a social tradition.

These anthropological observations do not get us very far, however. It is not the balancing of central against marginal principles or of significant against trivial ones that causes moral perplexity. It is the balancing of central and significant ones against each other. It is possible to demonstrate that individualism, with its consequent ethical principle of respect for persons, is central in American culture. However, it is also possible to demonstrate that beneficence, the duty to help others, has played a consistent role in Western culture and American life. Similarly, justice and fairness are central and significant notions. The problem of balancing arises when respect for autonomy must be balanced against other principles, such as beneficence. These notions all have, in the abstract, equivalent gravity, or, put less surely, it is difficult to show by theoretical argument how one should prevail over the other.

In the first instance, then, the weight of any principle derives from the gravity that pulls it into the center of any cultural and critical deliberations about a moral issue. The pull comes from the collective attraction that an idea exerts on a social community existing within a moral tradition and from the moral character endorsed in that tradition. If that community's history or social complexion fosters a certain idea, it will, when issues summon it, appear in the public discussion; if the idea is absent or marginal, it will be invisible or silent. Thus, "holy war" and "ethnic cleansing" do not appear as weighty moral notions in certain cultures, while they have powerful attraction in others. Much more needs to be said about the problems that arise if one accepts this explanation of the first source of moral weight: What about relativism? What about societies in which invidious principles (such as, in the American view, "holy war" and "ethnic cleansing") prevail? What about societies in which critical reflection repudiates central cultural concepts? How do competing, critical, innovative moral notions force their way into a moral tradition (Hauerwas 1983)?

The critical reflection of the scholars within the culture provides a second way in which a moral principle acquires weight. In some cultures there is a formal intellectual enterprise that is called philosophy; in other cultures, intellectual life runs in other courses, but there is, nonetheless, a recognized cultural wisdom that articulates ideals and announces priorities for social and personal life. Whenever this happens, respected thinkers select certain principles, ideals, and virtues for special attention. These principles are drawn from those available in the cultural tradition; the philosophers promote them to the center of the system of reflective thought that they construct. Their gravity becomes apparent when other ideas are drawn into their orbit and circle around them as implications. Thus, the notion of the individual as autonomous subject enthralled the thinkers of the Enlightenment and gradually attained a central place in the thought of leading philosophers such as Hobbes, Locke, Rousseau, Kant, and Mill. The philosophical reflections of British liberalism and American pragmatism elaborate and refine these central ideas. The principle of respect for persons becomes a familiar, indeed, indispensable notion among those who read and write in the Western philosophical traditions; those who ignore it do so at peril of exclusion from the philosophical society and those who criticize it must fight an uphill battle.

This sort of weight, however, is somewhat illusory. A system of moral philosophy is not a morality. While those who read and write philosophy may give great weight to a principle because it has made a system of thought coherent and convincing, that principle may not be as weighty in the lives of those who live the morality of the culture. Even if they do acknowledge its importance, they may not give it the preeminence or the priority accorded to it within the system of thought. For example, in recent years, we have seen the principle of respect for autonomy become the weightiest of principles in medical ethics. It is congenial to American moral tradition; it is central to much of Western moral philosophy. However, we are beginning to hear protests from those who speak with other voices within the dominant moral tradition and who are in the process of elaborating alternative moral philosophies, emphasizing community rather than individual, or a gender-balanced ethic. The scholarly authority of authors and the elegance of their argument may give weight to their notions; yet they may hardly be heard outside the scholarly world.

Weighty principles, then, acquire some of their gravity from tradition and culture, as well as from systems of moral reflection, but this is incomplete. There is a third way in which the metaphor of weight might be employed. This third way refers not so much to principles as to the ultimate moral decision. A moral decision follows consideration of various features of a situation, including both principles and circumstances. In this third view, it is the considerations, rather than the principles themselves, that are weighty. Many moral principles coexist within a moral tradition; many of them seem of equivalent importance and, on their face, do not announce their superiority over their competitors. However, when the circumstances surrounding a moral problem are specified in some detail, a sense of priority begins to emerge and begs to be investigated more closely. For example, "thou shalt not bear false witness" is a revered principle within the cultures affected by Jewish and Christian religions; similarly both faiths strongly advocate the protection of the weak from harm. Both are weighty principles within the American moral tradition. However, St. Augustine and Immanuel Kant relate a story that poses a painful paradox: an innocent man hides in your home from the agents of a tyrant bent on arresting him and you are asked by those agents whether he is here. Which of the two weighty principles should prevail? Arguments can be made on both sides: Augustine and Kant argue for the absolute priority of truth-telling and reject any casuistic palliation of strict adherence to the principle (Augustine 1952, ch. 5–6; Kant 1978). Thousands of brave persons who protected heretics from Inquisitors and Jews from Nazis preferred the principle of protecting the innocent. It is not the weight of the principle itself that tips the balance; it is the accumulated weight of the variety of circumstances that cluster around the principles in question that does so. When we hear the story, we want to know more. Precisely who is this person and in what does his innocence consist? What is the nature of the tyranny and why do they seek him? What is the likelihood that he will be found regardless of what you say? What are the consequences to you and your family if exposed? Are there alternatives to disclosure? (Admittedly, the example limps because, in critical situations, such prudential reflection is often impossible and may even be repugnant; still, the example is a historical one over which many good minds have puzzled.)

We might therefore change the terms of the metaphor: the principles are the scales on which the burdens of circumstances are placed. Principles do weigh on a final decision, but the scales dip, not under the principles' weight, but under the accumulated circumstances that pull on one or the other principle. Moral judgments bear on whole cases, the principles and maxims are welded together with the circumstances. Principles, values, circumstances, and consequences must be seen as a whole. The judgment about them comprises them all together: we do not, in Platonic fashion, turn our eyes from a vision of moral principle down to the nonmoral facts of a case. We sweep facts, values, consequences, and principles into a single vision.

A return to the National Commission deliberations will provide two instances that illustrate this idea. First, in "The Children's Report," the maxim "do no harm," while not explicitly cited, is all pervasive. Since children generally cannot give consent (a circumstance), the principle of respect for autonomy is of less weight than the principle of nonmaleficence. However, the maxim "do no harm" must be refined in the context of research. It is necessary to clarify what constitutes harm and how research might do harm. Although much of that clarification was tacit and implicit, the commission's conclusions bear witness to the realization that there are harms of many sorts and many degrees and that most research maneuvers do not do harm, but pose risks of harm, and that these are of many sorts and degrees. A harm such as deliberate death or maiming, such as took place in the Nazi research, is unquestionably unethical; how should the harm that comes from a needle stick to draw blood be judged? Is it more harmful or risky if the child is healthy and normal than if the child is a leukemia patient for whom needle sticks are routine? Is a change of daily activities for research observation a harm or risk of harm? Would it be so if the change involved placing the child for a day in the care of strangers rather than familiar caretakers? Should it be considered a harm to be randomly assigned into a treatment regimen that turns out at the conclusion of the study to be the less effective? These and many other variations on the theme of harm and risk are essential to any reasonable judgment that the maxim "do no harm" is being honored or violated. It is the total picture in the instant case that allows such a judgment to be made. The moral weight of "do no harm" is manifested only amidst the greater and less, the probables and the possibles of quite particular circumstances.

Paradigms and Analogies

One more step in casuistic reasoning must be noted. If the casuistic mind does not move immediately from cases to principles for resolution of moral perplexity, where does the casuist find the grounds for testing his conclusions in the particular case? The casuist seeks those grounds in other cases. The conclusions in a contested case are compared to conclusions in similar cases in which the relation between maxims and circumstances suggests an obvious resolution. The casuist reflects on the similarities and differences between the contested case and the uncontested cases—similarities and differences that are manifested in the actual circumstances of each case. In the uncontested case, the maxim and the circumstances are such that no other maxim has the weight to challenge or to uphold an exception to the rule. The casuist, like the jurist in Anglo-American law, always notes, "This case is very like, or somewhat like, the previous case of X," and then asks what it is about the instant case that might call for a different judgment than did the prior case (in Anglo-American jurisprudence, this process is canonized in the use of precedents). For example, the maxim that parents should determine what is best for their children is, in the usual circumstances of familial life, an uncontested maxim, even though many parents may make ill-considered judgments. However, given the circumstance that the parents are devoted believers in a sect that forbids medical care for children, another maxim, the protection of a vulnerable human being, grows strong enough to challenge the first maxim. Cases can then be lined up in which the uncontested case stands as a paradigm and other cases stand at various distant removes: at the first remove, the parents' faith does not forbid medical care but rather recommends that prayer be the first recourse; at the second remove the belief forbids all but emergency treatment; at the third remove, it forbids all medical attention without exception. At each remove, the danger to the child increases and the moral challenge to parental authority grows stronger. This simple example (which in reality might be very complex) shows how the circumstances change the case, modify the moral judgment about it, and justify different practical responses to it. The contested case is an analogy, a similar yet relevantly different instance in a series of cases in which the paradigm case is the most clear and compelling.

Reasoning by analogy is quite different than reasoning by logical deduction from premise to conclusion. Although philosophers assert that the logical properties of either form of reasoning are different, both are valid forms of reasoning. However, analogous reasoning is more problematic: it does not move in a straight line between propositions and its terms are not primarily conceptual. Rather, it moves back and forth within a myriad of empirical details as well as conceptual propositions. It is rather like an art critic comparing two (or more) paintings. One detail on one canvas is noticed and evaluated in view of another detail on the second canvas. The comparison highlights certain features of both paintings and only then can the critic render a judgment about the painting as a whole. Obviously, the details compared must be similar to each other in some respect—in both paintings, the intensity of the color of the sky might be the point of comparison—sky color is the similarity; intensity is the difference. The casuist is a sort of art critic, glancing at several cases, their maxims and circumstances, in order to compare one to the other and to render a judgment about the value of each.

The difference between the casuist and the critic, however, is that one sort of case serves as a paradigm, a prime example, or test case. True, an art critic may have in mind certain paintings or painters who are paragons against which all other creations can be judged, but so strong a preference might be judged a prejudice in a critic. The casuist needs relatively clear tests of right and wrong. These are found in cases rather than in principles or theories. The judgment in one case, with its pattern of circumstances and maxims, is clearly and incontestably right, and so becomes the paradigm against which other similar cases, with diverging patterns of circumstances and maxims, can be tested. In classical casuistry, for example, a "just war" was a military action that was launched after timely declaration, justified by a clearly just reason, carried out with due proportion between aggression and the goal, and that provided protection of innocent noncombatants. The just war casuists were not so foolish as to believe that such a war had ever, or ever would, be fought. Rather, they were proposing maxims that conscientious rulers or generals could attempt to realize in the circumstances of their political and military maneuverings. These maxims found their way into international rules of war and, while certainly never perfectly realized, went far to keep warfare within humane limits. Certain actual wars attain paradigmatic status in some respects: the Allies fought World War II for a just cause, the obliteration of Nazi aggression. In other respects, clear departures from the paradigm can be properly condemned: saturation bombing in World War II violated the maxim of noncombatant immunity.

Some paradigm cases are, as is the just war paradigm, an imaginative construction. They arise from real cases on which the casuist might reflect. During the Thirty Years War, for example, many horrors and injustices were committed by all sides. If human aggression seems inevitable, can it be carried out so as to diminish the horrors and enhance the moral rectitude of aggression? The actual examples reveal the evils of war without requiring proof: an instinctive response to the slaughter of innocent aged, women, and children is enough. The casuist may attempt to answer the question by referring to an example in which extreme aggression seems justified with as little proof. The case of self-defense against a potentially lethal and unprovoked attack provides such a paradigm. The casuist goes on to build the paradigm case for war on this paradigm for justified aggression. In all such construction, the question is "What circumstances could possibly justify attacking humans, which under most conditions is morally reprehensible?" In casuistry, no case stands alone; all cases stand within contexts of similar cases. The casuistic mind circulates among these contexts, seeking places of relative certainty about moral rightness and wrongness, and uses these places as testing grounds for questionable cases.

CRITIQUE OF CASUISTRY

Casuistry hardly needs another critique. It and its practitioners have been the object of the most scathing criticisms over the centuries. One of the world's most renowned satires is *The Provincial Letters* by the great French mathematician and philosopher, Blaise Pascal. This book demolishes the classical casuists (Pascal 1967). *The Abuse of Casuistry* contends that Pascal's critique was justified but that it demolished not the methods of casuistry but rather the abusive use of those methods. Casuistry is, as noted above, a form of rhetoric. Rhetoric becomes accomplished at sharp distinctions and striking comparisons and those with such skills can make a case for anything. Pascal found such casuistry in which the outrageous act won casuistic approbation (an arsonist could be absolved of burning down a house because he set fire to the wrong one) and such casuistry exists even today (in a notorious political sex scandal, the accused exculpated himself by claiming that since fellatio had been performed on him, not by him, he had not engaged in sex!). Pascal's sarcastic criticism, however, does not reach to the casuistic method as such. Indeed, if it had, the human activity of moral judgment would itself be accused, since the essential methods of casuistry mirror the common, untutored process of moral judgment. Nevertheless, since Pascal's time, the word casuistry itself has come to mean the unscrupulous art of making groundless distinctions to defend obviously outrageous behavior.

The renewal of interest in casuistry that followed the publication of *The Abuse of Casuistry* stimulated criticisms quite different from those of Pascal. These modern critiques go to the essence of the contemporary exposition of the casuistic method. They touch the important elements of casuistic reasoning: topics, maxims, and paradigms. Since casuistry begins by designating the topics inherent in a particular enterprise, some critics have questioned whether any human enterprise has a structure so defined and permanent as to permit the identification of a finite number of topics. All human enterprises, from marriage to medicine and from economics to education, are fluid and shift their constituent features over time and in different settings. The casuist who wishes to hang a particular case on a permanent structure will not find that structure in the human institutions. A second criticism touches topics: the purpose of designating topics is to create the boxes into which multitudes of heterogeneous circumstances can be filed. Although it is useful in any ethical discussion to get one's facts sorted out, the casuistical sorting is deceptively simple: one may sort circumstances into the wrong topics, particularly when many circumstances are open to several interpretation, and, even worse, one sorts in some circumstances and sorts out others. This latter fault arises from biases in the casuist and obviously biases the case. How can the casuist know that all the relevant circumstances have been collected and sorted? How can the casuist assure that the right circumstances are in the right boxes? Another casuist might construct the case quite differently, using different circumstances or topics and combining them in different ways. Similarly, those presenting the case might, consciously or unconsciously, select certain details to the detriment of others (Kopelman 1994).

Critics challenge the casuist's manner of relating maxims and circumstances. The maxims or principles that give the case its moral identity are, in the casuist's view, embedded in the case. They bear little meaning when stated in the abstract and without illustrating instances, which will always be cases. Yet the critic can ask, "What is the origin and nature of maxims and principles?" It is not enough to assert that they are embedded in cases and need case-specificity for their meaning; principles and maxims do appear to have at least general meaning on their own: we say without hesitation that lying is wrong or superiors should not exploit the vulnerability of their inferiors. Also principles and maxims are often used as critical tools to attack a practice or an institution. Respect for persons, fairness, and equity, we might say, show that sexual harassment is immoral. Principles and maxims, then, appear to have some logical, epistemological, and ethical function apart from cases. Casuistry does not offer an account of that function. Indeed, it seems not only to ignore it, but also to undermine it, since maxims and principles are always open to revision as new cases arise, and, as they are revised in the light of circumstances, they lose their power as critical tools of moral discourse (Arras 1991). It is this feature of casuistical reasoning that leads some to assert that casuistry is a form of situation ethics.

Finally, casuistry's reliance on paradigm cases for analogous reasoning has attracted criticism. The casuist maintains that moral reasoning moves not from theory and principle down to judgment but that it moves sideways from clear to less clear cases. This leaves open what makes a case clear enough to be a paradigm. In general, the casuist might say that a clear case is one in which the circumstances are such that the relevant maxim can be readily realized in choice and action and no other maxims contest for primacy. However, this still leaves many questions. One casuist's paradigm may not be that of another, since cases can be viewed under different perspectives: the same facts can constitute a case of assisted suicide and a case of medical manslaughter, but one casuist comes at those facts from the stance of personal autonomy and another from the perspective of protection of the vulnerable. Also, paradigm cases are not Platonic Ideas, free of earthly connections. They are instances found in quite real cultural settings imbued with custom and history. The moral judgment made about their paradigmatic status cannot be isolated from those earthly connections. Moreover, in the culture of contemporary moral pluralism, it is unlikely that everyone or even many will settle on a set of paradigms satisfactory to all. Finally, if paradigms are the final testing ground for moral judgments about analogous cases, the certitude of the paradigm must be guaranteed in some fashion. If casuistry declines to refer its judgments to some prior ethical theory, then the paradigms themselves must be the locus of certitude. This appears to invoke the questionable moral epistemology of intuitionism, moved from its usual place among principles to the realm of paradigm cases (Wildes 1991; Juengst 1989).

These are reasonable questions that must be posed to the casuist. If the casuist is more than a moral mechanic, fiddling with the machinery of cases, the questions will be taken seriously. As attempts to answer them are made, a theory of casuistry will appear, ironic as it may seem for those who eschew theory in moral reasoning. Yet even the dedicated casuist must admit that the work of casuistry is, as one critic said, "an engine of thought" (Arras 1991, 41). It is a technique of examining what ought to be done in the occasion, as Aristotle said. It is a tactic of bringing the circumstances into the moral evaluation of the case. Techniques and tactics are never the whole story; they work within a larger context of understanding. So the techniques of casuistry, topics, maxims and circumstances, paradigms and analogy, work within a broader understanding of the nature of the moral life, of moral reasoning, of the history of ethics, and of cultural and institutional values. Any theory of casuistry that might emerge would refer the critical questions noted above to this broader understanding.

CONCLUDING COMMENTS

In conclusion, casuistry is not "a much less respectable" study than theoretical ethics. Professor Moore, who wrote those words, was an Oxford don for whom respectability came from lineage and who probably left details of daily life to the college servants. The lineage of classical casuistry was, unfortunately, tainted by some of its practitioners, and so must have gained Moore's disdain. However, today we can trace that lineage back to more reputable ancestors, including Aristotle. Even more important than ancestry, however, we find contemporary casuists who are honest ethicists working with difficult problems. Also, the details of daily life are no longer beneath the notice of respectable people. Those details are the stuff of ethical judgment and they come to us in the form of cases, episodes, real or imagined, of human action. Casuistry is ethics respecting the moral dimensions of the gritty stuff of daily life and, as such, deserves respect. But its ultimate title for respect derives from the ability of its practitioners to elucidate sufficiently the obscurities of particular cases to enable persons to make responsible decisions; that is, decisions that are responsive not only to the needs, desires, exigencies, and hopes that generate the case, but also to the principles and values that sustain human dignity. To the extent that casuistry achieves this end, it deserves respect as (as Professor Moore admits) a study and activity that "ethics is not complete without."

NOTES ON RESOURCES AND TRAINING

Learning to use casuistry can be challenging. In part, this is due to the role of virtue in casuistry. Aristotle remarks, "Prudence is not concerned with universals only; it must also take cognizance of particulars, because it is concerned with conduct, and conduct has its sphere in particular circumstances." Those circumstances are, he says, "the agent, the act, the object of the act, the instrument, the aim and the manner." The prudent person, he says, is one who can deliberate well about particulars. And again, he says, "The field of deliberation is that which happens for the most part, where the result is obscure and the right course not clearly defined; and for important decisions we call in advisors, distrusting our own ability to reach a decision" (Aristotle 1976, VI, vii, 1141; III, i, 1110; III, iii, 1112). The casuist should be such an advisor.

The casuist should "be cognizant of particulars," that is, should have a solid, even scientific understanding of the topics within the endeavor in which advice is given (thus, a medical ethicist must know a modicum of medical science and clinical medicine; a business ethicist must understand economics, banking, investment, and commerce). He or she should recognize the obscurity of the situation and thus depend on other involved parties to illuminate as best they can. He or she must be able to hear and hold in mind a variety of arguments about the maxims appropriate to complex situations. He or she should be able to tolerate uncertainty about the right course and, within that uncertainty, find a reasonable course of action; that is, the course recommended by the most persuasive argument in the circumstances, with due recognition of other arguments that are plausible. A good casuist must, then, have all the intellectual virtues recommended by Aristotle: science, prudence, intuition, wisdom. Can someone be taught to be a casuist, then, or must one be born to the trade?

Casuistry can be taught by outlining the technique and by inviting the student to apply it to cases again and again. Persons more adept can criticize the adequacy of the application. However, the casuist must constantly argue his or her analysis with others both from and outside the world of ethics. The initial framing and analysis of a case must be subject to other views and sources of information. Casuistry should not be a solitary reflection but a vivid interchange of facts and ideas. This sort of exercise is training for casuistry. Another aspect of training is the broadening education about ethical theory, history of ethics, and the ethos of the culture (or cultures) where casuistry is being performed.

A final characteristic of a casuist is a controversial one: the casuist must be a person of probity. As Pascal brilliantly exposed, casuistry can be a cleverness that makes convincing arguments in defense of reprehensible behavior. The casuist must be able to control his or her cleverness, or ethical virtuosity, and link it to serious moral intent. Aristotle recognized this, saying, "if the aim of action is noble, cleverness is praiseworthy but if the aim is ignoble, cleverness is unscrupulousness . . . now since only a good person can discern the good for humans and because wickedness can distort this vision and cause serious error about the principles of conduct, it is evident that one cannot be prudent without being good" (Aristotle

1976, VI, xii, 1144). This is a strong proposition and unwelcome to many modern hearers, yet it is worth pondering. Even if we cannot conceive a model of virtue, or demand that every person be a paragon of all virtues, at least we can recommend honesty, truthfulness, fidelity, compassion, and responsibility and hope that ethical advisors possess these moral characteristics. Whether these virtues come by nature or nurture remains a perennial question.

The principal resources for the study of casuistry lie hidden in rare book libraries. The casuistic books of the era of "high casuistry," 1550–1650, contain the full panoply of cases and analyses that lay the foundations for the methodology proposed by contemporary commentators. A list of the major casuistic books of that era can be found as an appendix to *The Abuse of Casuistry.* Contemporary resources for the study of casuistry are both historical and analytic. In the opinion of this author, an adequate understanding of casuistry and a sound criticism of its strengths and weaknesses must be informed by both its history and the critical analyses employed by philosophers, theologians, and rhetoricians. A collection of informative essays, *Conscience and Casuistry in Early Modern Europe* (Leites 1988), exposes the social and religious changes in the seventeenth century that radically modified the perceived relationship between personal conscience and law, and the consequent shifts in the ways in which morality was conceived and taught, stimulating the growth of casuistic thinking. Unfortunately, this volume was in press at the same time as *The Abuse of Casuistry;* otherwise its scholarship would have informed the writing of that book. The acute crisis of conscience that the English Reformation forced on many religious persons was a significant source of much seventeenth-century casuistry; that story is told in detail in Elliot Rose's *Cases of Conscience: Alternatives Open to Recusants and Puritans under Elizabeth I and James I* (1975). Pascal's critique of casuistry is itself criticized by Richard Parish in *Pascal's* Lettres Provinciales*: A Study in Polemic* (1989), a book that sustains in substance the analysis of Pascal's attack made by Jonsen and Toulmin in *The Abuse of Casuistry.*

The contemporary literature that is cited previously in this essay, particularly the essays mentioned in "Critiques of Casuistry," constitute the principal resources for the current reflections on the use of the casuistic method. However, much of that literature is polemical rather than systematic. Efforts to explain the nature of casuistic reasoning more systematically are rare, but several are worthy of notice. One of these, Kenneth Kirk's *Conscience and Its Problems,* was written many years ago (1927) but a recent re-edition, with introduction by David Smith, makes available a learned and literary exposition of classical casuistic ethics. Kirk's remark, "The abuse of casuistry is properly directed, not against all casuistry, but only against its abuse," suggested the title for Jonsen and Toulmin's *Abuse of Casuistry* and many of Kirk's insights informed the theses of that book (Kirk 1999). *The Abuse of Casuistry* surveyed rather summarily the ancient and medieval precursors to the "high casuistry" of the Renaissance. A volume of essays edited by James Keenan and Thomas Shannon, *The Context of Casuistry* (1995), goes more deeply into that earlier literature, particularly the writings of the late scholastic nominalist theologians who immediately preceded the neoscholasticism of the Renaissance. Several essays explore the work of the Anglican casuists and the effect of casuistry (or its abuse) in the moral theology manuals of the nineteenth century. This volume is a valuable addition to the history of casuistic thinking. Richard B. Miller, in *Casuistry and Modern Ethics* (1996), has written a book about casuistry that would be dear to any casuist's heart: he has explained casuistic methodology as he works through particular cases. He moves beyond the problems in medical ethics that have absorbed the attention of modern casuistic analysts and turns to cases raised by modern warfare, politics, and social issues. His use of the casuistic method is insightful and imaginative, balanced and provocative, all virtues required in the contemporary casuist. In *Fragmentation and Consensus* (1999), Mark Kuczewski explores the similarities and differences between two approaches to moral philosophy, casuistry and communitarianism, and in so doing, explicates several of the most difficult problems inherent in casuistic reasoning, the selection of paradigms, and the role of consensus. He, like Miller, does so with reference to cases but remains within the moral world of medical ethics. Kuczewski also contributed to the *Encyclopedia of Applied Ethics* an excellent article comparing various modern approaches to casuistic reasoning (Kuczewski 1989). Baruch Brody's *Life and Death Decision Making* (1988) is the major exposition of a form of casuistic reasoning that gives a larger place to ethical theory than does the method explained above. Carson Strong has written many essays in defense of a paradigm-based casuistry and lucidly applied his own version of casuistic method in the analysis of difficult cases in pediatrics, obstetrics, and reproductive medicine (1988; 1997; 2000). Finally, collections of cases in medical ethics can be found in many textbooks and anthologies. Among these are the cases that have appeared in the *Hastings Center Report* from its beginnings in the 1970s and Gregory Pence's narrative of many of the major cases that have engaged medical ethicists (Crigger 1998; Pence 1994).

NOTES

1. For a more detailed and referenced history of philosophy's turn from cases to theory see Jonsen (1998), chapter 3.
2. For a detailed exposition of the development of casuistry in Catholic moral theology, see Keenan and Shannon (1995) and for the place of casuistry within Roman Catholic moral theology generally, see Mahoney (1987).
3. On the work of the National Commission, see Jonsen (1998), chapters 4 and 5.

REFERENCES

Aristotle. 1976. *The Ethics of Aristotle*, ed. and trans. J. A. K. Thomson and H. Tredennick. London: Penguin Books.

Arras, J. 1991. "The Revival of Casuistry in Bioethics." *Journal of Medicine and Philosophy.* 16:9–51.

Augustine, Saint. 1952. "Lying." In *Early Christian Biographies*, ed. and trans. R. Deferrari. New York: Fathers of the Church.

Beauchamp, T., and J. Childress. 1994. *Principles of Biomedical Ethics*. 4th ed. New York and Oxford: Oxford University Press.

Bellah, R., R. Madsen, W. Sullivan, A. Swidler, and S. Tipton. 1985. *Habits of the Heart.* New York: Harper and Row.

Brody, B. A. 1988. *Life and Death Decision Making*. New York: Oxford University Press.

Crigger, B. J. 1998. *Cases in Bioethics. Selections from the Hastings Center Report*. 3rd ed. New York: St. Martin's Press.

Hauerwas, S. 1983. "Casuistry as a Narrative Art." *Interpretation* 37:377–88.

Jonsen, A. R. 1993. "Casuistry, Situationism and Laxity." In *Joseph Fletcher: Memoir of an Ex-Radical. Reminiscence and Reappraisal*, ed. K. Vaux. Louisville, KY: John Knox Press, pp. 10–24.

———. 1998. *The Birth of Bioethics*. New York: Oxford University Press.

Jonsen, A. R., and S. Toulmin. 1988. *The Abuse of Casuistry: A History of Moral Reasoning*. Berkeley and Los Angeles: University of California Press.

Jonsen, A. R., M. Siegler, and W. Winslade. 1998. *Clinical Ethics*. 4th ed. New York: McGraw-Hill.

Jonsen, A. R., R. Veatch, and L. Walters, eds. 1998. *Source Book in Bioethics: A Documentary History*. Washington, D.C.: Georgetown University Press.

Juengst, E. 1989. "Casuistry and the Locus of Certitude in Ethics." *Journal of Medical Humanities* 3:19–27.

Kant, I. 1978. "On the Supposed Right to Tell Lies from Benevolent Motives." In S. Bok, *Lying: Moral Choice in Public and Private Life*. New York: Pantheon Books, pp. 267–74.

Keenan, J., and T. Shannon, eds. 1995. *The Context of Casuistry*. Washington, D.C.: Georgetown University Press.

Kirk, K. E. 1999. *Conscience and Its Problems: An Introduction to Casuistry*. Louisville: Westminster/John Knox Press.

Kopelman, L. 1994. "Case Method and Casuistry: The Problem of Bias." *Theoretical Medicine* 15:21–37.

Kuczewski, M. G. 1989. "Casuistry." In *The Encyclopedia of Applied Ethics,* ed. Ruth Chadwick. San Diego: The Academic Press, pp. 423–32.

———. 1999. *Fragmentation and Consensus: Communitarian and Casuist Bioethics*. Washington, D.C.: Georgetown University Press.

Leites, E., ed. 1988. *Conscience and Casuistry in Early Modern Europe*. Cambridge: Cambridge University Press.

Mahoney, J. 1987. *The Making of Moral Theology*. Oxford: The Clarendon Press.

Miller, R. B. 1996. *Casuistry and Modern Ethics*. Chicago: University of Chicago Press.

Moore, G. E. 1903. *Principia Ethica*. Cambridge: Cambridge University Press.

National Commission for the Protection of Human Subjects of Biomedical and Behavioral Research. 1979a. "The Belmont Report." In *Source Book in Bioethics: A Documentary History,* ed. A. R. Jonsen, R. Veatch, and L. Walters. 1998. Washington, D.C.: Georgetown University Press, pp. 22–28.

———. 1979b. "Research Involving Children." In *Source Book in Bioethics: A Documentary History,* ed. A. R. Jonsen, R. Veatch, and L. Walters. 1998. Washington, D.C.: Georgetown University Press, pp. 41–53.

Oakeshott, M. 1975. *On Human Conduct*. Oxford: The Clarendon Press.

Oxford English Dictionary. 1989. 2nd ed. Vol. II. Oxford: The Clarendon Press, pp. 933, 935.

Parish, R. 1989. *Pascal's* Lettres Provinciales*: A Study in Polemic.* Oxford: The Clarendon Press.

Pascal, B. 1967. *The Provincial Letters*, trans. A. Krailsheimer. London: Penguin Books.

Pence, G. E. 1994. *Classic Cases in Medical Ethics: Accounts of Cases that Have Shaped Medical Ethics, with Philosophical, Legal, and Historical Backgrounds.* New York: McGraw Hill.

Rose, E. 1975. *Cases of Conscience. Alternatives Open to Recusants and Puritans under Elizabeth I and James I.* Cambridge: Cambridge University Press.

Ross, W. D. 1930. *The Right and the Good.* Oxford: The Clarendon Press.

Strong, C. 1988. "Justification in Ethics." In *Moral Theory and Moral Judgments in Medical Ethics*, ed. B. Brody. Dordrecht, The Netherlands: Kluwer Academic Publishers, pp. 193–211.

———. 1997. *Ethics in Reproductive and Perinatal Medicine: A New Framework.* New Haven, CT: Yale University Press.

———. 2000. "Specified Principlism: What Is It and Does It Really Resolve Cases Better than Casuistry?" *Journal of Medicine and Philosophy* 25:323–41.

Tallmon, J. M. 1993. "How Jonsen Really Views Casuistry: A Note on the Abuse of Father Wildes." *Journal of Medicine and Philosophy* 18:33–49.

———. 1995. "Casuistry and the Role of Rhetorical Reason in Ethical Inquiry." *Philosophy and Rhetoric* 28:377–87.

Wildes, K. 1991. "The Priesthood of Bioethics and the Return of Casuistry." *Journal of Medicine and Philosophy* 18:33–49.

8

History

Darrel W. Amundsen

I shall begin this chapter by defining the most pertinent terms and delineating the parameters of the history of medical ethics. After briefly surveying the history of medical history with a view to discerning medical ethics' place in that field, I shall examine the nature of the historian's craft and then suggest where the historically uninitiated may begin, providing some important caveats. I then give two examples of scholarship on issues of medical ethics. I end the chapter with some concluding observations and a description of useful resources.

DEFINING TERMS AND DELINEATING THE TERRAIN

In everyday usage the nouns "ethics" and "morality" and the adjectives "ethical" and "moral" are often employed interchangeably, although they are not, of course, precisely synonymous. These two word groups have specialized meanings in various disciplines, especially in philosophy. Even philosophers are not always in agreement about their exact definitions, but typically they use the word "ethics" to refer to the systematic and rigorous examination of moral norms.

Scholars who regard ethics as the systematic and rigorous examination of moral norms tend to distinguish historically between medical ethics and medical morality. When they speak of the genre of medical ethics as it existed prior to the mid-twentieth century, they may label it medical morality. By this they mean that it was nothing more than principles of etiquette and decorum informed by commonly held morality and circumscribed by religion and law. To such scholars medical ethics is a quite recent development, at which there had been only rare, spasmodic, and largely unnoticed earlier attempts. Thus understood, medical ethics, as a social and intellectual phenomenon, was initially but an adumbration of bioethics, of which it is now a subdivision.

A neologism datable to at least as early as 1971, bioethics has yet to achieve lexical stability. A quick and unsystematic survey of readily available dictionaries published between 1974 and the present reveals a wide range of nuances, but a primary emphasis on the ethical problems arising from advances in the biological sciences. Perhaps the much fuller definition given by Warren Reich in the revised edition of the *Encyclopedia of Bioethics* will influence lexicography: bioethics "can be defined as the systematic study of the moral dimensions—including moral vision, decisions, conduct, and policies—of the life sciences and health care, employing a variety of ethical methodologies in an interdisciplinary setting" (Reich 1995, 1:xxi). But as the field of bioethics, which has been transmogrified so marvelously in the decades since its inception, will likely continue to undergo unpredictable permutations, so also will the definitions of the word itself.

It is impossible to foresee the changes that will affect the definitional parameters of medical ethics as it continues to evolve as a subdivision of bioethics. One thing, however, appears to be reasonably certain: Medical ethics, vitalized by a diverse scope of issues and perplexities, will remain both the focus of debate among people from a wide variety of professions and academic disciplines and a vigorous component of the public consciousness. Such, of course, was not the state of medical ethics (or, if you prefer, medical morality) prior to the late twentieth century. Nevertheless, throughout history people have enjoyed health and have endured sickness, dysfunction, injury, and death. Usually there have been those who provided what may be loosely termed medical care. Insofar as evidence has survived, we may gain some understanding of the moral contexts in which people of diverse cultures have sought to understand and confront at least some of the most fundamental issues of life and death that, at present, are placed under such rubrics as medical ethics or bioethics.

The author of Ecclesiastes asserted that there is nothing new under the sun (1:9). However much one may qualify that statement, there are two senses in which those who seek to gain some understanding of the history of medical ethics and bioethics should apply that adage.

First, nothing in the increasingly broadening domain of bioethics lacks roots in the history of ethics, religion, politics, and law, i.e., in the nearly all-encompassing realm of social and intellectual history. Even the most spectacular scientific and technological achievements have built upon earlier scientific developments that themselves cannot be adequately understood if separated from their own broader social and intellectual contexts. Such virgin territory as cloning and genome mapping did not arise in a moral vacuum but in a moral environment that, however pluralistic and muddled, is merely the present phase of developments that have a complex history. The same may be said about those rubrics of bioethics that are alien or at least tangential to traditional medical ethics, e.g., deep ecology, land ethics, ecofeminism, and animal welfare and rights (in every realm and condition in which animals occur). The quantity of literature that the bioethics movement has generated is enormous. The variety of topics subsumed under the rubric of bioethics ranges from the most minutely specialized considerations to elaborately crafted philosophical systems of bioethics. In the decades since the advent of the bioethics movement, few realms of historical inquiry have been as rich with opportunities for both reinterpretation and groundbreaking investigations as bioethics (including medical ethics since the mid-twentieth century).

Second, although ethical dimensions of birth and death, health and sickness, caring and curing have been rendered more complex and perplexing by scientific advances and social changes of the last several decades, they have been and remain virtually timeless features of the human experience. A wealth of source material, much of which is outside the mainstream of medical ethics literature, awaits scholarly analysis. Such analysis could provide a much fuller picture than is presently available of the moral environments in which patients and physicians of the past encountered realities as personally poignant as any that we encounter today. Most of the history of medical ethics prior to the mid-twentieth century is sketchy and uneven and essentially remains to be researched and written. And that is because the potential boundaries of historical investigations of earlier medical ethics have been so enormously broadened by the bioethics movement that any history of medical ethics written henceforth that focuses primarily on already well-known sources composed by individual physicians for their fellow physicians or formulated by medical organizations would be parochial, narrow, and passé.

I mean by medical ethics the moral environment in which birth, sickness, and death occurred and medical care may have been sought and provided. At most times and in most places those moral environments were not subjected to such a degree of systematic and rigorous examination as that in which philosophers have recently been engaged as bioethicists. Hence the purist may insist that it is improper to apply the expression medical ethics to any era prior to the mid-twentieth century. By force of habit, and with a degree of conviction, I shall continue to employ that expression when addressing the history of those moral environments, however lacking in philosophical self-examination the participants may have been.

The history of medical ethics is itself a field of historical inquiry and those who write on the history of medical ethics are either trained as historians or are "amateurs." The history of medical ethics may be regarded as a subdivision of both the history of philosophy and the history of medicine. Histories of philosophy, whether broad in temporal and thematic scope or limited by topic or time, are usually written by philosophers who typically are not trained in history.

A BRIEF SURVEY OF THE HISTORY OF MEDICAL HISTORY

Arguably, the scholars best qualified to write on the history of medical ethics are historians whose major area of expertise is the history of medicine, especially the social history of medicine. Some historians regard history as a social science, others as a branch of the humanities. Typically historians are trained in methods of historical research and analysis, and, depending on the extent to which their graduate programs emphasize the social sciences, in how such disciplines as anthropology, sociology, linguistics, and psychology can contribute to historical understanding. Training in complementary disciplines in the humanities (e.g., philosophy, literature, and philology) is emphasized to a lesser or greater extent, depending primarily on the principal and secondary specialties within history that the graduate student chooses to pursue. These will typically involve both specific regions (e.g., European, American), eras (e.g., Renaissance/Reformation, early modern), areas (e.g., political, social, intellectual history), and perhaps methodologies for gathering and analyzing of sources such as those for oral history. The number and difficulty of the languages of which the graduate student in history must acquire a functional reading knowledge will depend on his or her fields. The history of medicine most commonly is a secondary area of specialization.

Until the second half of the twentieth century, the history of medicine was primarily the purview of physicians and professors of medicine.[1] As long as the writings attributed to Hippocrates and, even more importantly, Galen's voluminous adaptations of earlier medical literature were venerated as authoritative, and much subsequent medical discourse was simply commentary on, or relatively minor corrections of, these giants, the history of medicine was the primary vehicle for the teaching of medicine itself. Gradually, as the humoral theory gave way to new models, from Sydenham's and Bichat's *historiae morborum* and Koch's postulates to modern bacteriology, the function of the history of medicine was transformed.

This new history of medicine continued to be written by doctors for doctors and was primarily about doctors; that is, about the "great men" of the history of medicine. Biographies of the medical giants of the past were primarily narrative histories of "progress" in the science of medicine that only occasionally detoured, intentionally or inadvertently, into largely anecdotal accounts of medical practice or the art of medicine. Hence, typically the history of medicine was written as the history of the science of medicine, its more human and humane aspects appearing only fleetingly. Its primary source material was essentially medical texts written by doctors for doctors, the grist for later narrative medical history, which was also written by doctors for doctors.

Nonetheless, the histories of medicine written by physicians were more than the fruits of narrow amateurism. Many of these scholars were classically educated and urbane humanists of the first rank who conceived of medicine as combining the most rewarding features of theoretical and applied science. Their acquaintance with the history of medicine reached beyond the scientific texts of medicine. Proud to be members of a high calling, these physicians were imbued with a veneration of what they esteemed as the timeless ethics of their profession. Throughout the history of Western medicine, beginning with the writings attributed to the semilegendary father of medicine, Hippocrates, until the late nineteenth century, physicians had written occasional treatises on physicians' character, deportment, and relations with patients and colleagues. Various medical oaths were composed, the most influential, of course, being that attributed to Hippocrates. They were not simply esoteric documents to be subjected to historical scrutiny, but vital and living texts essential for physicians' self-identity as professionals. Only well into the twentieth century did these texts become the objects of critical historical analysis.

More than any other individual, the Swiss physician Henry Sigerist transformed traditional medical history and opened its portals to scholars from a variety of fields outside medicine. In the early 1930s, Sigerist was appointed director of the newly founded Institute for the History of Medicine at Johns Hopkins University. Under the auspices of the Institute, the American Association for the History of Medicine and its organ, the *Bulletin of the History of Medicine*,[2] were soon inaugurated. A staunch admirer of the Soviet Union and an avowed Marxist, Sigerist asserted that "Medicine is not a *branch of science* and will never be. If medicine is a science, then it is a social science" (Sigerist 1936). In the words of Charles Webster,

> If any dimension was needed to make the subject more complete, it was integral reference to political history, social history, economic history and the history of religion. [Sigerist] called for social history of medicine, not as a complement or supplement to the history of medical science, but as a substitute for it. He wanted the history of medicine not to "limit itself to the history of science, institutions, and characters of medicine, but [to] include the history of the patient in society, and that of the physician and the history of the relations between physician and patient. History thus becomes social history" (Webster 1983, 39).[3]

Sigerist's change in orientation to social history from the philological emphasis of his mentor, Karl Sudhoff of Leipzig, was influenced by a variety of trends in historical inquiry. Several schools of historiography were determined, as it were, to turn history on its head—i.e., to research and write history "from the bottom up" rather than "from the top down"—and, in doing so, to avail themselves of the insights and methodologies of such social sciences as anthropology and sociology. The enormous broadening of the scope of history, traditionally dominated by political history has been and continues to be increasingly felt in the history of medicine as new topics of critical inquiry contribute to a fuller appreciation of how much of the human experience is related to issues of birth and death, health and sickness, caring and curing, and their ethical, religious, political, and legal dimensions.

By the last quarter of the twentieth century the majority of scholars who either regarded themselves as medical historians or focused primarily on aspects of the history of medicine within the parameters of their realm of scholarly competence had doctorates in the humanities and social sciences. The preponderance of these were trained as historians. All brought to their research and writing their own views of the nature, purpose, and possibilities of history that tempered all aspects of their scholarship.

THE HISTORIAN'S CRAFT

Although both professional historians and those who, though not trained in history, write either directly or incidentally on the history of medical ethics or of bioethics, all approach the past with differing preconceptions that affect their understanding and interpretation of history and its relevance for the present, there are three very significant differences between professional and amateur historians.

First, professional historians, as graduate students, have been trained in methods of historical research and analysis, have read broadly and deeply in their chosen areas and eras, and have acquired the research skills necessary to apply to increasingly narrower and more specialized realms of historical inquiry until they have proven themselves competent to embark on researching and writing their dissertations under the tutelage of supervisors and committees of scholars, some of whom may be drawn from ancillary disciplines. By the time they have finished their dissertations, doctoral candidates in history typically have become more knowledgeable than their mentors, probably more than any other scholars in the world, about the minutely refined focuses of their dissertations. The distinguished Cambridge historian Richard Evans remarks,

> The reason for this is that the materials left to us by the past are so extensive that all the historians who have ever worked have done little more than scratch the surface of the deposits which have accumulated, and continue to accumulate, over time. Of course, the farther back we go in time, the less evidence there is, and the more thoroughly what there is has been worked over by previous generations of historians. Even in medieval or ancient history, however, there are still many new things to discover, which do not necessarily depend on a reworking of old material. Indeed, despite the emphasis of university teaching on controversy, debate, and interpretation, the majority of working historians probably consider that adding to our knowledge

of the past—"filling in a gap"—is just as important as transforming our understanding of what is already known, if not more so (Evans 1999, 41–42).

Doctoral candidates in history must be able to deal with the intricacies of often highly technical materials usually from distant and often quite alien cultures and eras in which they have begun to feel at home through extensive reading and research, especially through the languages of those times and places. Such an experience should imbue historians with a sense of caution against speaking authoritatively regarding eras and cultures about which their knowledge is comparatively superficial. Such an awareness is salutary.

Second, professional historians are acutely aware of the extent to which their discipline is fraught with divisions and how disparate are the answers that they or their colleagues would give to some basic questions about the very nature of their discipline. Is history a "science" at all similar to the natural sciences, at least in the sense that it is reasonable to strive in historical analysis for a distinct separation between the researcher and the object of his or her research? Is historical knowledge cumulative, resting, as in the natural sciences, upon empirical foundations laid by earlier research? Can the "scientific method" be employed in historical research since historians' conclusions cannot be experimentally replicated? But since some sciences (e.g., astronomy) are based on observation and postulation rather than on experimentation, cannot history thus qualify as a science and at least postulate theoretically defensible principles of causation? If so, should not history be able to establish rules of predictability? Furthermore, is history even a social science, since social sciences tend not to frame general laws but rather to describe norms based largely on quantification, which only the most statistically oriented historians do? Or is history an art only somewhat less driven by emotions and subjectivity than belles lettres? Is history, perhaps, as some have suggested, *sui generis*, combining its at least quasi-scientific research with a speculative and imaginative mode of interpretation conveyed through literary presentation? If so, can its disciplinary strictures be defined meaningfully enough to apply to the enormously diverse range of its specialties and to the immense breadth of its temporal and geographical scope? Although professional historians can engage in their research, which typically involves, to use Evans's phrase, "filling in a gap" in our knowledge of the past, without rethinking these issues again and again, such questions will continue to generate debate among historians that ideally should render them more sensitive to the strengths and limitations of their discipline.

Third, professional historians are divided on other fundamental questions. For example, what is ultimately knowable about the past? Is objectivity possible about the past (since, some would argue, it is not possible even, or perhaps especially, about the present)? Hence, historians ought to be considerably more aware than others of the extent to which their ideologies, philosophy of history, and personal motives can condition their historiography (though some may see this only in the work of other historians and not in their own). Some historians are committed, e.g., to a political ideology that is itself an historical paradigm. A Marxist has a very distinct view of reality, past, present, and future. Hence, when one reads history written by a Marxist, one should not be surprised to find a Marxist interpretation, whether subtly nuanced or conspicuously ideological. Likely, when those who are unaware of the reverberations that postmodernism has been causing within many disciplines first encounter history written by postmodernists, they experience something akin to

Alice's stepping through the looking glass. Wading through the subjective hyperrelativism of much postmodernism, especially that driven by linguistic deconstructionism, may make the uninitiated abandon any hope that there is any objective basis for knowledge.

Those historians who do not ally themselves with any faction (of which there is a plethora besides Marxism and postmodernism) may at least strive for objectivity by seeking to write history as a descriptive and not prescriptive enterprise. Making explicit moral judgments about the past, especially with a view to drawing lessons for the present and future while claiming objectivity, smacks of presumptuous arrogance. Historians should, if they are honest and do not have a hidden agenda, take special care to seek to create an interpretive grid cleansed as much as possible of their own ideological preconceptions and presuppositions. And this is said in deference to cynics whose derisive laughter is directed at anyone who might even appear to claim that objectivity is possible.

The greater the "relevance" to the present of the subjects that historians pursue, the greater the likelihood that their interpretations of the past will be marred by myopia. This is not to suggest that historians should not bring their knowledge and expertise to the history of issues of immediate interest and concern. It is simply to state what should be self-evident: that when investigating and writing about the history of contemporary issues, there is a compounded potential for the present to distort the past. First, we are all creatures of our own time and culture. This alone will influence historians' vision of the past irrespective of the specific focus of their research. Second, if a current issue of popular interest so intrigues historians that they determine to investigate its past, their attraction to the current nature of the problem can condition their approach to its history. Properly cautious historians will strive to subdue the distorting influence of both. This is particularly important if one is attracted to the history of medical ethics by the ethical dilemmas of the contemporary scene.

Some historians refuse to make the available sources address questions of current bioethical interest unless the primary sources themselves have specifically dealt with these issues. This approach is the most historically tidy and responsible. Numerous ethical issues of contemporary concern have been raised and discussed in the genre of medical ethics for over two and one half millennia. Historians can talk intelligently about these matters, especially if they discuss them within the broader context of social and intellectual history. Numerous issues of medical ethics that were not raised in the literature of medical ethics during certain periods appear in other sources, either anecdotally or as the objects of religious, philosophical, or legal attention. These sources need to be plumbed in order to provide a fuller picture of most eras.

Historians may legitimately address some questions to past environments in which such questions could have been raised but were not addressed by the extant or known sources. It is reasonable to assume that the broad ethical framework of any society informs the ethics of the healing arts and human encounters with birth and death, health and sickness. Hence, historians may pose cautious questions that historically informed common sense suggests as relevant to a period for which no pertinent evidence has survived. It is also then very appropriate to ponder the significance of the absence of certain issues from the extant sources of various cultures. But historians should exercise considerable care to ensure that they rigorously refuse to read issues peculiar to contemporary medical culture into a past environment in which they could never have arisen.

WHERE TO BEGIN: SOME CAVEATS

If one wishes to embark on serious reading in the history of medical ethics or bioethics, where and how should one begin? The best introduction to the kinds of concerns raised in the preceding section, to the caveats that I shall introduce in the present section, and generally to the historian's craft, is Richard Evans's *In Defense of History* (1999), which is accurately described on its dust jacket as "an entertaining and instructive tour of the historian's workshop and, along the way, a spirited defense of the search for historical truth." Perusing this intriguing volume will not only acquaint the reader with the entire range of approaches to history, but will also encourage him or her that there is a reasonable course to navigate between the Scylla of positivism and the Charybdis of relativism. One need not acquire the specialized skills of a professional historian to profit from the study of any aspect of history for which primary documents are available if one consults competent scholarly surveys and specialized analyses of the milieus from which these sources come. This certainly applies to the history of medical ethics and bioethics.

There are many surveys of the history of medical ethics prior to its current blurring with that broad and nearly amorphous phenomenon known as bioethics. The section entitled "Medical Ethics, History of," in the revised edition of the *Encyclopedia of Bioethics* (Reich 1995), consists of 208 large, double-columned pages and contains thirty-four discrete articles arranged chronologically under geographical rubrics. There is no better introduction to the field yet available than this book-length collection of highly compact articles, each of which is accompanied by a bibliography. The editorial board of this encyclopedia invited scholars recognized as leading authorities in the history of medical ethics to write the articles on the eras of their specialties. Particular editorial care was taken not only in selecting the authors, but also in refereeing and editing the manuscripts through their various stages to ensure that the kinds of special pleading and ideological biases that are such impediments to historical objectivity be eliminated as much as possible without attempting to force these scholars to write against their best historical judgments.

Those who wish to pursue some specialized topic will likely find an article, or a series of articles, in the *Encyclopedia of Bioethics* on that exact subject. Many articles that are not specifically historical in their focus contain some historical background or analysis, although the encyclopedia is somewhat uneven in that regard. It is important to be aware that most of those articles that are not primarily addressed to history were written by scholars from fields other than history. And, of course, in such an encyclopedia, articles on specialized topics, even if they contain some history, are addressed to a specific aspect of a recently created and evolving phenomenon; that is, bioethics.

Nearly everything written about bioethics is, with considerably varying significance, primary source material for those who limit their inquiry to the history of bioethics and contemporary medical ethics. Most of this literature was written by philosophers and members of the health care professions (especially physicians), as well as theologians, lawyers, sociologists, and journalists. Some of this literature seeks to provide some historical background, context, or analysis.

The history provided by such literature varies from the superficial and historically naive to the insightful and historically sophisticated. There are numerous articles in professional journals written by scholars who believed that a brief historical introduction would be a useful propaedeutic to the specialized focus of their study. And there are also many books written about the bioethics movement by scholars who helped to make the very history about which they are writing. The titles of some of these books may not explicitly signal that they contain an historical component. And some, in fact, briefly acknowledge the history of medical ethics prior to the advent of the bioethics movement, only to dismiss it as ultimately irrelevant because of its inadequacy to meet today's moral conundra before becoming enmeshed in the tangle of history of the bioethics movement itself (e.g., Veatch 1981; Beauchamp and Childress 1989). More commonly, however, major studies of bioethics are much concerned with the history of medical ethics extending back well before the beginning of bioethics. And their authors typically interpret the past quite differently from each other to provide verification of their disparate understandings of the present (e.g., Emanuel 1991; Engelhardt 1996; Pellegrino and Thomasma 1993; Morreim 1995; Jonsen 1998). This is not to suggest that they approach history dishonestly and selectively include only that which would support their conclusions. Rather they have a vision of the present that affects their perception of the past that, in turn, reinforces their understanding of the present. These scholars, however, are not historians but primarily philosophers and physicians.[4]

Now some caveats for anyone who intends to read about or investigate any aspect of the history of medical ethics or bioethics. Two tendencies against which one should guard in one's own analysis and be vigilant to detect in secondary literature on the history of medical ethics or bioethics, whether written by amateurs or professional historians, are essentialism and presentism.

Essentialism is the tendency to see ideas (in the broadest sense of the word) as free-floating in time and space; i.e., to view them metaphysically without reference to any temporal context other than the present, and then, when looking at the culture of any era, to see whatever idea one is examining as essentially the same everywhere and at all times. When seeking to understand any feature of the present as it has ostensibly manifested itself in the past, one must be sensitive to the likelihood that a multitude of cultural differences will, when informed by an appreciation of that culture's distinct character, reveal a significantly modified version of one's initial preconceptions.

Similar in some respects to essentialism, but yet distinct from it, is presentism, or anachronism, which is a failure to recognize the extent to which the past typically differs fundamentally from the present. It is the natural but naive tendency to ascribe to earlier periods contemporary values, structures, and interpretive categories. Some degree of presentism is unavoidable, since even in conceiving and formulating one's research one cannot avoid imposing present categories on the past, at least in some measure. Hence a sensitivity to presentism is a defining feature of a mature historical consciousness.

A variety of presentism that should be comparatively easy to avoid is the *deliberate* interpretation of the past through the grid of one's own values. This interpretation of history, however, can take many forms and may sometimes be so subtle that it is not recognized by those who employ it, in which case it is not deliberate and hence not easily avoided. Commonly held at virtually a subconscious level and hence often consciously denied are the twin assumptions that the past tells a story of improvement and that the social structures and values of the present are the results of progress. These assumptions easily insinuate themselves into the historical reasoning even of those who excoriate many defining characteristics of the present. Although an effort to overcome this form of presentism is essential for the writing of competent history, such an effort may lead to an opposite and by no means subtle extreme, namely a flagrant denial of the very idea of progress. While this extreme should be avoided, it is undeniable that the awesome advances in science and technology are mixed blessings. And skepticism about the idea of progress is splendidly salutary in the history of ethics, especially in the history of medical ethics.

As old schools of historical interpretation fade into oblivion, new ones continue to arise and thus sustain the bewildering diversity and fragmentation of the historical profession. The most radical ones typically hold an explicitly relativistic view of reality in general and history in particular. They tend to attack what they regard as an "establishment" interpretation of the past by the political and intellectual (and medical) elites who ostensibly hold the reigns of power. As byproducts of contemporary trends especially in academe, they are as presentistic as those whom they deprecate. They would, of course, heatedly deny that their methodologies are presentistic. Yet their various methodologies are designed to break through the alleged facade of objectivity of contemporary power brokers to expose it as an intellectually indefensible instrument for the oppression of those very groups whom these new historical presentists exist to empower. And their particular brands of historical revisionism are one of their major tools.

This is not to say that such movements as social constructionism, postmodernism, and standpoint epistemology have nothing positive to contribute to the historical dialogue, especially through the writings of some of their more moderate advocates. They at least prove to be a restraining influence against the proclivity of historians to slip into an epistemologically complacent positivism. It is important for the reader who is uninitiated in the disparately diverse approaches to history that one is liable to encounter in reading modern historical scholarship to be cautious regarding the reliability of any form of historical revisionism that is dogmatic in its advocacy of a partisan position and has the tone of special pleading. And it is also useful, when reading historical surveys or specialized studies written during earlier eras, to be aware of what schools of historiography were then in vogue, for the writing of history has always been conditioned by contemporary social and intellectual conditions, some of which are quite alien to the present. But having one's critical senses tuned to detect agenda-ridden historical scholarship of the past or present can make one too suspicious of any reinterpretations of the past. It is a delicate balance that one strives to achieve through extensive reading, guarded openness to new ideas, and cautious reflection on the comparative merits of differing views, all tempered by an increasingly refined historical common sense.

TWO PERTINENT EXAMPLES

In this section I shall first give an example of historical analysis gone awry and then an example of the need for balanced historical inquiry into a variety of related issues.

Physician-Assisted Suicide

Physician-assisted suicide is an especially controversial issue that will continue to arise in public, legislative, and judicial fora. Research into the history of physician-assisted suicide in the West will inevitably bring inquirers into the history of both Christianity and suicide. Whether student or professor, law clerk or judge, physician or patient, their quest could well start with a seminal work that has had a greater impact on modern conceptualizations of suicide than any other. It is by the father of French sociology, Émile Durkheim: *Le suicide: étude sociologique*. Although published in 1897, it was not translated into English until 1951.

Durkheim created three categories of suicide that he explained with reference to social structures: (1) egoistic (resulting from a lack of social integration); (2) anomic (precipitated by the destabilizing effects of sudden negative or positive social change); and (3) altruistic (resulting from overintegration, especially when the individual is completely controlled by religious or political groups). Durkheim thus defined suicide: "All cases of death resulting directly or indirectly from a positive or negative act of the victim himself, which he knows will produce this result" (Durkheim 1951, 44).

Durkheim was determined to avoid the question of motivation or even whether the individual actually desired to die. It was suicide if one believed that one's actions or passivity would eventuate in one's own death. Hence, he classified the death of Christian martyrs as (altruistic) suicide since,

> . . . though they did not kill themselves, they sought death with all their power and behaved so as to make it inevitable. To be suicide, the act from which death must necessarily result need only have been performed by the victim with full knowledge of the facts. Besides, the passionate enthusiasm with which the believers in the new religion faced final torture shows that at this moment they had completely discarded their personalities for the idea of which they had become the servants (Durkheim 1951, 227).

According to Durkheim, dying for one's beliefs was suicide. Since those who committed suicide were, in Durkheim's construct, victims of pathological social phenomena, martyrs were victims not of the people who killed them but of their own religious group's demand for excessive integration, control, and regimentation.

Some popular authors and scholars who adopted Durkheim's definition of suicide have argued passionately in favor of various forms of voluntary euthanasia. They support their position, in part, by presenting a highly distorted view of early Christianity's position on suicide. By far, the most influential of these is the poet and literary critic Alfred Alvarez. Writing for a more scholarly audience, the philosopher and legal theorist Glanville Williams and the philosopher Margaret Pabst Battin have also had a significant impact on current understanding of suicide in early Christianity. These three authors (Alvarez 1970, 51, 68, 73; Williams 1957, 254–55; Battin 1982, 29, 71–73, 89) paint the following picture:

1. Not only does the Old Testament nowhere condemn suicide, it records several suicides without any hint of disapproval.
2. The New Testament nowhere forbids suicide. Indeed, the one suicide that it relates, that of Judas, is presented as a mark of his repentance rather than as a further sin. Even Jesus' death was, in a sense, suicide.

3. So eager were many early Christians to realize their fullness of joy in heaven that they committed suicide if they were unable to provoke pagans to put them to death as martyrs.

4. So depressing was the burden of sin and guilt of many early Christians that they killed themselves in despair.

5. So intensely did many early Christians despise their sinful flesh that they killed themselves, often through severe asceticism.

6. So low a regard did early Christians have for their lives that they were willing to die for their faith, some even volunteering for or provoking martyrdom. And martyrdom, of course, is suicide.

7. Augustine was the first Christian to denounce suicide as a sin. His negative influence has subsequently tempered the Christian attitude to suicide, including both active and passive euthanasia.

In 1993 and 1996, two judges ruled on the constitutionality of physician-assisted suicide: Michigan appellate court judge Andrew Kaufman, in one of the numerous prosecutions of retired pathologist Jack Kevorkian for assisting the suicide of the chronically ill (1993 WL 603212 [Mich. Cir. Ct.]), and Stephen Reinhardt of the 9th Circuit U.S. Court of Appeals in California (*Compassion in Dying v. Washington*, 79 F. 3d 790 [9th cir en banc 1996]). Both judges relied primarily on Alvarez and hence both reached the same conclusions regarding the position of early Christianity on suicide as summarized in the seven points given above.

Judges Kaufman and Reinhardt (or their law clerks) could have availed themselves of a book published in 1992. When two theologians, Arthur J. Droge and James D. Tabor, both trained in history and in patristics, wrote *A Noble Death: Suicide and Martyrdom among Christians and Jews in Antiquity*, one could reasonably have anticipated a more perspicacious historical analysis than that provided by Alvarez, Battin, and Williams, none of whom were historians or theologians, all of whom have argued passionately in favor of various forms of voluntary euthanasia. But Droge and Tabor have added confusion to inaccuracy. Rejecting for their purposes the word suicide as "a recent innovation and pejorative term," they prefer the designation "voluntary death." "By this term we mean to describe the act resulting from an individual's intentional decision to die, either by his own agency, by another's, or by contriving the circumstances in which death is the known, ineluctable result." They concede that their definition of voluntary death is quite similar to Durkheim's definition of suicide and assert that theirs is "intended to be morally neutral, since our enterprise is not one of moral (or clinical) judgment but an attempt to understand the ways in which voluntary death was evaluated in antiquity" (Droge and Tabor 1992, 4).

Emphasizing that both "suicide" and "martyrdom" are semantically and conceptually ambiguous, Droge and Tabor think that they have reduced the ambiguity and confusion by providing the concept of voluntary death as a much more objective grid for the historian. They, of course, convey a positive view of voluntary death; after all, a voluntary death is a noble death, as the title of their book declares. They acknowledge in their conclusion that their purpose had been "to deconstruct the 'linguistics of suicide' by examining the precise terms and formulations employed in antiquity to denote the act of voluntary death" (Droge and Tabor 1992, 187).

Droge and Tabor maintain that, "Despite the claim of Augustine and later theologians, the New Testament expresses no condemnation of voluntary death. . . . Yet, to say only that the writers of the New Testament did not condemn voluntary death is to miss the positive significance they attached to the act. The authors of the Gospels created a Jesus who died by his own choice, if not by his own hand" (Droge and Tabor 1992, 125). They are especially fascinated with the apostle Paul's supposed "fascination with death and his desire to escape from life" and suggest that "for Paul, an individual could kill himself and be 'glorifying God with his body' by doing so. . . . In a world-negating system like the apostle Paul's, the question became how to justify continued existence in the world rather than voluntary death" (Droge and Tabor 1992, 119, 124, 187). "Voluntary death," as they conclude in their book, "was one of the ideals on which the church was founded" (Droge and Tabor 1992, 189).

Droge and Tabor begin and end their book with reference to the current debate regarding physician-assisted suicide. Although they insist that "when the conventional distinction between 'suicide' and 'martyrdom' is read back into antiquity, it conceals rather than reveals the issues" (Droge and Tabor 1992, 187), it is actually their own faddish linguistic deconstructionism and historical revisionism that are blatantly presentistic and do violence to the texts that they "deconstruct." Their determination to label such a diverse variety of motives and actions "voluntary death" is conspicuously special pleading and hence entangles them in contradictions and inconsistencies. A recurring theme in their book is that Augustine condemned "voluntary death." Nevertheless, they maintain that he attempted to "draw a distinction between two kinds of voluntary death: 'self-homicide' and 'martyrdom.' The former was condemned as reprehensible; the latter was praised as noble and ennobling" (Droge and Tabor 1992, 179). It appears, then, that although Augustine ostensibly condemned "voluntary death," nevertheless, since he made a distinction between "self-homicide" (sc., "suicide"), which he condemned, and "martyrdom," which he praised, he did not actually condemn Droge and Tabor's meaningless category of "voluntary death" per se. Labeling as "voluntary death" everything that Durkheim calls "suicide" proves nothing other than that it is, at the best, as meaningless, or, at the worst, as tragically a misleading grid to apply to any period of history (not to speak of the present) as is Durkheim's. Both have in common, and as their Achilles' heel, their inclusion of martyrdom and self-sacrificial death as suicide or voluntary death.

Did Augustine formulate the Christian position on suicide? The answer must be an unequivocal no. He based his condemnation of suicide most fundamentally on the same presuppositions and values that had caused earlier church fathers to condemn the act. Furthermore, Augustine's influence has been minimal in Eastern Christianity. Indeed, it has long been fashionable in some quarters of Eastern Orthodoxy virtually to excoriate Augustine as the veritable font of fundamental theological errors. Hence, it should be troubling to those who credit Augustine with introducing a negative attitude to suicide into Christian theology and practice that the same position that Augustine articulates on suicide also prevails in Eastern Christianity.

Although early Christians lived in a secular milieu in which suicide by the ill was frequently practiced and its probity seldom questioned, not only is there no discussion of the issue in patristic literature, but there is also not a single example of Christians committing suicide, asking others' assistance in doing so, or requesting others to kill them directly in order to escape from the grinding tedium of chronic, or the severe suffering of terminal, illness. Repeatedly the church fathers emphasized that in death it was God who issued the summons; God who was the active party. Christians were to yearn for heaven and to pray, if God so willed, for an early departure from life. Clinging desperately to life when ill was condemned by Augustine and other church fathers as a tragic contradiction of the most fundamental spiritual values. The care of the body was never to be at the expense of the soul's health. Indeed, one must mortify the flesh. Yet Christians were to care for their own bodies and seek healing when ill. Christianity had introduced an imperative to care for the sick, Christians and pagans alike, an obligation incumbent upon all Christians. There was no room here for suicide. Patient endurance of all afflictions, perseverance to the end, final resignation to God's will in the midst of those very circumstances that God used to test and refine the Christian: such thought is antithetical to the taking of one's own life. And such thought permeates patristic literature. So foundational are the goodness of God and his sovereignty in patristic theology and patient endurance of affliction so regularly and consistently stressed as an essential Christian virtue that it is not in the least surprising that patristic texts are void of any reference to suicide by the ill.[5]

Whether ancient Christian attitudes toward suicide should influence American judicial decisions regarding physician-assisted suicide is not here at issue. But distorting history to support any position is hardly defensible.

Commercialism in Medicine

Another example of the need for balanced historical inquiry involves the very nature of the medical profession in its socioeconomic dimensions. The exemption of the learned professions from the ban on monopolization in the Sherman Antitrust Act of 1891 ended in 1975 with the U.S. Supreme Court's decision in *Goldfarb v. Virginia State Bar*. That same year the Federal Trade Commission sued the American Medical Association (AMA) because its code of ethics prohibited advertising. Although the AMA removed this prohibition in its revised code of ethics in 1980, the U.S. Supreme Court heard the case and barred the AMA from prohibiting advertising and solicitation of patients. The Court also directed the AMA to obtain prior permission from the Federal Trade Commission before formulating, adopting, and disseminating any new ethical guidelines. The door had definitely been thrown open for imaginative entrepreneurialism in medicine unprecedented in American history. I shall highlight one aspect that raises a variety of ethical issues.

Although the preponderance of the myriad health-related websites as of late in 1997 had not been created by the health care industry but rather by patients or patient groups (Ferguson 1997), some have been established by entrepreneurial physicians who diagnose and prescribe medications online (Greene 1997). Even disregarding websites established by unlicensed physicians and outright quacks, most objective observers would likely agree that the diagnostic and therapeutic limitations of a patient-physician "interface" are self-evident and the opportunities for abuse readily apparent. Legal and ethical problems abound that include "a physician's duty of confidentiality, a patient's right to informed consent, the components of a medical record, customary usage and practice standards, state licensing, and product endorsement" (Spielberg 1998, 1355).

Litigation will continue to arise that will regulate and refine the parameters of various features of American medical culture of the Information Age. Federal regulatory agencies will be both proactive and reactive in their bureaucratic capacities. Professional medical organizations will adopt ethical guidelines, as the AMA already did in 1997, regarding some of these issues. And historical analyses will be written by professional historians and amateurs alike.

As legal battles are fought, a diverse range of litigants on all sides of the issues will argue their cases from law, ethics, and history. Bioethicists will haunt the print and broadcast media and speak with varying degrees of dogmatism or equivocation about a broad spectrum of pertinent ethical issues. It is likely that a few people will explore the history of these issues earlier than the inception of the bioethics movement. The backgrounds, competence, and motivations of such investigators will vary considerably, as will the scope and quality of their contributions to the dialogue.

What are the historical precedents for online doctors, virtual house calls, and cyberspace prescriptions? In a sense, there are no historical precedents for many of those aspects of life that are defining features of the unique ethos of mass media, of the Information Age, of technoculture, and of the incessant demand for the empowerment of consumers and instant gratification. But in another sense, there are historical precedents that are already part of the flow of the history of medical ethics. They cannot be fully appreciated without reference to the history of numerous issues, some of which have always been central to the history of medical ethics, others that have been so only intermittently or recently— e.g., medical paternalism, munificence, and cupidity; professional self-regulatory rights and responsibilities; society's ostensible obligation to restrict professional freedoms for the common good; and patient's rights and autonomy.

Diverse approaches or grids may be used for historical analysis of these issues. Simply for illustrative purposes, I shall very briefly describe one that organizes the issues under the three rubrics of physicians' relationships with (1) their patients, (2) their fellow physicians, and (3) the state or other external regulatory authorities.

Before beginning, however, it is reasonable to pose some preliminary questions:

1. Is there a discrete tradition in Western history regarding these issues?
2. Is the evidence for countertraditions plentiful enough to discard the concept of "tradition" in these areas?
3. If a discrete tradition may be identified, to what extent is that tradition affected by social peculiarities of a given time and place?
4. If a discrete tradition may be identified, how has that tradition affected the behavior of physicians?
5. When the behavior of disparate individual physicians or groups of physicians seems to have been at variance with tradition, does that represent a countertradition or simply the reality of inconsistency between ideals and practice?

There are other questions that one who pursues the history of medical ethics may already have settled in his or her mind. But even if a discrete tradition may be identified, what ethical value do historical traditions have? In other words, should history be used to justify ethical claims? Historians' reaction may be that such questions are irrelevant to their historical analysis. Indeed, it can be argued that, if researchers begin their inquiry with the firm conviction that history should be used to justify ethical claims, their objectivity may be hampered by a desire to find in history the specific data that will be the grist for their interpretive mill. The negative implications should be obvious.

At the outset, it should be noted that the illustrative grid given above focuses on physicians. The words "physician," "doctor," and "surgeon" may seem quite unambiguous. We typically use them to refer to those who, after requisite training, are licensed to practice aspects of medicine and surgery, including prescribing governmentally regulated drugs, which are privileges denied to those not thus trained and licensed. Those thus trained but never licensed to practice may still be casually referred to as physicians, doctors, or surgeons, as may those who have lost their license to practice. The word "physician" blurs somewhat when we speak of naturopathic physicians, typically called "doctor" by their patients, as are, e.g., optometrists, chiropractors, podiatrists, and acupuncturists, some of whom, in some jurisdictions, are permitted to prescribe a tightly circumscribed range of drugs. These ambiguities, common throughout the languages and practices of the Western world, appear very trivial when compared to the semantic and conceptual challenges that arise when considering the very diverse range of "healers" in contemporary Asian and "third world" cultures and in the not too distant past in Western history.

Needless to say, when attempting to deal with an aspect of the history of medicine as central as the relationships of physicians, semantic and conceptual parameters must be clearly and reasonably delineated in order to determine whom one may responsibly label as physicians in different times and places. One cannot competently approach the history of medical ethics without the realization that, by labeling various people as physicians, one has applied to them a wide range of modern social and professional assumptions that may well not be historically warranted. Hence, both caution and precision are necessary as one begins and, of course, a sensitivity to the ubiquitous specters of presentism and essentialism.

The history of physicians' relationships with their fellow physicians typically focuses on efforts of groups of practitioners to exclude other practitioners from the marketplace by whatever mechanisms were then available. Especially before the advent of medical licensure, the literature of medical ethics often was a vehicle for articulating standards of training and practice that were designed to ostracize alleged "charlatans" and "quacks" from the ranks of "qualified" practitioners. After medical licensure, whether imposed by the state or won through negotiations for monopolies, the protection of this monopoly was supported by frequently rearticulated standards of training and practice. Whether before or after licensure, the arguments were consistently made that excluding the unqualified from practice was *pro bono publico.* Standards of collegiality consistent with a professionalism that was restricted to a limited number who met stringent criteria not only reinforced popular perceptions of the dignity and value of the profession, but also enabled those within to avoid the very competition that threatened from outside by forbidding or severely limiting competition within. Hence, throughout the history of Western medicine, even as early as the time of Hippocrates, any form of advertising was characteristically castigated in the literature of medical ethics as typical of quacks and charlatans and unworthy of physicians. In medieval medical and surgical guild regulations, advertising and other forms of overt competition were strictly proscribed, as they have generally been by later medical associations and societies until such restrictions recently were banned by courts. Indeed, the distinct impression is that entrepreneurialism consistently has been excoriated as prejudicial to the good of the profession and accordingly prejudicial to the common good as well. On closer scrutiny, however, the record is not as consistent as usually presented in surveys of the history of medical ethics. Primary documents from some parts of Renaissance and early modern Europe suggest that historical precedents for physicians' treating virtually anonymous, possibly pseudonymous, patients vicariously are not so rare as to be properly dismissed as aberrant. Hence, whether online doctors are taking advantage of antitrust court rulings to break free from the restrictive protectionism of professional elitism or rather blatantly violating a principle of professional ethics consistently honored for twenty-five hundred years is a matter about which more historical inquiry is needed.

Passions flair between people of opposite convictions on the legitimacy of the "traditional" claims of organized medicine. Vocal critics castigate organized medicine in general and the AMA in particular for ostensibly having acted from the most consistently transparent mercenary and selfish motives designed to protect income, status, and nearly autonomous self-regulation. These avowed enemies of the medical establishment rejoice in recent antitrust judicial activism and yearn for the demise of medical "Mandarinism" to which they will eagerly contribute through historical revisionism. The opposite extreme maintains that organized medicine in the United States has been and remains resistant to various forms of government regulation and movements from "below" because the medical profession stands on the time-honored and venerable ethics and ideals of medical professionalism, without which the most fundamental principles of medicine as an altruistic calling will fall.

Historians who are critical of the medical establishment as the systematizer of authority fault bioethicists and fellow historians for their "shallowness (or absence) of socio-economic and political understanding" and their histories of medical ethics as a "rather bloodless substitute for the political and social history of medical power, practices, and epistemology" (Cooter 1995, 259, 263). Hence, social historians should be focused on what apparently is the task ostensibly inherent in social history "of demystifying rhetorics, representations, and power relations in medicine . . . defrocking doctors and 'unmasking' medicine as a 'political enterprise' [and of] exposing the cultural relativity of truth, rationality, ethics, and morals" (Cooter 1995, 260).

Many social historians would disagree that such is their task. But even social historians who are not avowed revisionists do tend to write history "from the bottom up." In the process they look at groups often ignored by those historians who write "from the top down." These two different orientations will often result in different conclusions regarding the issues here under consideration. Those writing "from the bottom up" will often unearth material that has not been subjected to historical scrutiny that will then shed a sometimes very different light on conditions of which those who write "from the top down" would have remained unaware, for the latter often have limited their primary sources to the "classic texts" that appear, in the absence of other evidence, to reveal one discrete, continuous tradition. There is a high level of objectivity in much of the available scholarship. But at the opposite ends of the ideological spectrum the lines are clearly drawn. The self-righteous hauteur of traditionalists and the equally self-righteous vitriol of revisionists rarely nurture historical objectivity.

CONCLUDING COMMENTS

History should be descriptive, not prescriptive. Since ethics involves values, the history of ethics, medical or otherwise, is the history of values. The history of medical ethics is vast in its purview and cannot be separated from the history of the relation of medicine (in the broadest sense of the word to include the entire realm of birth and death, caring and curing, wellness and illness) with religion, philosophy, law, politics, and numerous other facets of society.

Since the history of medical ethics is part of the history of values, one should be particularly cautious and circumspect about sitting in judgment on the past. Nevertheless, as Richard Evans says regarding moral issues, "historical judgment" need not "be neutral. But . . . the historian has to develop a detached mode of cognition, a faculty of self-criticism, and an ability to understand another person's point of view" (Evans 1999, 219). And historians, he remarks earlier, must "make the effort to understand in a cognitive sense the actions, ideas, and motivations of people in the past without direct reference to their own beliefs in the present" (Evans 1999, 165–66).

Total objectivity in history, as in everything, is impossible. But that does not mean that one should not strive for it. In doing so, however, self-criticism, self-doubt, and humility will at least temper, if not entirely subdue, proclivities to dogmatism.

NOTES ON RESOURCES AND TRAINING

As described above, the revised edition of the *Encyclopedia of Bioethics*, published in 1995, is the first source to which one should have recourse regarding any aspect of the history of medical ethics or bioethics.

The National Endowment for the Humanities is funding a research project that will eventuate in the publication by Cambridge University Press of a 925-page book entitled *A History of Medical Ethics*. Edited by Laurence B. McCullough and Robert B. Baker, this volume will consist of twenty-one chapters and several appendices. The projected publication date is fall, 2002, to coincide with the World Congress on History of Medical Ethics.

Databases, electronic information sources, and websites are rapidly proliferating. The National Library of Medicine (NLM) provides access through *Internet Grateful Med*, a WWW Server interface, to several bibliographical databases including BIOETHICSLINE and HISTLINE. BIOETHICSLINE is maintained by the NLM and the Kennedy Institute of Ethics of Georgetown University, with coverage from 1973 and more than 50,000 records. My most recent search of "history" generated 3,522 citations. HISTLINE is maintained by the NLM with coverage since 1965 and nearly 200,000 records. My most recent search of "ethics" yielded 2,627 citations.

Numerous hard copy bibliographies are helpful. Many are going online. I shall only mention the two that I find most useful. *Current Work in the History of Medicine* is published quarterly by the Wellcome Institute for the History of Medicine. The subject index contains a section labeled "Ethics, Medical" as well as various relevant sections such as "Euthanasia." Since 1975 the Center for Bioethics of the Kennedy Institute has published an annual *Bibliography of Bioethics*, although only the first six volumes contain under "Subject Entries" a section entitled "Historical Aspects." Ferreting out from subsequent volumes references to historical materials is more challenging and will drive even the most reluctant user of computers to BIOETHICSLINE.[6]

NOTES

1. There is a steadily increasing literature on the historiography of medical history. See, e.g., Temkin (1971), Rosenberg (1971), Webster (1983), Brieger (1993), and Porter (1998).
2. Initially named the *Bulletin of the Institute of the History of Medicine*.
3. The quotation is from Sigerist (1940); see further Fee and Brown (1997), especially "Part 2: Sigerist as Medical Historian," and "Part 4: Sigerist's Legacy."
4. For a provocative analysis of several histories of bioethics, see Chambers (1998).
5. On suicide in early Christianity, see, e.g., chapter 4 of Amundsen (1996) and chapters 2–4 of Larson and Amundsen (1998).
6. I wish to thank Dr. Gary B. Ferngren, Oregon State University, for his insightful criticisms of earlier versions of this chapter.

REFERENCES

Alvarez, A. 1970. *The Savage God: A Study of Suicide*. New York: Random House.

Amundsen, D.W. 1996. *Medicine, Society, and Faith in the Ancient and Medieval Worlds*. Baltimore, MD: Johns Hopkins University Press.

Battin, M. P. 1982. *Ethical Issues in Suicide*. Englewood Cliffs, NJ: Prentice Hall.

Beauchamp, T. L., and J. F. Childress. 1989. *Principles of Biomedical Ethics*. 3rd ed. New York: Oxford University Press.

Brieger, G. 1993. "The Historiography of Medicine." In *Companion Encyclopedia of the History of Medicine*, ed. W. F. Bynum and Roy Porter. London: Routledge, pp. 24–44.

Chambers, T. 1998. "Retrodiction and the Histories of Bioethics." *Medical Humanities Review* 12:9–22.

Cooter, R. 1995. "The Resistible Rise of Medical Ethics." *Social History of Medicine* 8:257–70.

Droge, A. J., and J. D. Tabor. 1992. *A Noble Death: Suicide and Martyrdom among Christians and Jews in Antiquity*. San Francisco: Harper.

Durkheim, E. 1951. *Suicide: A Study in Sociology*. Trans. J. A. Spaulding and G. Simpson. Glencoe, IL: The Free Press.

Emanuel, E. J. 1991. *The Ends of Human Life*. Boston: Harvard University Press.

Engelhardt, H. T., Jr. 1996. *The Foundations of Bioethics*. 2nd ed. New York: Oxford University Press.

Evans, R. J. 1999. *In Defense of History*. New York: Norton.

Fee, E., and T. M. Brown, eds. 1997. *Making Medical History: The Life and Times of Henry E. Sigerist*. Baltimore, MD: Johns Hopkins University Press.

Ferguson, T. 1997. "Health Care in Cyberspace: Patients Lead a Revolution." *The Futurist* 31 (Nov.–Dec.): 29–33.

Greene, J. 1997. "Sign On and Say 'Ah-h-h-h-h-h.'" *Hospitals and Health Networks* 71 (April 20): 45–46.

Jonsen, A. R. 1998. *The Birth of Bioethics.* New York: Oxford University Press.

Larson, E. J., and D. W. Amundsen. 1998. *A Different Death: Euthanasia and the Christian Tradition.* Downers Grove, IL: InterVarsity Press.

Morreim, E. H. 1995. *Balancing Act: The New Medical Ethics of Medicine's New Economics.* Washington, D.C.: Georgetown University Press.

Pellegrino, E. D., and D. C. Thomasma. 1993. *The Virtues in Medical Practice.* New York: Oxford University Press.

Porter, R. 1998. "Medicine, Historiography of." In *A Global Encyclopedia of Historical Writing,* ed. D. R. Woolf. New York: Garland, pp. 607–08.

Reich, W. 1995. *Encyclopedia of Bioethics.* Rev. ed. New York: Simon and Schuster Macmillan.

Rosenberg, C. E. 1971. "The Medical Profession, Medical Practice and the History of Medicine." In *Modern Methods in the History of Medicine,* ed. E. Clarke. London: Althone, pp. 22–35.

Sigerist, H. 1936. "The History of Medicine and the History of Science." *Bulletin of the Institute of the History of Medicine* 4:1–13.

———. 1940. "The Social History of Medicine." *Western Journal of Surgery* 48:715–22.

Spielberg, A. R. 1998. "On Call and Online: Sociohistorical, Legal, and Ethical Implications of E-mail for the Patient-Physician Relationship." *Journal of the American Medical Association* 280:1353–59.

Temkin, O. 1971. "The Historiography of Ideas in Medicine." In *Modern Methods in the History of Medicine,* ed. E. Clarke. London: Althone, pp. 1–21.

Veatch, R. 1981. *A Theory of Medical Ethics.* New York: Basic Books.

Webster, C. 1983. "The Historiography of Medicine." In *Information Sources in the History of Science and Medicine,* ed. P. Corsi and P. Weindling. London: Butterworth Scientific, pp. 29–43.

Williams, G. 1957. *The Sanctity of Life and the Criminal Law.* New York: Knopf.

9

Qualitative Methods

Sara Chandros Hull, Holly A. Taylor, and Nancy E. Kass

Qualitative research methods are particularly well suited for understanding values, personal perspectives, experiences, and contextual circumstances, all of which are concerns of medical ethics. The term "qualitative research" is used broadly to refer to any non-quantified, nonstatistical method. Generally, qualitative methods involve asking open-ended questions of a relatively small number of informants to gather data to address particular research questions. Although qualitative data can be gathered to test hypotheses, more typically the research questions addressed by qualitative methods are discovery oriented, descriptive, and exploratory in nature. Qualitative methods expand understanding of what types of experiences, beliefs, or attitudes might exist.

This chapter provides an overview of frequently used qualitative data collection techniques and explains when it is appropriate to use each technique. Drawing upon our own qualitative research experiences, as well as published studies of qualitative research in medical ethics, we focus on several specific examples of research in medical ethics, including informed consent in research and genetic testing; medical information privacy; reproductive decision making; and end-of-life decision making. We also present a critique of qualitative research, including its advantages and limitations, to help researchers maximize the quality of their own work and readers critique research conducted by others. Finally, we review the skills and training needed by qualitative researchers and suggest additional resources for those interested in using qualitative methods for empirical research in medical ethics.

THE TECHNIQUES OF QUALITATIVE EMPIRICAL RESEARCH

A researcher must make several decisions before embarking on an empirical study in medical ethics. These decisions can be broken down into five steps. First, the researcher must select a topic to study. Second, depending on the nature of the study topic, the researcher needs to decide whether qualitative or quantitative methods (or some combination of these methods) are warranted. Third, if a qualitative approach is selected, the researcher must decide whether to follow a traditional qualitative research approach, such as phenomenology, ethnography, or grounded theory, to guide the overall study design, or whether a "hybrid" of approaches is more appropriate. Fourth, the researcher should determine which specific data collection techniques would be best for addressing the study's specific aims and research questions. Fifth, the researcher must decide upon an analytic plan to make sense of the data collected. The following sections review these steps in more detail.

Selecting a Research Topic

The choice of a research topic may be stimulated by personal or professional experience, a review of the literature, or a specific assignment or charge. A researcher may want to explore why particular experiences, beliefs, or attitudes exist, or to estimate the proportion of individuals with those particular experiences, beliefs, or attitudes. Research can be initiated when a previous understanding of a phenomenon is lacking, or gaps appear in results from previous work.

Empirical Approaches

Once the research topic has been identified, the next decision facing a researcher is what kind of research approach to undertake. The phenomenon under study, the goal of the study, and the experience and expertise of the researcher direct the selection of the most appropriate approach for a particular project. First, a broad decision regarding the use of qualitative and/or quantitative approaches must be made. If a qualitative approach is appropriate, the next decision involves the specific type of qualitative approach to take. These two decisions frame the overall design of the study, guiding the data collection and analysis stages of the research.

Deciding between Qualitative and Quantitative Approaches

Qualitative and quantitative methods are quite different from each other both in terms of their outcomes and in the specific steps taken to achieve those outcomes. Qualitative methods help to explain why certain experiences, beliefs, or attitudes exist. Asking respondents to use their own words often reveals new concepts relevant to the research question that were previously unknown to the researcher. In contrast, quantitative methods are appropriate for estimating the proportion of individuals with particular experiences, beliefs, or attitudes, and for exploring statistical associations between these experiences, beliefs, and attitudes and both various sociodemographic factors and other factors. Accurate estimates generally require conducting research with large numbers of respondents. Quantitative methods, which are most appropriate when some previous understanding of a phenomenon exists, can specify how many and what types of respondents have experienced previously recognized phenomena or hold previously recognized beliefs. As brief examples, one might do a quantitative study on advance directives by interviewing all patients newly admitted to a certain hospital to find out what proportion have heard of advance directives and what proportion already have one. Alternatively, or in addition, one could do a qualitative study, interviewing a much smaller number of informants to learn why those who chose to complete an advance directive have one and why those who do not have one say they do not.

TABLE 9.1 *Comparison of Qualitative and Quantitative Methodologies[a]*

Category	Qualitative Research	Quantitative Research
General research focus	Description, documentation, and analysis of patterns; values, worldview, meanings, beliefs, and attitudes. Totality of experiences in natural or particular contexts.	Measurement of controlled or manipulated variables by experimental and other methods. Causal and measurable relationships.
Scope	Generally broad, holistic, and comprehensive; worldview.	Particularist, narrow, and limited focus. Controlled. Excludes more than includes.
Research goal	Development of understandings and meanings of what one sees, hears, experiences, and discovers through a variety of sensual observation-participation modes. Obtain a full and accurate "truth" from people.	Testing hypotheses to obtain measurable outcomes among variables under study. Precision and objective findings.
Sources of data	Participants, informants, role takers, and respondents.	Objects, subjects, cases, data banks, code numbers, and figures.
Domains of analysis	Can reformulate and expand focus of study as one proceeds. No predetermined, *a priori* judgments. Open discovery. Flexible and dynamic. Moves with people, context, situation, or events.	Predetermined. A fixed design. Prejudgments and *a priori* position taken. Rigid and fixed categories. Non-dynamic. Fixed and planned sequence of research design to reduce variances.

Table 9.1 compares the relative purposes and goals of each method. The decision to use qualitative research enables a researcher to answer "how" or "what" questions, to explore, to present a detailed view, and to study individuals in their natural setting (Creswell 1998, 17–18). It can provide an understanding of context and environmental factors, meaning, process, and consequences.

Numerous topics in medical ethics are amenable to exploration using qualitative research methods. A review of journal articles in the online search engines MEDLINE (National Library of Medicine 1999b) and BIOETHICSLINE (National Library of Medicine 1999a) revealed many publications using qualitative methods to address issues in ethics. Some examples include the perspectives of health care providers (Musser 1997; Asai et al. 1997); cultural aspects of care (Jecker, Carrese, and Pearlman 1995); cultural feasibility studies prior to implementing a study or a program of care (Coreil et al. 1998); ethical issues faced by providers (Homenko 1997); ethics committees, consultations, and guidelines (Kelly et al. 1997; Stovall 1996; Rowan et al. 1996); and the development of ethics curricula for medical or nursing students (Hundert, Douglas-Steele, and Bickel 1996).

Quantitative research, by contrast, enables a researcher to ask "how many" questions, including how many respondents believe in certain previously identified phenomena, how many make decisions based on previously identified reasons, or how many have had certain types of previously identified types of experiences. Quantitative approaches are described in chapters 11, 12, and 13 of this volume in greater detail.

Deciding between Various Qualitative Research Approaches

That a particular research question is best addressed by qualitative methods still leaves open many choices for the researcher. Multiple qualitative research approaches have been developed by a variety of academic disciplines. Philosophers, anthropologists, and sociologists, among others, have developed empirical approaches (also known as "paradigms" or "traditions") that reflect their philosophical background and the intended goal of their inquiry. Though there are numerous approaches, we consider here the three that influence the majority of qualitative research conducted today: phenomenology, ethnography, and grounded theory (Creswell 1998; Morse and Field 1995). The parent academic discipline, type of research questions, methods, and other data sources corresponding to each of these approaches are displayed in Table 9.2.

Phenomenology

Phenomenology has its roots in philosophy. As applied to qualitative research, phenomenology seeks the essence of lived experience. A researcher engaged in a phenomenologic study relies heavily on in-depth interviews with individuals familiar with the phenomenon of interest. The individuals identified as appropriate subjects would be asked to describe fully their experience regarding that phenomenon. The goal of the researcher taking a phenomenologic approach is to produce a narrative that allows the reader to share in the experience described by the participants in the study.

For example, a researcher may want to draw on the phenomenologic approach to better understand the experiences of pregnant women who discover they are carrying fetuses with life-threatening genetic disorders. Using this approach, the researcher would talk in-depth with several women who have experienced this phenomenon in order to learn enough to describe it accurately. A reader of the final product of the study would have an appreciation of the women's lived experience.

Ethnography

Ethnography has its roots in anthropology and has as its goal the description of a particular culture. A researcher engaged in traditional ethnography would become immersed in a culture as a participant observer. The researcher may also conduct interviews and collect documents that allow him or her to fully understand and describe that culture. The product of these activities is a full and rich description of cultural beliefs and practices. As compared with the product of a phenomenologic approach, the reader of an ethnographic

TABLE 9.2   *Comparison of Major Qualitative Research Approaches*[a]

Tradition/ Approach	Parent Discipline	Type of Research Questions	Methods	Other Data Sources
Phenomenology	Philosophy (phenomenology)	Meaning questions— eliciting the essence of experiences.	Audiotaping conversations; written anecdotes of personal experiences.	Phenomeno- logical literature, philosophical reflections; poetry; art.
Ethnography	Anthropology	Descriptive questions—of values, beliefs, and practices of a cultural group.	Unstructured interviews; participant observations; field notes.	Documents; records; photographs; maps; genealogies; social network diagrams.
Grounded Theory	Sociology (symbolic interactionism)	"Process" questions— experience over time or change; may have stages or phases.	Interviews (tape recorded).	Participant observations; recording of memos; diary.

[a]Abstracted from Morse and Field 1995.

report would know about how individuals in a particular culture carry out their daily activities but would not know how those individuals felt participating in a particular task or their experience of a particular cultural tradition.

A classic example of an ethnographic approach to a question in medical ethics is found in Renee Fox's *Experiment Perilous,* a book that reports on the lives of patients with metabolic disorders and the physicians who care for them in an academic hospital (Fox 1959). Based on months of observation and informant interviews, Fox describes the culture of academic medicine.

Grounded Theory

Grounded theory has its roots in sociology, specifically *symbolic interactionism,* and has as its goal the exploration of the social and psychological processes involved in a particular experience. A researcher uses a grounded theory approach to discover and develop a theory that explains the particular process of interest. To this end, the researcher would conduct in-depth interviews with those familiar with the process of interest, asking questions about steps and/or components that are relevant to that process. Additional interviews are conducted as the researcher identifies and defines the core of the theory. Data collection is completed when the theory is fully elaborated. As compared to the product of an ethnographic study, the reader will be introduced to a theory that attempts to explain a single process relevant to a particular individual or group, but will know little about the cultural context within which the process occurs.

For example, a researcher interested in the process by which cancer patients make decisions regarding their enrollment in an early phase clinical trial may want to consider an approach guided by grounded theory. The researcher might conduct successive open-ended interviews with patients until a theory regarding patients' decision-making patterns begins to emerge. The product of the investigation will be a decision-making theory that can be tested among other groups of patients.

Data Collection

Qualitative research involves a variety of data-gathering techniques. The decision to collect existing data or create one's own depends largely on the types of research questions being asked. (See Table 9.2.) In this section we describe three general sources of data for qualitative research: existing documents, observation, and interviews. For each, we provide an overview of the purpose and characteristics of the technique and actual examples of empirical research using each of these techniques.

Document Review[1]

Documents are an important source of data for qualitative research because they provide a stable, written record of events and decisions. Public documents that may be relevant to research in medical ethics include official correspondence, legislation, minutes of meetings, written reports, proposals, progress reports, consent forms, newspaper editorials, films, videos, and advertisements. Private documents, such as personal correspondence, diaries, and autobiographies, are also potential sources of data for qualitative research.

By way of example, the Advisory Committee on Human Radiation Experiments (ACHRE) reviewed and analyzed documents from federally funded research proposals involving human subjects. The documents that were reviewed in this study included the original grant proposal and the corresponding Institutional Review Board (IRB) documents, such as the research protocol, consent forms, and IRB correspondence. The purpose of ACHRE's review was to evaluate how well these documents described (1) informed consent procedures, (2) the balance of risks to potential benefits for the subject, and (3) subject selection and recruitment. An evaluation form was used by ACHRE researchers to rank how well each of these aspects was addressed in the available documentation (ACHRE 1995).

A study that examined how written pamphlets convey information about carrier testing for cystic fibrosis (CF) and reproductive options utilized aspects of both quantitative and qualitative methods. The study reviewed twenty-eight published pamphlets and counted the number of neutral, positive, and negative textual descriptions of CF that were contained within the pamphlets. In addition, this study produced examples of descriptive statements about CF and the kinds of language used to discuss life expectancy and reproductive options (Loeben, Marteau, and Wilfond 1998).

Document review also can be used to complement other sources of qualitative or quantitative data. Yin explains that an important use of documents "is to corroborate and augment evidence from other sources" (1994, 81). For example, a study on reproductive decision making among adults with genetic conditions compared the language contained in educational pamphlets to the language used in interviews with affected adults and their health care providers in discussing reproduction (Hull 1999). In another study using interviews to learn about health insurance and the privacy of medical information, informants who reported that they had been denied health insurance were asked to provide documentation as additional evidence of this denial. When such documentation is available, it validates the self-reported interview data that might otherwise be viewed skeptically (Kass 1997).

Observation

In observational research, the researcher visits a site where an activity or behavior of interest is occurring. This might include on-site clinic observations of interactions between patients and their clinicians, or of how researchers engage in an informed consent process with potential research participants. Two techniques used in observational research include *participant observation* and *direct observation*. In participant observation (see chapter 10), the researcher becomes an "insider" and plays an active role in the activity or behavior being observed. For example, a participant observer might be a member of a committee or a care provider. This is not intended to be deceptive—all members of a group being observed should understand that research is occurring.

In direct observation, on the other hand, the researcher is an "outsider" and attempts to observe behaviors passively without contributing to them. The goal of direct observation is to "watch a subject, or group of subjects and record their behavior as faithfully as possible" (Bernard 1995, 311). Although the researcher does not become involved in the activities and behaviors being observed, subjects are often aware that the researcher is recording their behavior. Field notes are recorded by the researcher in both kinds of observational research—concurrent with the observation, if possible.

Direct observation can serve as a formative data collection stage to orient the researcher to the topic under study. We have used this technique in the preliminary phases of research to learn more about the clinical settings in which the subsequent phases of the research were to be conducted. This involved spending many hours observing the various activities that occurred in the clinic in preparation for conducting interviews with clinic patients and staff (Taylor 1999; Hull 1999).

A variation of observational research involves tape recording "naturally occurring" interactions between physicians and patients. This method of data collection differs from direct observation because the researcher need not be present while the behavior of interest is taking place. For example, to examine how information about early phase oncology trials is presented to patients and what patients understand, conversations in which a physician offers a patient the option to enroll in an early phase clinical trial are recorded (Kass, Sugarman, and Taylor 1999).

Interviews

Interviews allow researchers to ask individuals about their beliefs and experiences and what they think and feel about particular issues. The interview is a kind of conversation between a researcher and an informant (or group of informants) that seeks to elicit the informant's understanding, knowledge, and insights about a particular topic (Rubin and Rubin 1995). Personal interviews and focus groups, two types of interviews commonly used in research in medical ethics, are explored in this section.

Personal Interviews A personal, in-depth interview involves an interaction between two people: a researcher and an interviewee, or *informant*. Informants are often people who have a common background or experience, such as patients with a particular condition, health care providers, or research subjects. In-depth interviews vary in the degree to which they are structured because different purposes are achieved with the various degrees of structure. *Unstructured interviews* begin with a topic and perhaps a few specific questions, allowing the interviewer to identify and explore new questions and topics throughout each interview and the research process. *Structured interviews*, on the other hand, use a specific set of open-ended questions that is identical for all study participants. Between these two extremes, a *semi-structured interview* balances structured and less-structured components. The semistructured interview tends to be interactive, with the interviewer asking follow-up questions based on the specific comments of each informant.

The semistructured *interview field guide* includes a basic set of questions that should be covered in the course of an interview. The field guide is particularly useful when more than one interviewer is involved in a study to ensure that the same general topics are covered by different interviewers. Although the field guide includes a basic set of questions to be asked of everyone, it often does not specify a particular order in which these questions need to be asked. It also leaves room for the interviewer to ask extensive follow-up questions. Because of the iterative nature of qualitative data collection and analysis, the interview field guide evolves over time, based upon findings from emerging data. It may be desirable to conduct follow-up interviews with previous study participants when new or more focused questions emerge during the course of a study.

A recent interview study examined the perspectives of health care providers and HIV-infected women about reproduction. One part of the study sought to understand health care providers' beliefs and attitudes concerning HIV infection and childbearing and how they counsel HIV-infected women about reproduction. Another part of the study sought to understand HIV-infected women's intentions concerning childbearing and how their providers discussed reproduction and childbearing with them. In these interviews, women sometimes said that they both did and did not want to have children, a finding related to their own internal conflict (Faden and Kass 1996). This finding illustrates one of the major values of using qualitative research methods; this conflict would likely not have been captured using standard quantitative surveys. For example, a quantitative survey that asked women, "Do you want to have children?" would require a "yes" or "no" response, leaving no room for the possibility that both answers could be true.

Both quantitative/close-ended and qualitative/open-ended questions can be included within a single interview. In the interview study on privacy, confidentiality, and health insurance mentioned above, interviewees who answer affirmatively the close-ended question, "Have you ever been denied health insurance?" are then asked in an open-ended question to explain in detail the circumstances under which this occurred (Kass 1997). Similarly, a study on genetic testing might first ask an at-risk informant, "Do you plan to be tested for the gene in question?" followed by the open-ended question, "Why/why not?"

The location of the interview is an important consideration. To the extent possible, interviews should be conducted in a setting that is comfortable for the informants. While it may be ideal to conduct interviews with physicians within the clinic or their offices, the clinic may seem formal, sterile, and intimidating to patients who would be more comfortable being interviewed at their homes. However, it may not always be feasible to travel to informants' homes to conduct interviews for logistical, safety, and/or cost-related reasons. At a minimum, an interview location should be convenient, private, distraction-free, and comfortable.

The use of telephone interviews, which may be logistically simpler than in-person interviews, has both potential benefits and drawbacks. Participants may feel more comfortable sharing sensitive information in the more anonymous format of the telephone interview. However, it is more difficult for the interviewer to establish rapport with participants without the ability to shake their hands and make eye contact. Personal interviews, both telephone and in person, typically are tape-recorded and transcribed for analysis.

Focus Groups   Focus groups, or group interviews, allow researchers to gain insights into the behaviors of groups of people and to learn why they feel certain ways about specific issues. Originally used for marketing research, the focus group has been defined as "a research technique that collects data through group interaction on a topic determined by the researcher" (Morgan 1997, 6). Focus groups are advantageous for several reasons. They allow researchers to obtain input from a large number of people in a short amount of time and to produce concentrated amounts of data. In contrast to one-on-one interviews, the group setting may encourage participants to discuss issues that they might not think of on their own (Morgan 1997). In addition, a practical benefit of focus groups is that they generally are less expensive than survey research (Bernard 1995, 226).

Focus groups may stand alone as a self-contained method of data collection. For example, focus groups were conducted with families affected with Alzheimer's disease (AD) to examine their arguments for and against predictive genetic testing for AD. The results from the study were used by a consensus group to make policy recommendations (Post et al. 1997).

Alternatively, focus groups can be used to supplement other methods of data collection. They often are used to collect preliminary data that is then used to develop interview guides or questionnaires for later stages of the research. Focus groups can identify substantive areas to be explored further in the interviews. In addition, focus group data can provide insight into the language used by the study populations regarding the issues of interest. Bernhardt et al. (1997) conducted a series of focus groups as the first stage of a project to develop a model informed consent process for BRCA1 genetic testing. Eight focus groups, of nine to ten women each, were convened to discuss beliefs about the causes of breast cancer, their expectations of health care providers, what they would want to know if offered a genetic test, and their understanding of the benefits and risks of genetic testing.

Focus groups can be conducted with "naturally occurring" groups of previously acquainted persons, such as support groups, committees, or students in a class. In many cases, however, focus group participants are strangers who are recruited solely for the purpose of the research via a flyer, newspaper advertisement, or other method. Ideally, focus groups include between six and twelve participants and the group moderator (Bernard 1995, 225). In addition, a notetaker/research assistant is often included as a second moderator.

Composition of focus groups is also an important consideration. It is generally thought best for participants in focus groups to be in some way homogeneous so that respondents will feel comfortable voicing their views. Homogeneous focus groups also facilitate analysis of differences in perspective among groups (Morgan 1997). For instance, focus group participants are often from the same background, all women or all men, or homogenous on factors relevant to the research question, such as having the same medical condition.

The choice of moderator should be made with sensitivity to the composition of the group (gender, age, race, ethnicity, etc.) A moderator with a similar background will generally make people feel more comfortable revealing personal or sensitive information. A skilled focus group moderator will draw out the quieter participants and limit the more outspoken ones. The moderator's goal is to guide the topic of the conversation.

Focus groups typically are audiotaped and transcribed for analysis. Though expensive, the use of a stenographer can be helpful in focus groups, since voices can be hard to distinguish on an audiotape. The stenographer attends the focus group and by using specialized equipment is able to record a verbatim transcript while attributing each comment to the specific person who said it.

Analysis

The specific analytic techniques chosen are influenced by the qualitative approach taken by the researcher, the phenomenon under study, and/or the goal of the study. However, there are three basic steps followed in virtually all qualitative analysis: immersion, data reduction, and synthesis.

One of the ways in which qualitative and quantitative research methods differ is related to the researcher's role in the data analysis process. While the researcher strives to remain detached and objective during the analysis of quantitative data, the researcher becomes *immersed* in the data during qualitative analysis. In qualitative analysis the researcher routinely reviews the data as it is being collected in order to identify what additional data are needed and when *saturation* has been achieved (i.e., no new information is emerging, so the data set is complete). Immersion is the necessary first step that enables the researcher to complete the remaining analysis tasks.

The next step in the data analysis process usually involves data reduction. *Data reduction*, a term used by Miles and Huberman (1994), refers to the process of dividing the data into more manageable units and labeling or coding the units. For example, a large interview transcript may be reduced into smaller units according to the different topics covered within the interview (e.g., views about genetic testing; views about disability; views about abortion). The mechanics of data reduction typically involve labeling topically related units of data with *codes* that help identify and sort the data. Codes are generated either from topics identified in advance (e.g., questions included in a semistructured interview guide) or from topics that emerge from the data itself. Coding of data can be done by hand (e.g., highlighting on an interview transcript the passages related to a particular topic or "code") or in conjunction with qualitative data analysis software.

Once the data have been reduced, themes and patterns can then be explored to re-shape and *synthesize* the data into a more coherent whole. Conclusions and/or hypotheses generated during this process of data synthesis are then tested within the data set. For exam-ple, a hypothesis about the relationship between two or more themes identified during data reduction is tested by reexamining the data in search of instances that contradict the pro-posed hypothesis. Qualitative data analysis is an iterative process: while data reduction and synthesis usually follow one another, the sequence is often repeated to create a feedback loop that continues throughout the data analysis process.

The final product of data synthesis is determined by the qualitative approach taken and/or the phenomenon under investigation and the goals of the study. For example, the product of a project guided by grounded theory will be an inductive theory about a process related to the phenomenon under study. Maintaining a record of each decision made dur-ing the data analysis process to arrive at the theory is helpful both to the researcher and to the readers of the research (Koch 1993). An analysis roadmap can facilitate the replication of the study and allow readers to assess whether they agree with the researcher's synthesis and interpretation of data. In addition, when developing the final product, it is important for researchers to aim for an appropriate balance of substance (e.g., quotes) and interpreta-tion (e.g., synthesis) to allow the reader to follow the reasoning behind the analysis and de-termine whether they share the researcher's conclusions (Morse 1999).

Summary of Steps in Qualitative Research

Table 9.3 introduces a potential topic for a qualitative research project—women at risk for breast cancer seeking genetic testing—and provides examples of the research ques-tion/focus, potential participants or informants, data collection methods, and type of re-sults that projects guided by each of the three qualitative approaches discussed would produce.

CRITIQUING QUALITATIVE RESEARCH IN MEDICAL ETHICS

In the following section we present a critique of qualitative research, including its scope, advantages, and limitations. Our goals are to provide researchers with tools to help maximize the quality of their own work and to assess the quality of research conducted by others. The quality or *rigor* of an empirical study refers to how confident one is that the findings and conclusions from that study are accurate. Methodological rigor occurs at each stage of a qualitative research project, including selection of a topic, data collection, analy-sis, and writing/presentation. The concept of *validity* in qualitative research generally refers to the credibility of the study findings, while *reliability* refers to the consistency and de-pendability of the research process over time and across researchers and methods (Miles and Huberman 1994).

Qualitative researchers have several techniques available to them to improve the re-liability and validity of their research, and critical readers of qualitative research will want to see that these techniques have been utilized. For example, *peer* or *colleague review* and *mem-ber checking* improve the reliability of qualitative research findings. Peer review involves so-

TABLE 9.3   *Comparison of Approaches in a Hypothetical Qualitative Project*[a]

Approach	Research Question/ Focus	Participants/ Informants	Data Collection Methods	Type of Results
Phenomenology	What is the meaning of seeking genetic testing?	Women at risk of breast cancer; phenomenological literature; art; poetry; and other descriptions.	In-depth conversation	In-depth reflective description of the experience of "seeking genetic testing."
Ethnography	What is the setting like when women come to seek out genetic testing?	Women at risk of breast cancer in the clinic; families; genetic counselors; clinic staff; other clinic staff who work in the setting.	Interviews; participant observations; direct observations; other records such as medical charts.	A description of the day-to-day events and relationships at the genetic testing clinic.
Grounded Theory	What is the process like when women seek out genetic testing?	Women at risk of breast cancer; families.	In-depth interviews; observations.	Description of the social, psychological process in the experience of seeking genetic testing.

[a]Abstracted from Morse and Field 1995.

liciting the help of colleagues or peer researchers to analyze a subset of the data and compare their findings with those of the researcher. Member checking involves sharing emerging findings with study participants to see if the researcher's interpretation of the data is consistent with those of the participants (Creswell 1998).

The use of multiple sources of data or analytic techniques, which is known as *triangulation*, increases the validity of qualitative research by using complementary methods and data sources to produce converging conclusions. When different conclusions emerge from related data sources, the researcher needs to reconsider the entire data set until all of the evidence corroborates a single set of conclusions, or a reasonable explanation is discovered for the apparent divergence. Although it is common to defend the merits of one empirical research method over another (Carr 1994; Kvale 1996), different types of qualitative and quantitative research methods should be treated as interactive and complementary rather than mutually exclusive. A qualitative study may involve the use of both observational and interviewing techniques, for example, to look at a particular issue in several ways. Alternatively, the use of one kind of method may follow from the other. For example, qualitative research can be used to identify new variables and develop hypotheses that can then be tested using more quantitative research methods. In addition, qualitative research can provide data to explain the statistical findings of quantitative studies.

Empirical researchers in medical ethics who use qualitative methods (ourselves included) tend to identify their projects in ways that focus on the data collection technique, such as *qualitative interview studies* or *focus group studies*, rather than as being characterized by a broader approach, such as phenomenology, ethnography, or grounded theory. Some methodologists argue that a qualitative project undertaken without clear, informed commitment to one of these broad approaches is ill advised (e.g., Morse 1991). We take a less stringent view, and believe that qualitative research is not invalid in absence of such commitment or, indeed, with a clear commitment to a "hybrid" of approaches, as long as researchers appreciate the limitations of the methods they choose. For example, a study that relies solely on focus group data will generate more tentative conclusions than a study that draws upon well-established ethnographic techniques and includes multiple sources of data. At the same time, an in-depth ethnographic study requires substantial resources and time, whereas a focus group study is a more efficient and feasible approach to examine a narrow set of issues within a short timeframe.

The Strengths of Qualitative Methods

The primary strengths of qualitative research include its ability to uncover new concepts, its exploratory and explanatory roles, and its ability to provide illustrative examples of quantitative phenomenon. By having informants describe phenomena in their own voices, the researcher may be less likely to impose a preconceived understanding on the results of the research. The benefits of qualitative research have been summarized in four points by Gittelsohn et al. (1998, 369): explorative flexibility; going in-depth; validation of information; and taking a holistic perspective.

Explorative flexibility refers to the researcher's ability to acknowledge assumptions and biases about the topic to be studied, enter data collection with an open willingness to learn from the study participants, and to explore new questions that are likely to emerge throughout the study. Detailed information is acquired in qualitative research by *going in-depth* and conducting increasingly specific data collection, while *validation of information* occurs through the use of multiple data collection methods, and sometimes returning to the same participants/informants to validate conclusions. *Taking a holistic perspective* using qualitative methods permits an elucidation and examination of the contextual conditions under which the topic of study occurs.

In addition to the general benefits of qualitative research, each specific data collection technique contains its own unique advantages. Documents are stable and precise, and their retrieval for research purposes is generally unobtrusive. Observation allows the researcher to examine actual events and behaviors as they occur in their natural context. Interviews allow the researcher to ask participants directly about a specific topic of interest. The strengths of the specific data collection techniques reviewed in this chapter are summarized in Table 9.4.

TABLE 9.4   *Strengths and Weaknesses of Qualitative Data Techniques*[a]

Technique	Strengths	Weaknesses
Documentation	• stable; can be retrieved repeatedly • unobtrusive • exact; contains exact names, references, and details of an event • broad coverage; long span of time, many events, and many settings	• access may be blocked • may not convey what actually occurs in practice
Observation	• covers events in real time • covers context of events	• time consuming • event may proceed differently because it is being observed
Interviews	• targeted; focuses directly on the topic of interest • provides insight into participant's perspectives	• potential biases related to: —how researcher frames the questions, choice of vocabulary —subject's ability to recall events accurately —interviewee gives what interviewers want to hear —which informants are willing to be interviewed

[a]Adapted from Yin 1994.

The Weaknesses of Qualitative Methods

Qualitative research methods are also characterized by several weaknesses or limitations. These limitations can be placed into one of three categories: the general limitations of qualitative research, the limitations of individual qualitative research techniques, and limitations related to the research climate. An oft-referenced limitation of qualitative research is its lack of *generalizability*. The term *generalizability*, as it is commonly used, refers to the applicability of a study's findings beyond the research context, and is the gold standard to which the findings of quantitative research are held. Quantitative research is designed to be generalizable, typically through selecting a random sample of subjects that represents a larger population of interest. Qualitative research is not generalizable in the same sense because it involves selecting a smaller, nonrandom, purposive sample of individuals who contribute to the generation of theories and hypotheses. One cannot be certain that the findings from an individual qualitative study are applicable outside of the narrow research population and context; additional research is required to establish whether these findings are indeed generalizable to other settings.

As an example, a qualitatively derived theory that predicts how a small sample of purposively selected parents of HIV-infected children make decisions about enrollment in a clinical trial may also predict the behavior of parents of children with asthma, cancer, or other childhood illnesses faced with similar decisions. However, one cannot be certain that this is true without first testing this theory among parents of children with conditions other than HIV infection. By contrast, a single quantitative study could accommodate a representative sample of parents of children with varying conditions, with the goal of testing (rather than producing) a theory about enrollment decisions.

It is also important to note that a weakness inherent in the qualitative approach is that collection and analysis of qualitative data are influenced by the subjectivity and biases of researchers. The personal worldviews of the researchers, including biases of which they might be unaware, are reflected in how qualitative studies are conducted.

Each of the qualitative data collection techniques reviewed in this chapter is characterized by specific limitations as well. For example, ACHRE's document review of federally funded research was limited in that consent documentation may not be a good surrogate for learning about the consent process (ACHRE 1995). In both observational and interviewing research, the research participants may react to the researcher's presence and provide inaccurate or modified information. The limitations of these methods are summarized on p. 159 in Table 9.4.

In addition to these methodological limitations, some barriers to the acceptance of qualitative research in medical ethics also exist. Qualitative methods are not yet a dominant approach to empirical research at many medical institutions. Unfamiliarity with the overall goals and methods of qualitative research may lead to a lack of its acceptance among more quantitatively oriented researchers. For example, we have heard anecdotes from our colleagues suggesting that some Institutional Review Boards (IRBs) have been resistant to approving qualitative research proposals, or have questioned the small sample sizes inherent in qualitative methods. Graduate students in schools with a strong statistical orientation may find it difficult to identify dissertation committee members who understand and accept the use of qualitative research methods. Groups of researchers who are called upon to review grant applications in a particular content area (study sections) may exhibit a similar resistance or lack of understanding of qualitative research.

CONCLUDING COMMENTS

Numerous topics in medical ethics are appropriate to explore using qualitative methods, particularly those that seek a better understanding of values, personal perspectives, experiences, and contextual circumstances. In this chapter, we have provided an overview of qualitative research methods that might serve as a starting point for those interested in using qualitative methods to conduct research in medical ethics, or those interested in becoming a more critical reader of qualitative ethics research. The decisions facing any researcher begin with selecting a topic and appropriate research questions, which lead to decisions regarding what kind and how much data to collect. For researchers who seek to gain an understanding of the meaning of a phenomenon, of the context in which an event occurs, or why individuals act in certain ways or hold certain beliefs, qualitative research is appropriate. Qualitative researchers then must decide how best to organize and synthesize the collected data and create a product with an appropriate balance of substance and interpretation.

NOTES ON RESOURCES AND TRAINING

A well-trained qualitative researcher possesses *theoretical sensitivity.* Although this term derives from the grounded theory research tradition (Glaser 1978; Strauss and Corbin 1990), theoretical sensitivity generally applies to a researcher's ability to recognize the subtleties of meaning in qualitative data. This ability to recognize what is important in the data and give it meaning develops through personal and professional experience. An increased understanding of the phenomenon under study develops during a researcher's interaction with data collection and analysis.

Qualitative research that involves group or personal interviews requires a researcher to have excellent communication skills. Qualities like empathy, sensitivity, and sincerity are central. The ability to build rapport, inspire trust, and ask questions in a sensitive manner will enable a researcher to acquire more accurate and detailed responses from interviewees. Furthermore, because qualitative researchers serve as the primary data gathering instruments in interview research, they do not play a neutral role in data generation and analysis. Personal experiences and biases shape the kinds of questions a qualitative researcher asks. Therefore, one of the most important skills for qualitative researchers is to recognize and openly describe personal perspectives and biases that might influence the research. Achieving balance, rather than neutrality, is a goal of qualitative research (Rubin and Rubin 1995).

The role of mentoring in qualitative research should not be underestimated. Training with a mentor who is experienced in a particular kind of qualitative methodology is a critical step in becoming a good qualitative researcher. Many of the skills required to conduct qualitative research may be better conveyed through one-on-one communication, rather than in written texts (Burns 1989). Although referring to methodological texts is an important component of learning how to conduct qualitative research, it is not sufficient training in itself. Sole reliance on methodological texts, without the guidance of a mentor, has been analogized to learning how to drive from reading a car manual, or learning how to write from reading a computer manual (Morse 1997). Mentors may be identified among colleagues who are doing qualitative research at one's institution, at professional conferences, or from courses, workshops, and seminars.

Coursework in qualitative research offers a more formal way to review methodological texts, conduct fieldwork in a supervised setting, and develop relationships with potential research mentors and collaborators. Precise data on the extent to which courses on qualitative research methods are offered at universities and medical schools are lacking. However, schools seem to vary on the extent of courses available on qualitative research. Schools of nursing seem to offer a wider range of qualitative methods courses compared with schools of medicine and public health. The most comprehensive qualitative research training program for health professionals of which we are aware is offered by the University of North Carolina at Chapel Hill School of Nursing. This program, called the Summer Institutes in Qualitative Research, features a series of courses on qualitative methods, analysis, and evaluation. The educational objectives of this particular program, displayed in Table 9.5 below, represent a comprehensive set of goals for qualitative methods coursework in general.

TABLE 9.5   *Educational Goals in Qualitative Research Coursework*[a]

	Objectives
Methods	1. Describe the implications of competing paradigms of inquiry on the practice of qualitative research.
	2. Compare commonly used qualitative methods in health professions research.
	3. Describe the typical design features of each of these methods, including staging and scene setting, strategies for sampling, and techniques for data collection, preparation, analysis, interpretation, and representation.
	4. Describe major data collection techniques and sources, including interviews, observations, documents, and artifacts.
	5. Describe prevailing orientations to, and techniques for, validation of qualitative research findings.
	6. Describe the features of a "good" qualitative research proposal and completed project.
Analysis	1. Differentiate among data preparation, analysis, and interpretation.
	2. Differentiate between analysis approaches aimed at informational content and narrative/discursive features of data.
	3. Compare approaches to qualitative analysis.
	4. Explain the varied uses of "theory" in qualitative analysis and interpretation.
	5. Compare interpretive products, including qualitative descriptions, grounded theories, ethnographies, and phenomenologies.
	6. Describe the use of data displays in analysis and re-presentation.
	7. Differentiate between case- and variable-oriented analysis.
	8. Describe various templates for re-presenting qualitative data, including approaches emphasizing time, theme, and sensitizing concept.
	9. Describe the role of computerized text management systems in qualitative analysis.
Evaluation	1. Describe frameworks for qualitative evaluation, especially utilization-focused evaluation, and their utility for assessing health care practices, programs, and policies.
	2. Describe templates and techniques for combining qualitative and quantitative methods.
	3. Describe the use of qualitative methods in intervention and outcome studies.
	4. Describe issues related to triangulation in qualitative research.
	5. Describe issues relating to and techniques for putting qualitative findings directly into practice.

[a] Adapted from University of North Carolina at Chapel Hill School of Nursing 1999.

For students or faculty at institutions that do not offer extensive coursework in qualitative research methods, there are several alternatives. It is advisable to look to other divisions within their institution for methodological courses. For example, departments of anthropology, sociology, and political science, as well as schools of nursing, are good places to look for qualitative coursework. However, we want to reiterate here that coursework is not the only manner in which to receive methodological training, which can occur through mentorship, collegial support, independent reading, and participation in qualitative research methods discussion groups.

Although we have presented a broad overview of qualitative methods in medical ethics research, we were not able to go into detail on any particular aspect of these methods. Those interested in conducting qualitative research should consult methodological texts that review the overall approaches, data collection, and analysis in greater detail. The references cited throughout this chapter represent a cross-section of the literature available on qualitative research, including methodological texts and journal articles. A list of general texts that we have found to be quite helpful in our research is included in Appendix A.

A review of published literature on MEDLINE (National Library of Medicine 1999b) and BIOETHICSLINE (National Library of Medicine 1999a) revealed increasing numbers of journals that are receptive to publishing qualitative research. Appendix B provides a selection of medical and/or ethics journals that have published reports using qualitative research methods. This list includes traditionally more quantitative journals (such as the *Journal of the American Medical Association*), which are increasingly likely to consider qualitative research, particularly manuscripts for research in which qualitative methods are used in a complementary way with quantitative methods. We also reviewed recent editions of journals that are most likely to publish research in medical ethics to examine the extent to which such research was qualitative in nature. We found the following journals have published qualitative research in medical ethics within their five most recent editions: *AIDS and Public Policy Journal; American Journal of Law, Medicine, and Ethics; Cambridge Quarterly of Health Care Ethics; Journal of Clinical Oncology; Journal of Medical Ethics;* and *Social Science and Medicine* (Hull, Burger, and Otero 1999). The *Hastings Center Report* often provides annotated bibliographic information on qualitative empirical research in medical ethics.

Professional conferences are yet another resource for learning about the types of qualitative projects on topics in medical ethics. The number of presentations of qualitative empirical research at professional conferences seems to have increased in recent years. For instance, the majority of empirical research presentations and poster sessions at the first annual meeting of the American Society for Bioethics and Humanities (ASBH) in 1998 reported the results of qualitative research that utilized either focus group or personal interviewing techniques (ASBH 1998).

Finally, the Internet is an excellent resource for current information about qualitative research. Qualitative methods course syllabi, information about current qualitative textbooks and journals and their publishers, and online discussion groups devoted to qualitative research are all available via the Internet. Because of the dynamic and ever-changing nature of the Internet, information about any specific websites has not been included in this chapter.

NOTE

1. The term *document review* is used to refer specifically to the review and analysis of previously existing documents. The term *content analysis* also may be used to refer generally to the analysis of written materials. Bernard explains that "Content analysis is a catch-all term covering a variety of techniques for making inferences from 'texts'" (1995, 339). According to this definition, content analysis can be used for interview transcripts that were generated as part of a research project, as well as documents that existed outside of the research project. Because the term *content analysis* is somewhat ambiguous, we avoid using it in this chapter.

REFERENCES

Advisory Committee on Human Radiation Experiments. 1995. *The Human Radiation Experiments*. New York: Oxford University Press.

American Society of Bioethics and Humanities. 1998. *First Annual Meeting: Program Book*. Glenview, IL: American Society of Bioethics and Humanities.

Asai, A., S. Fukuhara, O. Inoshita, Y. Miura, N. Tanabe, and K. Kurokawa. 1997. "Medical Decisions Concerning the End of Life: A Discussion with Japanese Physicians." *Journal of Medical Ethics* 23:323–27.

Bernard, H. R. 1995. *Research Methods in Anthropology: Qualitative and Quantitative Approaches*. Walnut Creek, CA: AltaMira Press.

Bernhardt, B. A., G. Geller, M. Strauss, K. Helzlsover, M. Stefanek, P. M. Wilcox, and N. A. Holtzman. 1997. "Toward a Model Informed Consent Process for BRCA1 Testing: A Qualitative Assessment of Women's Attitudes." *Journal of Genetic Counseling* 6:207–22.

Burns, N. 1989. "Standards for Qualitative Research." *Nursing Science Quarterly* 2:44–52.

Carr, L. T. 1994. "The Strengths and Weaknesses of Quantitative and Qualitative Research: What Method for Nursing?" *Journal of Advanced Nursing* 20:716–21.

Coreil, J., P. Losikoff, R. Pincu, G. Maynard, A. J. Ruff, H. P. Hausler, J. Desormeau, H. Davis, R. Boulos, and N. A. Halsey. 1998. "Cultural Feasibility Studies in Preparation for Clinical Trials to Reduce Maternal-Infant HIV-Transmission in Haiti." *AIDS Education and Prevention* 10:46–62.

Creswell, J. W. 1998. *Qualitative Inquiry and Research Design: Choosing among Five Traditions*. Thousand Oaks, CA: Sage Publications.

Faden, R. R., and N. E. Kass. 1996. *HIV, AIDS, and Childbearing: Public Policy, Private Lives*. New York: Oxford University Press.

Fox, R. C. 1959. *Experiment Perilous: Physicians and Patients Facing the Unknown*. Philadelphia, PA: University of Pennsylvania.

Gittelsohn, J., P. J. Pelto, M. E. Bentley, K. Baltacharyya, and L. Jensen. 1998. *Ethnographic Methods to Investigate Women's Health: Rapid Assessment Procedures (RAP)*. Boston: International Nutrition Foundation.

Glaser, B. 1978. *Theoretical Sensitivity*. Mill Valley, CA: Sociology Press.

Homenko, D. F. 1997. "Overview of Ethical Issues Perceived by Allied Health Professionals in the Workplace." *Journal of Allied Health* 26:97–103.

Hull, S. C. 1999. Sickle Cell Disease, Cystic Fibrosis, and Reproduction: A Qualitative Study of Affected Adult and Health Care Provider Perspectives. Unpublished dissertation manuscript. Baltimore, MD: Johns Hopkins University.

Hull, S. C., I. Burger, and I. Otero. 1999. *Review of Qualitative Research in Medical Ethics Journals.* Unpublished data.

Hundert, E. M., D. Douglas-Steele, and J. Bickel. 1996. "Context in Medical Education: The Informal Ethics Curriculum." *Medical Education* 30:353–64.

Jecker, N. S., J. A. Carrese, and R. A. Pearlman. 1995. "Caring for Patients in Cross-Cultural Settings." *Hastings Center Report* 25:6–14.

Kass, N. E. 1997. "Experience and Attitudes of Persons with Genetic and Other Serious Illnesses Concerning Privacy, Confidentiality, and Access to Health Insurance." Paper presented at Visions for Ethics and Humanities in a Changing Health Care Environment: The Joint Meeting of the American Association of Bioethics, Society for Bioethics Consultation, and Society for Health and Human Values. 5–9 November, Baltimore, MD.

Kass, N. E., J. Sugarman, and H. Taylor. 1999. "Improving Understanding of Early Phase Clinical Trials." Panel Session on Results from the NIH Informed Consent Initiative. Second Annual Meeting of the American Society for Bioethics and Humanities. 28–31 October, Philadelphia, PA.

Kelly, S. E., P. A. Marshall, L. M. Sanders, T. A. Raffin, and B. A. Koenig. 1997. "Understanding the Practice of Ethics Consultation: Results of an Ethnographic Multi-Site Study." *Journal of Clinical Ethics* 8:136–49.

Koch, T. 1993. "Establishing Rigour in Qualitative Research: The Decision Trail." *Journal of Advanced Nursing* 19:976–86.

Kreuger, R. A. 1994. *Focus Groups: A Practical Guide for Applied Research.* 2nd ed. Thousand Oaks, CA: Sage Publications.

Kvale, S. 1996. *InterViews: An Introduction to Qualitative Research Interviewing.* Thousand Oaks, CA: Sage Publications.

Leininger, M. M. 1985. "Nature, Rationale, and Importance of Evaluative Research Methods in Nursing." In *Qualitative Research Methods in Nursing,* ed. M. M. Leininger. New York: Grune & Stratton, Inc., pp. 1–25.

Loeben, G. L., T. M. Marteau, and B. S. Wilfond. 1998. "Mixed Messages: Presentation of Information in Cystic Fibrosis—Screening Pamphlets." *American Journal of Human Genetics* 63:1181–89.

Miles, M. B., and A. M. Huberman. 1994. *Qualitative Data Analysis.* Thousand Oaks, CA: Sage Publications.

Morgan, D. L. 1997. *Focus Groups as Qualitative Research.* Thousand Oaks, CA: Sage Publications.

Morse, J. M. 1991. "Qualitative Nursing Research: A Free-for-All?" In *Qualitative Nursing Research: A Contemporary Dialogue,* ed. J. M. Morse. Newbury Park, CA: Sage Publications, pp. 14–22.

———. 1997. "Learning to Drive from a Manual?" *Qualitative Health Research* 7:181–83.

———. 1999. "Silent Debates in Qualitative Inquiry." *Qualitative Health Research* 9:163–65.

Morse, J. M., and P. A. Field. 1995. *Qualitative Research Methods for Health Professionals.* Thousand Oaks, CA: Sage Publications.

Musser, L. E. 1997. "Using a Feminist Framework for Investigating Staff Nurses' Philosophies of Nursing." *Seminars for Nurse Managers* 5:194–201.

National Library of Medicine. 1999a. BIOETHICSLINE® BIOETHICS onLINE. Internet Grateful Med V2.6.3. http://igm.nlm.nih.gov/

———. 1999b. MEDLINE® MEDlars onLINE. Internet Grateful Med V2.6.3. http://igm.nlm.nih.gov/

Post, S. G., P. J. Whitehouse, R. H. Binstock, T. D. Bird, S. K. Eckert, L. A. Farrer, L. M. Fleck, A. D. Gaines, E. T. Juengst, H. Karlinsky, S. Miles, T. H. Murray, K. A. Quaid, N. R. Relkin, A. D. Ross, P. H. St. George-Hyslop, G. A. Sachs, B. Steinbock, E. F. Truschke, and A. B. Zinn. 1997. "The Clinical Introduction of Genetic Testing for Alzheimer Disease: An Ethical Perspective." *Journal of the American Medical Association* 277:832–36.

Rowan, M. S., M. Toombs, G. Bally, D. J. Walters, and J. Henderson. 1996. "Qualitative Evaluation of the Canadian Medical Association's Counseling Guidelines for HIV Serological Testing." *Journal of the Canadian Medical Association* 154:665–71.

Rubin, H. J., and I. S. Rubin. 1995. *Qualitative Interviewing: The Art of Hearing Data.* Thousand Oaks, CA: Sage Publications.

Stovall, E. L. 1996. "Practice Guidelines: Patients' Perspectives." *Oncology* 10:255–60.

Strauss, A., and J. Corbin. 1990. *Basics of Qualitative Research: Grounded Theory Procedures and Techniques.* Newbury Park, CA: Sage Publications.

Taylor, H. A. 1999. The Recruitment of HIV-Infected Children into Clinical Research: An Exploration of Factors that Influence Decision Making. Unpublished dissertation manuscript. Baltimore, MD: Johns Hopkins University.

University of North Carolina at Chapel Hill School of Nursing. 1999. Summer Institutes in Qualitative Research. http://www.unc.edu/~msandelo/homeisnt.htm#methods

Yin, R. K. 1994. *Case Study Research: Design and Methods.* Thousand Oaks, CA: Sage Publications.

APPENDIX A

Recommended General Qualitative Research Methodological Texts

Bernard, H. Russell. 1995. *Research Methods in Anthropology: Qualitative and Quantitative Approaches.* Walnut Creek: AltaMira Press.

Creswell, John W. 1998. *Qualitative Inquiry and Research Design: Choosing among Five Traditions.* Thousand Oaks, CA: Sage Publications.

Kreuger, R. A. 1994. *Focus Groups: A Practical Guide for Applied Research.* 2nd ed. Thousand Oaks, CA: Sage Publications

Miles, Matthew B., and A. Michael Huberman. 1994. *Qualitative Data Analysis.* Thousand Oaks, CA: Sage Publications.

Morgan, David L. 1997. *Focus Groups as Qualitative Research.* Thousand Oaks, CA: Sage Publications.

Morse, Janice M., and Peggy Anne Field. 1995. *Qualitative Research Methods for Health Professionals.* Thousand Oaks, CA: Sage Publications.

Rubin, Herbert J., and Irene S. Rubin. 1995. *Qualitative Interviewing: The Art of Hearing Data.* Thousand Oaks, CA: Sage Publications.

APPENDIX B

Examples of Medical and Ethics-Related Journals that Publish Qualitative Research

Advanced Nursing Science

American Behavioral Scientist

Archives of Family Medicine

Cambridge Quarterly of Health Care Ethics

Culture, Medicine and Psychiatry

European Journal of Cancer Care

Family Medicine

Family Practice Research Journal

Hastings Center Report

Health Communication

Heart and Lung

HEC (Health Care Ethics Committee) Forum

Holistic Nursing Practice

Humane Health Care International

IRB

Journal of the American Medical Association

Journal of Applied Behavioral Science

Journal of Clinical Ethics

Journal of Genetic Counseling

Journal of Medical Ethics

Journal of Medicine and Philosophy Journal of Pediatric Nursing

Journal of Public Health Medicine

Journal of Social and Behavioral Sciences

Neonatal Network

Nursing Ethics

Nursing Management
Nursing Research
Patient Education and Counseling
Psychiatry: Interpersonal and Biological Processes
Psychotherapy
Qualitative Family Research
Qualitative Health Research
Qualitative Inquiry
Qualitative Sociology
Research on Social Work Practice
Social Science and Medicine
The Gerontologist
The Qualitative Report
Western Journal of Nursing Research

10

Ethnographic Methods

Patricia Loomis Marshall and Barbara A. Koenig

In recent years, qualitative research approaches, including ethnographic methods, have been used to examine issues in medical ethics such as decisions at the end of life (Orona, Koenig, and Davis 1994; Koenig 1997; Hern et al. 1998); decision making in neonatal intensive care units (Anspach 1993; Levin 1986; Lock 1995); human organ and tissue replacement therapies (Sharp 1995; Hogle 1999; Marshall and Daar, 2000); informed consent (Kaufert and O'Neil 1990; Barnes et al. 1998); and human genetics (Bosk 1992; Rabinow 1999; Rapp 1999; Press and Browner 1998).

Ethnography refers to the description of cultural systems, or an aspect of a culture, based on fieldwork in which the investigator is immersed in the ongoing, everyday activities of the designated cultural community for the purpose of describing the social contexts, networks, relationships, and processes relevant to the topic under consideration. In its broadest articulation, ethnographic inquiry focuses attention on beliefs, values, rituals, customs, and behaviors of individuals interacting within socioeconomic, religious, political, and geographic environments.

In their reviews of the foundational schema of bioethics, anthropologists who typically take an ethnographic approach have criticized work in medical ethics for its lack of attention to the lived experience of illness, suffering, and death (Marshall 1992b; Kleinman 1995; Muller 1994; Marshall and Koenig 1996). Kleinman (1995) argues that an anthropological—in particular an ethnographic—approach to medical ethics has the potential to expand conventional perspectives through cultural analysis of moral conflicts found within unique local worlds. Marshall, Koenig, Levin, Brown, and other anthropologists illustrate how ethnographic approaches to ethical questions can both elicit and help clarify the uncertain, ambiguous, and contextual features that are intrinsic to problematic moral issues that arise in clinical care and medical research (Koenig 1988; Marshall 1996; Marshall et al. 1998b; Levin 1999; Brown 1994).

In the field of medical ethics, there is a heightened awareness of the importance of ethnographic attention to moral dilemmas encountered in the social worlds in which scientific technologies are conceived and applied. A small number of scholars (Hoffmaster 1992; Jennings 1990; Conrad 1994) have begun to challenge ethicists to incorporate ethnographic approaches in their philosophical research. Hoffmaster (1992,1421), for example, argues that, "What is needed is a different brand of moral theory, one that is more closely allied with and faithful to real-life moral phenomena. Ethnography has a vital role to play in developing a more empirically grounded theory of morality."

Indicative of the appreciation for contextualized and meaning-centered perspectives on medical morality, a number of medical ethicists have argued that ethics is essentially an interpretive enterprise (Carson 1990; Churchill 1990; Thomasma 1994). Advocates of hermeneutical explorations of medical morality make explicit the interpretive nature of understanding ethical issues in science and medicine. Carson (1990), for example, proposed a multifaceted framework for considering moral questions in medical care. His framework incorporates elements of hermeneutics, casuistry, practical reasoning, and "thick description" (see Geertz 1973) of cases. The development of contextual models in medical ethics has the potential to bridge some of the fundamental tensions between the context-rich perspectives of the humanities and social sciences and the abstract reasoning associated with traditional philosophical approaches to ethical questions in medicine. Ethnographic and other qualitative approaches employed in medical ethics research provide methodological opportunities for achieving greater sensitivity to social context. In this chapter, we describe the relevance of ethnography to medical ethics research. We begin with a brief comparison of quantitative and qualitative methodologies in research. We then identify ethnographic research strategies and discuss the strengths and weaknesses of ethnographic methods. Finally, drawing on our own research experiences, we summarize two ethnographic studies exploring issues in medical ethics. One study examines end-of-life decision making among ethnically diverse cancer patients; the other study explores the process of implementing clinical ethics consultation in hospital settings. These studies demonstrate the power of ethnographic inquiry to reveal the meaning attached to beliefs and behavior, thus enhancing our understanding of the moral dimensions of medical care. We argue that ethnography in medical ethics research—either alone or in combination with other methods—has the capacity to reveal contextual issues and the deep-seated complexity of moral dilemmas in human lives.

QUANTITATIVE AND QUALITATIVE METHODS IN RESEARCH

Quantitative and qualitative research approaches are often described in oppositional terms. *Quantitative* data gathering methods are characterized as mechanistic, positivistic, deductive, precise, and objective. *Qualitative* research methods, on the other hand, are represented as interpretive, hermeneutical, phenomenological, inductive, imprecise, and subjective. Quantitative research has the goal of examining phenomena apart from the subjective state of the individual researcher, and apart from historical, cultural, and environmental contexts. The results of quantitative research methods are used to test hypotheses and make generalizations using statistical analysis. In contrast, qualitative research methods provide an understanding of social phenomena from an individual's or a community's perspective and offer explanations of human behaviors in the local and historical context in which they occur.

While quantitative methodologies are commonly utilized in experimental designs and survey research, qualitative methods are characteristic of ethnography, textual analysis, and historical studies. Indeed, despite differences in underlying theoretical orientations (Geertz 1983; Clifford and Marcus 1986; Denzin and Lincoln 1994; Bernard 1994; Gupta and Ferguson 1997; Denzin 1997), scholars involved in qualitative research rely on similar techniques, including ethnographic methods such as participant observation, individual or group interviews conducted in informal or formal interactions, and analysis of historical or other types of relevant documents (Denzin and Lincoln 1998; Fetterman 1998; Emerson, Freta, and Shaw 1995; Lofland and Lofland 1995; Krueger 1997). The essential phenomenological concern for investigators who use qualitative techniques in their research is recognizing and understanding behavior and beliefs in particular social contexts; intepretation is the primary goal.

In quantitative research, deductive reasoning is used; definitions of specific variables being investigated in a study are determined before the investigation begins. Large sample sizes are necessary to generate statistical power in order to make generalizations across similar populations. In qualitative research, inductive reasoning is used to analyze patterns that emerge from the data collected. Precise definitions of the phenomena under study evolve over time. Because in-depth data are collected, sample sizes tend to be smaller, limiting the potential for generalizability to larger populations.

The conceptual split between quantitative approaches and qualitative, interpretive-phenomenological approaches is pervasive within the biological and social sciences. However, emphasizing the differences between the approaches is neither useful nor productive. Instead, quantitative and qualitative research methods may be used in complementary ways to develop an in-depth and robust understanding of a problem. For example, a study of advance care planning in a hospice program might include a survey of a random sample of patients, their families, and their health providers. In addition, researchers might want to initiate an ethnographic investigation to explore how the evolving relationships among patients, families, and health care staff explain preferences about end-of-life care. In-depth semistructured interviews also might be conducted with a subsample of patients, families, and providers in order to examine in greater detail the issues addressed in the survey. This type of multifaceted research design demonstrates the strategic use of both quantitative and qualitative methods; findings from the ethnographic study and in-depth interviews with survey respondents augment and contextualize survey results (Blackhall et al. 1995; Frank et al. 1998).

ETHNOGRAPHY

The breadth and scope of traditional ethnography illustrates the importance early anthropologists placed on obtaining a holistic view of cultural worlds. In addition, ethnographers emphasize the importance of an *emic* (native) perspective, a perspective that privileges the worldview of members of the "culture" being studied. An important goal of ethnography is to provide a comprehensive and coherent description of cultural practices, symbols, and ideas associated with a particular group or problem at a particular historical moment in time.

A defining feature of ethnography is that it provides an analytical framework for assessing the relationship between practices observed at the local level (e.g., at an institutional, programmatic, or community level) and broader sociocultural, political, and economic phenomena. For example, an ethnographic examination of ethical problems associated with clinical practices observed at a health maintenance organization would take into account the increasing regulatory demands of managed care at the macro-level of organization of medicine in the United States.

Specific definitions of ethnography have been the subject of debate among social scientists for many years. At the heart of the controversy is an ideological divide that separates those investigators for whom ethnography represents a broad philosophical paradigm and others who view it simply as a methodology that is used when appropriate (Hammersley and Atkinson 1995; Atkinson 1994). Early in the twentieth century, under the considerable influence of Bronislaw Malinowski in Great Britain and Franz Boas in the United States, ethnographic fieldwork became the methodological foundation of cultural anthropology. Malinowski (1961), renowned for his ethnographic descriptions of the Trobriand Islands in the South Pacific, was clear about the ethnographer's task: "Find out the typical ways of thinking and feeling, corresponding to the institutions and culture of a given community and formulate the results in the most convincing way." Thus, documenting, analyzing, and reporting the relationship between meaning and observable action in the context of local worlds is the core of an ethnographer's job. In the development of the field of anthropology throughout the twentieth century, scholars have emphasized various aspects of the enthnographic enterprise, including the focus of its inquiry and the nature of its underlying purpose (Tyler 1996; Geertz 1973; Marcus and Fischer 1986; Harris 1968). In 1973, Clifford Geertz published *The Interpretation of Cultures*, in which he argued that ethnographers practice what he called "thick description"—descriptions of events, beliefs, and behavior, with sufficient attention to *local background and meaning*, so that they are comprehensible from the perspective of the people involved (Geertz 1973).

In the last two decades, increasing attention has been given to the importance of critical self-reflexivity in writing ethnographies. Scholars such as Clifford and Marcus (1986) and, more recently, Denzin and Lincoln (1994), argue that it is impossible to write an "objective" account of someone else's cultural world because ethnographers bring to an investigation their own cultural constructions and their own worldviews and assumptions about the meaning of cultural practices and beliefs in particular social contexts. Thus, an ethnographer's account is necessarily a second-hand account—a description of a cultural problem filtered through the interpretive lens of the ethnographer. Given the inevitability of our own cultural socialization, it is imperative that ethnographers maintain a reflective posture concerning their own beliefs and values. The researcher openly reveals how his or her background shapes interpretation.

Hammersley and Atkinson (1995) suggest that, practically speaking, ethnography refers to forms of social research that include the following features:

> a strong emphasis on exploring the nature of particular social phenomena, rather than setting out to test hypotheses about them; a tendency to work primarily with "unstructured" data, that is data that have not been coded at the point of data collection in terms of a closed set of analytic categories; investigation of a small number of cases perhaps just one case, in detail; analysis of data that involves explicit interpretation of the meanings and functions of human actions, the product of which

mainly takes the form of verbal descriptions and explanations, with quantification and statistical analysis playing a subordinate role at most.

Researchers utilizing ethnographic methods employ a combination of different approaches, including participant observation, various kinds of ethnographic interviews, focus groups, archival research, life histories, diaries, and other personal documents. In this chapter, we focus on participant observation and ethnographic interviews (see chapter 9 for further discussion of some of these other qualitative methods issues).

Participant Observation

Participant observation is the cornerstone of ethnographic research and is characterized by a period of intense social interaction and engagement between the researcher and individuals involved in the study, during which time data (e.g., field note observations, interview results, archival materials) are systematically collected. There are several examples of classic medical ethnographies in which participant observation was used to examine moral dimensions of clinical care and biomedical practice. In 1959, Renee Fox used participant observation with patients and staff on a hospital ward, focusing particularly on the work of physicians involved in refining treatments for metabolic diseases. Charles Bosk's (1979) classic text *Forgive and Remember* is based on intensive participant observation during fieldwork conducted with surgeons to understand the nature of medical mistakes in the process of professional socialization. During his fieldwork, Bosk spent considerable time with the surgeons and surgical residents, in formal and informal settings, attending rounds, and observing surgical operations.

More recently, ethnographies of neonatal intensive care units have incorporated participant observation techniques to demonstrate how moral dilemmas evolve within the cultural framework of biomedicine in caring for critically ill newborns (Guillemin and Holmstrom 1986; Anspach 1987; Jennings 1990). These investigations have shown that, despite the emphasis on an idealized partnership between parents and the health care team, physicians' opinions about therapeutic interventions often override the views of parents. Moreover, these ethnographies illustrate that evaluative judgments of an infant's diagnosis and prognosis are culturally and professionally situated. Anspach (1987) for example, observed that nurses' judgments of a baby's future condition were based on sustained interactions with the infant, while physicians relied primarily on diagnostic information from test results to determine the infant's prognosis.

Participant observation is characterized by a continuum of roles, depending upon the context of the research, the relationships developed in the process of conducting the research, and the experience and background of the ethnographer. In some investigations, observation, rather than participation, may be the dominant model applied. For example, in an ethnographic study of factors contributing to staff anger toward adolescent psychiatric patients hospitalized on locked wards, the investigators were primarily observers, documenting behavior and affect of staff and patients during routine activities such as group therapy sessions, meals, and "free" time (Scheinfeld et al. 1989). Although the ethnographers participated in informal conversations on the psychiatric units with staff and patients, they were not actively engaged as participants during group therapy or other formal activities.

In other situations, ethnographers may be more active as participants because of the nature of the research and the opportunities to develop relationships with participants, or because of the ethnographer's role in the community being studied. In a study of end-of-life decision making among ethnically diverse cancer patients, Koenig and the ethnographers involved in the study developed close personal relationships with a number of the participants and their families (Orona, Keonig, and Davis 1994; Hern et al. 1998; Barnes et al. 1998). Under these circumstances, it was not uncommon for the ethnographers to provide transportation to and from the hospital or to assist the families in other ways when possible.

A different articulation of the ethnographer as observer and participant is illustrated in a study conducted by Marshall on decision making surrounding which patients were considered to be appropriate candidates for heart transplantation. In weekly meetings of the Cardiac Transplant Team, it was decided who would be placed on the "list" to receive a cardiac transplant. Handwritten notes were taken during the meeting; additional comments were recorded after the meeting ended. Although Marshall was primarily an observer of the interactions that took place, because she was involved in the clinical activities of the medical center as an ethics consultant, occasionally she would volunteer or be asked for information, or an opinion, on a patient with whom she was familiar. In this sense, Marshall was both a participant and observer at the weekly meetings of the Cardiac Transplant Team.

Although ethnographers using participant observation may begin a research project with a substantive or theoretical question, the particular focus of their inquiry evolves as they become acclimated to the field. For example, in her exploration of decisions about heart transplantation, Marshall's ongoing analysis of the ethnographic field notes revealed an interesting dynamic that occurred in situations of medical ambiguity (Marshall 1992a). If a physician was invested in pursuing a cardiac transplant for a patient, but results of medical tests did not clearly support a heart transplant, then a process of "character construction" began to unfold. This process involved a systematic attempt to promote a view of the patient as someone of "good moral character," someone who was "worthy" of the transplant. In one case, a mother of four young children was being evaluated for a heart transplant. The medical evidence to support transplantation was marginal. Her cardiologist began to call upon others at the meeting—cardiology nurses, the social worker, the pastoral care counselor—to provide "evidence" that would support the image of a "good mother," a woman whose young children depended on her ability to provide for them in the future. The "evidence" presented was used to support a favorable decision for the patient. Marshall did not begin her fieldwork with the intention of examining the process of constructing a "virtuous" character in situations of medical uncertainty; instead, this process became evident through her systematic review and analysis of field observations of the meetings throughout the year. Ethnographers routinely move between analyzing ongoing field observations and using the results of analysis to go back to the "field" for further exploration of the issues that emerge.

Ethnographic Interviews

Ethnographic interviews are designed to elicit an individual's interpretation of events, beliefs, and behavior; special attention is given to the meanings attached to cultural symbols and activities. Different types of interviews may be used in an ethnographic study, depending upon the context and the kind of information the researcher seeks.

Informal Ethnographic Interviews

Informal ethnographic interviews are characterized by a lack of structure or control; these are conversations the researcher may have with individuals during the course of daily fieldwork. Informal interviewing may be used while getting settled in the field or can be used throughout the ethnographic study to build rapport or explore newly emerging topics of interest. Notes from informal interviews may be taken in the field, then fleshed out later in the day as one records more substantive descriptions.

Unstructured Ethnographic Interviews

Unstructured ethnographic interviews, in contrast to informal interviews, have a topical focus but are marked by minimal control over the informants' responses. An ethnographer working in the area of HIV prevention among injection drug users, for example, may use unstructured interviews to explore beliefs and practices associated with obtaining informed consent for participation in HIV prevention studies (Strenski et al. 2000). While the general topic has been defined, there is no attempt to follow a predetermined line of inquiry. In an unstructured ethnographic interview, the conversation follows the direction taken by the ethnographer based on the responses of the interviewee. Notes or audio recordings may be taken during the interview, or details of the discussion may be written following the interview.

Semistructured Interview

In a *semistructured interview*, a written guide is used to help the ethnographer in systematically reviewing a particular set of issues. Questions are preestablished and are often followed by leads (for probes) for exploring the topic in greater detail. Semistructured interviews might be used in situations in which the researcher has only one opportunity to interview someone or needs to be sure that the same data are collected from all informants. Marshall used semistructured interviews in a recent case study exploring the process of informed consent for genetic epidemiological research conducted in Nigeria (Marshall 2000). A set of questions was designed to elicit information on the procedures used by tribal chiefs to let the community know that a health care study would be taking place. Respondents often would begin by providing one approach to informing the community. Additional questions elicited a range of possible strategies for alerting the community about upcoming research. This information would not have been easily accessible using a survey or questionnaire with forced choice responses.

Structured Interviews

Structured interviews are characterized by asking all research participants an identical set of questions through the use of a detailed interview schedule. A set of explicit instructions is developed for interviewers who administer the questionnaires. Interviewers normally undergo a period of training in which they learn how to conduct the interview. Attention is given to the importance of adhering to the questions laid out in the instrument, collecting the data in a systematic fashion, and avoiding leading questions (i.e., the way in which the question is phrased suggests the answer).

Key Informant Ethnographic Interviews

Key informant ethnographic interviews are those interviews conducted with carefully selected individuals knowledgeable about the topic being explored. A semistructured interviewing guide is often used in these interviews. In the Nigerian case study mentioned above, a list of key informants was identified that included research investigators and physicians involved in the epidemiological studies, individuals who obtained informed consent from potential participants, and participants in the research. These interviews helped to identify ethical issues relevant to the process of obtaining informed consent for genetic epidemiological research from the perspective of individuals with diverse roles in the implementation of the studies. As research progresses, ethnographers often return frequently to key informants, using a series of informal interviews to aid understanding. Key informant interviews often are conducted in the early stages of an ethnographic or quantitative study to help clarify the focus of the inquiry and to provide useful information for the development of subsequent interview guides or surveys.

Focus Groups

Focus groups may also be useful early in a study. Focus groups involve conversations with small groups of individuals selected on the basis of specific criteria to discuss a particular topic (e.g., a sample of women with known risk factors for breast cancer; family members caring for an elderly parent with Alzheimer's disease; scientists involved in international collaborative health research; and so on). The number of individuals included in a focus group varies, although experts recommend that smaller numbers—between six and ten individuals—provide a comfortable environment for eliciting information from participants. A moderator facilitates discussion using a flexible interview guide. The discussion may continue for one to two hours and is audiotaped and transcribed. (See chapter 9 for more information on focus group interviews.)

VALIDITY AND RELIABILITY IN QUALITATIVE RESEARCH

Validity refers to the credibility and accuracy of the basic concepts used, the instruments developed, the data collected, and the findings obtained in a study. *Reliability* refers to the capacity to obtain the same findings in repeat measurements. A number of approaches are used in determining validity in research. Investigators applying either qualitative or quantitative methods determine *face validity* by examining the operational indicators of the concepts being examined to decide if they make sense "on the face of it." Another method of determining validity is *triangulation*; this involves the use of multiple methods and diverse data sources to cross-check data. For example, in an ethnographic study being conducted on practices associated with advance directives in a hospital intensive care unit, results of in-depth interviews with patients might be compared with the results of key informant interviews and reviews of medical records to determine the validity of the concepts used and the data collected. Investigators may also conduct *member checks* to determine validity.

Member checks refer to the process of feeding back results of analyses to key informants in order to verify and affirm interpretations of the data collected. This may be accomplished by informal interviewing. Validity is a particular strength of ethnographic research because the concepts developed are based on direct interaction with research subjects.

Ethnographers cross-check the validity of coding categories used in analyzing text data from interviews and field observations by involving several individuals working independently as judges in coding the data. *Interrater reliability* is high when thematic codes are applied in a consistent and similar pattern.

A threat to reliability in ethnographic research may occur when interview guides are revised in response to new developments in the field. Information may come to light in the course of conducting interviews that necessitates changing the interview guide; changes in instruments, such as the interview field guides, result in what is called *instrumentation confound.* Thus, careful attention must be given to patterns that emerge in data collected when instruments are revised.

An additional threat to reliability occurs when there are a number of different people conducting interviews. Individual styles of interviewing vary, even when an interview guide is used. If one interviewer consistently reports certain data while another interviewer consistently reports contrasting information, it might be an indication of *interviewer bias.* These problems can be diminished when interviewers are trained to conduct the interview similarly, to see things, ask questions, and record them in more or less the same way. In ethnographic research where there are multiple interviewers, careful attention to training enhances data reliability.

Tradeoffs between validity and reliability must always be made. Data collection techniques that change over time enhance validity but may sacrifice reliability, making both analysis and interpretation of data complex.

STRENGTHS AND WEAKNESSES OF
ETHNOGRAPHIC METHODS

Perhaps the strongest contribution that ethnographic methods make in medical ethics research is that they provide the investigator with tools for uncovering and illuminating the complexity of meanings underlying behavior. Ethnographic research strategies accommodate the complicated social interactions and experiences of everyday life. In this way, social process is highlighted. Ethnography allows the researcher to make an in-depth exploration of moral dilemmas. Ethnography and related qualitative methods also enable researchers to contextualize quantitative results, augmenting the findings with experiential reports and observations. Moreover, the exploratory nature of ethnographic techniques is hypothesis generating. In this way, ethnographic methods can be extremely useful in the preliminary stage of quantitative investigations of clinical issues with ethical implications. Results of ethnographic investigations inform the development of structured interviews, surveys, and other quantitative techniques.

Although ethnography is unquestionably useful in clarifying the nuanced and multifaceted realities of social life, ethnographic methods have a number of limitations. In conducting fieldwork, the investigator is unable to control contingent events. The ethnographer cannot regulate who is involved in activities or what occurs when he or she is observing or participating in ongoing social processes. Fieldwork in clinical settings, in laboratories, or in neighborhood communities is defined by its openness to social process, unconstrained and uncontrived by an investigator's experimental model. Similarly, ethnographic interviews allow for the emergence of new avenues of exploration even when the investigator is pursuing a clear direction using an interview guide. Study variables are not predefined to the extent that they are in quantitative research, and this limits the amount of control the investigator has over the specific factors examined.

Another limitation associated with ethnography is that study samples tend to be smaller than when quantitative methods are used to test hypotheses and generalize the results to similar populations. Ethnographers can speak in detail about a particular group of people in a specific social setting, but their ability to generalize beyond the study sample is limited. It is important to note that generalizable results are never the main aim of ethnographic inquiry. In addition, unlike quantitative methods, ethnographic approaches are time consuming to implement. Ethnographers spend considerable time familiarizing themselves with the study site, conducting field observations, recording field notes, and implementing in-depth ethnographic interviews. Analyzing transcript data from field notes is significantly more labor intensive than conducting statistical analyses of survey data. Even when computer software programs such as Ethnograph or NUD*IST are used to assist in the analysis, the ethnographer must develop coding categories for open-ended responses to questions or notes from field observations.

Finally, there is the challenge of objectivity. Some critics argue that the subjective and experiential nature of ethnography and the data it provides is "unscientific"—that ethnographic approaches lack the rigor of an experimental design. Ethnographers tend to be unapologetic about their methods, observing correctly that the purpose of ethnography is not to predefine a patient's experience or categorically to set limits on a social domain. Indeed, it is the very absence of these features that allows for the unique expression of a participant's perspective and for the study of social behavior in natural settings. Thus, ethnography offers a framework for collecting and interpreting data that is paradigmatically different from quantitative methods. A good ethnographer acknowledges the limitations that necessarily constrain and influence the study results. Experienced ethnographers do not attempt to overgeneralize from the data collected and actively maintain a posture of reflexivity to enhance their awareness of possible biases.

PROTECTION OF HUMAN SUBJECTS IN ETHNOGRAPHIC RESEARCH

The implementation of ethnographic research requires careful attention to the protection of human subjects. Ethnographers confront unique ethical challenges because of the unstructured nature of participant observation and because of the types of interviews conducted, which often involve the collection of sensitive information concerning an individual's personal life (Marshall et al. 1998a; Marshall 1992a; Kayser-Jones and Koenig 1994; Singer et al. 1999). The range of problems includes obtaining informed consent, respecting confidentiality and privacy, and determining whether or not to intervene in a situation that occurs while in the field.

A number of questions must be addressed regarding informed consent for ethnographic research: Is written consent necessary, or will oral consent suffice? When group observations are conducted, who should be asked to provide consent? Informed consent is an interactive process between investigators and potential subjects to insure voluntary participation based upon a clear understanding of the purpose of the research, the procedures and methods of data collection, and the risks associated with participation. Deciding whether or not to seek written or oral consent is a judgment based on the nature of the research, the context of the study, and the seriousness of the risks involved for participants, both risks arising from the research and those created by signing an informed consent document. In some cases, oral consent may be warranted (e.g., if participants are illiterate or vulnerable because of their legal status or involvement in illicit activities, or if the research is conducted in a cultural setting in which signing a document to participate in research is viewed as inappropriate). However, Institutional Review Boards (IRBs) unfamiliar with ethnography may require written consent for ethnographic studies, even when the circumstances require sensitivity to the vulnerability of participants or to the cultural context of the research. For example, in an ethnographic and epidemiological study of the indirect benefits of participating in a syringe exchange program, the IRB at the medical center sponsoring the study required signed consent forms for all injection drug users participating in the research (Strenski et al. 2000). Moreover, after conferring with legal representatives at the medical center, the IRB insisted that the consent form state that, although a federal "Certificate of Confidentiality" (Comprehensive Drug Abuse and Control Act of 1970, Public Law No. 91–513, Section 3[a]) had been obtained, confidentiality could not be guaranteed if there was a court order to secure research records. Despite the strong language included in the informed consent document, to date none of the more than two hundred injection drug users involved in this ethnographic study have refused to sign the form.

In ethnographic research involving direct observation of group activities, arrangements usually are made *before* the initiation of the study to inform group members that the ethnographer will be present in the course of routine activities. In closed systems such as a hospital unit, an outpatient clinic, or a laboratory, informed consent should be obtained from all those who are at the facility on a regular basis, including staff, patients, and family members. For example, in an ethnographic study of a cardiac transplant unit, informed consent should be obtained from all patients, members of their family, and staff. Other individuals who are not present on a regular basis, but whose behavior may be observed in public group activities, should be alerted to the presence of an ethnographer if it is feasible to do so. Informed consent always should be obtained from individuals in the group who are interviewed.

In some group observations, it may not be possible or necessary to obtain informed consent from every person present. For example, at informal gatherings of family members or staff at a nurses' station in a busy unit of a medical center, it would be intrusive to introduce the ethnographer and explain the study to every person who passed by. On the other hand, an ethnographer's presence at a family conference for an ethics consultation should be explained and permission should be obtained to observe the proceedings; if any of the family or members of the staff are uncomfortable with the observation, the ethnographer should leave. A good rule to follow is that in private interactions such as these, informed consent—not necessarily documented with a written form—should be obtained from everyone present. In public places where individuals interact informally, however, it is less important to obtain consent from everyone, and it may be impossible.

Protection of confidentiality and privacy for research participants is important in any investigation. The data collection strategies associated with ethnography require careful attention to the representation of individuals and communities in written transcripts derived from interviews and observations. Descriptive data collected by the ethnographer are recorded in field notes, daily logs, or diaries, using a coding system that protects the confidentiality of the research participants. Data collected in the field must also be secured out of the field setting to safeguard the identity of participants, especially if they are involved in deviant or illegal activities. In published manuscripts that include case narratives, pseudonyms are used rather than participants' names. This gesture, however, will not necessarily protect confidentiality because it may be possible to identify the individuals involved based on the details of the case and the research setting. At each stage of the research—data collection, data analysis, and data reporting—every effort should be made to protect the privacy of the study participants. Individuals participating in ethnographic research must be advised during the informed consent process about the methods being employed to protect their privacy.

The question of whether the ethnographer should intervene in a problematic situation that occurs in the course of conducting ethnographic observations can be difficult. Once again, it is a judgment based on the purpose of the study, the context, and the specific event that occurs (Kayser-Jones and Koenig 1994). If ethnographers were to intervene continually in field situations that are directly related to the issue being investigated, the possibility that their research will have an impact is jeopardized since they would be unable to document the events being studied.

In some ethnographic studies, however, intervention may be the correct course of action. For example, in her two-year investigation of the technological imperative in medical practice, Koenig (1988) conducted extensive observational fieldwork on the introduction and application of therapeutic plasma exchange (TPE), at that time an innovative treatment for autoimmune diseases. In addition to conducting interviews with key participants involved in therapeutic plasma exchange research and development, Koenig was a participant observer in TPE units and observed numerous treatments as they were carried out. An incident occurred in the course of her studies in which the TPE blood tubing broke while a patient was undergoing treatment. Koenig was the only other person in the room; she acted quickly and clamped off the machine, thereby preventing the patient from losing a large volume of blood. Her background in nursing, combined with her understanding of the TPE process, enabled her to prevent a crisis for the patient.

In addition to obstacles regarding informed consent, confidentiality, and interventions in ongoing field activities, ethnographers must address questions that arise in the course of obtaining approval from IRBs at local study sites. Most IRBs do not have members with expertise in ethnographic methods. This often leads to confusion and misunderstandings concerning the research design and the protocols for implementing the study. Individuals considering the use of ethnographic methods in medical ethics research should not make assumptions about the IRB's capacity to adequately evaluate ethnographic research. Instead, investigators might consider contacting the chair of the IRB to discuss questions that may arise in the IRB's discussion of the study. In preparing their research protocols, ethnographers need to be explicit about strategies for protecting participants from unintentional risks and harms associated with the study.

CASE EXAMPLES OF ETHNOGRAPHIC STUDIES IN MEDICAL ETHICS RESEARCH

In this section, two cases illustrate how ethnography can be used in exploration of issues in medical ethics. The first case demonstrates how ethnographic methods reveal intracultural variations in response to practices associated with end-of-life decision making among Latino cancer patients. The second case illustrates the power of ethnography for discerning the complex social processes surrounding ethics consultations. In both cases, all proper names have been changed to pseudonyms.

Case One: Decisions at the End of Life among Ethnically Diverse Cancer Patients

In the last decade, investigators have begun to examine the influence of ethnicity and cultural traditions on end-of-life decision making, including the disclosure of a diagnosis of terminal illness and approaches to advance care planning (Orona, Koenig, and Davis 1994; Blackhall et al. 1995; Carrese and Rhodes 1995; Murphy et al. 1996). Results of these studies suggest a consistent trend in which individuals from "minority" backgrounds are less likely to adopt the autonomy-based practices that have become standard procedure in many U.S. hospitals and clinics. These findings raise important questions concerning how clinicians and medical ethicists *should* take account of ethnicity and what often are perceived as "cultural barriers" in clinical settings. When treating a patient from a Korean, Chinese, or Mexican background, should the clinician infer that patients will not desire information about their prognosis, or that they will not want to execute a durable power of attorney for health care? Should clinicians assume that African Americans will want all medical interventions continued when the patient is near death, even when interventions might be considered by others to be futile? The use of empirical studies to predict patients' responses to medical decision making based on their ethnic background is problematic. Both quantitative and qualitative studies reveal consistent trends, yet only ethnography has the power to explicate the range of responses identified in survey data (Frank et al. 1998). In the worst case scenario, superficial stereotypes are perpetuated and can seriously undermine patient care. Not all individuals will follow a particular norm; intracultural variation is inevitable. The following ethnographic study on decision making among ethnically diverse cancer patients demonstrates that a patient's cultural background is of vital importance and must be carefully assessed.

Participants in the study were recruited from an outpatient clinic affiliated with a large, urban public hospital in California (Orona, Koenig, and Davis 1994). At the time of recruitment, all patients had been diagnosed with incurable cancer and their prognosis for survival was approximately six months. Individuals were assigned to cultural categories based on their self-identification as African American, Chinese-American, European-American, or Hispanic/Latino.

In this investigation, a case portfolio was prepared for each patient. Each case study included a set of in-depth, semistructured interviews with the patient, two family members, and two members of the health care team (one physician and one nonphysician, e.g., social worker, nurse). Interviews were audiorecorded and transcribed. Those interviews conducted in Cantonese or Spanish were translated into English for analysis. Interviews with patients, family members, and health care providers were designed to elicit an illness narrative, which was then followed up with specific questions and probes dealing with end-of-life decision making. Observational research was conducted during clinic sessions.

To illustrate the relevance of culture in making decisions at the end of life, two case narratives, one involving a man from El Salvador and the other a woman from Nicaragua, are presented (Marshall et al. 1998a).

Mr. Samuel Hurtado

Mr. Samuel Hurtado, a fifty-four-year-old Salvadorian, has lived in the United States for six years, has a high school education, and has worked in a variety of jobs, including tailoring and dish washing. Mr. Hurtado says he speaks some English but does not understand it very well. During his clinic visits, his daughter-in-law or someone from the clinic acts as his interpreter. Mr. Hurtado was diagnosed with multiple myeloma. He has used a variety of therapies to treat both the pain and the cancer, including visits to a chiropractor and acupuncturist, oral garlic and lemon juices, and intramuscular injections of pain medicine that he continues to buy in El Salvador. He has received repeated rounds of radiation and chemotherapy both in California and El Salvador.

Mr. Hurtado reports that it was extremely difficult for him to accept that his illness made it impossible for him to remain employed, as this has had serious consequences for his familial relationships and financial obligations. Mr. Hurtado displays a number of strategies for either maintaining hope or expressing denial when he discusses his prognosis. For example, he says that the doctors told him that there was no cure and he believes that he has accepted the cancer. Yet, at another point in the conversation he says, "The disease is not going to kill me. I am going to defeat the disease. I have faith."

Mr. Hurtado's daughter-in-law concurs with Mr. Hurtado's statements that his family refers to his illness as "cancer" and that everyone in the family knows about it. She goes on to relate what happened at the clinic visit when the oncologist first told her, as translator, to tell her father-in-law that he had approximately eight months to live. Because she was only a relative by marriage, she did not feel it was her place to give him that information, so she did not translate it, but instead went home and told her husband what the doctor had said. Her husband told his mother, the patient's wife, who then told the patient. Thus, Mr. Hurtado was eventually told what the physician had said, but only through channels considered appropriate and acceptable to the family. The daughter-in-law also states that although the family members know that the father's prognosis is short and they discuss it among themselves, they do not talk about the prognosis with Mr. Hurtado, believing that it is more merciful to withhold such painful information.

Mr. Hurtado states that no one has discussed resuscitation with him, but goes on to suggest that if he had a heart attack, he would want his doctor to let him die because he does not want to create problems for his family. Mr. Hurtado denies that anyone has discussed advance directives with him, and suggests the issue has not come up because, "Perhaps they haven't seen the need to do so." In fact, many patients in the study assumed that treatment would continue as long as they were alive, thus making resuscitation or advance directive decisions unnecessary from their perspective. On the other hand, it is not uncommon for health care providers to routinely postpone talking about advance directive issues until patients are hospitalized, at which time they may be too sick to discuss their wishes. Indeed, Dr. Green, Mr. Hurtado's oncologist, acknowledges that he has not discussed advance directives or resuscitation issues with Mr. Hurtado, stating repeatedly that resuscitation conversations do not come up at the clinic but usually are reserved for the hospital when the patient becomes critically ill. Dr. Green observes with some frustration that, "We convince people to say they do not want to be resuscitated." Many factors—not necessarily related to ethnic diversity—may contribute to the delay in speaking with patients about end-of-life decisions, including time pressures or the discomfort experienced by some physicians when faced with the possibility of discussing death and dying.

When interviewed, the daughter-in-law comments that no health care provider has discussed advance directives with Mr. Hurtado while she was present, but that resuscitation questions did come up during one visit. She says that Mr. Hurtado was first questioned about his resuscitation wishes without a translator being present, and that he was upset because he thought they were telling him that he was going to die. At a subsequent visit, the daughter-in-law asked about the incident and a nurse described her understanding of Mr. Hurtado's choice should he need to be resuscitated.

The conflicting reports of whether or not a discussion about advance directives occurred with Mr. Hurtado, and the conflicting views about what exactly was said, illustrate how complicated it is to "speak the truth" about advance care planning for death. There will always be multiple perspectives on events or discussions that take place in the course of planning for end-of-life care. Mr. Hurtado's case narrative reveals the complexity of cultural background and the complicated way it is expressed in the course of routine cancer treatment. Discussions about end-of-life care and treatment decisions are shown to be embedded in the constraints of his everyday life, including his relationship with his family.

Ms. Irene Guerrera

Irene Guerrera is a sixty-four-year-old woman from Nicaragua who has lived in the United States over twenty years. She has had no formal education, and worked in domestic service in a private home until diagnosed with breast cancer with bone metastasis. Ms. Guerrera's closest support person is her employer, whom she describes as "family." Her only other family members live elsewhere in the United States or remain in Nicaragua.

Ms. Guerrera describes herself as an "independent" decision-maker and discusses her diagnosis openly with clinic oncologists, nurses, and social workers. However, when her sister was coming to visit, Ms. Guerrera revealed that she had not told her family in Nicaragua that she was sick and that she did not want them to know that she had cancer. Ms. Guerrera believes she will die from the disease; she is active in a cancer support group, and is deeply religious, identifying herself as "very Catholic." She says that she will "die according to God's will." Ms. Guerrera has indicated she does not want to be resuscitated or kept alive on machines. In interviews with the project team, she names her former employer as the person to make decisions for her if she were unable to do so. Her last wish is that she be able to return to Nicaragua to die.

Ms. Rolinsky, Ms. Guerrera's former employer, agrees that Ms. Guerrera is an independent decision-maker, that she is aware of her grim prognosis, and that her deep religious faith is helping Ms. Guerrera to cope. Ms. Rolinsky says that the patient's family views her as the alternate decision-maker for Ms. Guerrera. However, to her knowledge, a legal document has not been signed naming her as Ms. Guerrera's durable power of attorney for health care. Ms. Rolinsky does not know if resuscitation has been discussed with the patient.

Dr. Carlson, Ms. Guerrera's oncologist, also acknowledges that Ms. Guerrera is an independent decision-maker. He understands that Ms. Guerrera does not want to be resuscitated and that her primary wish is to return to Nicaragua to die. Dr. Carlson says that they have discussed these decisions openly and that he agreed that he will tell her, "when the game is up . . . when it's not worth doing [treatment] anymore." Dr. Carlson indicates that durable power of attorney issues only have been discussed briefly and concedes that this issue is generally handled by the social worker. He says that Ms. Guerrera is unsure whom she would appoint as a proxy decision-maker.

Individual Differences

The narratives of Mr. Hurtado and Ms. Guerrera illustrate how cultural background influences end-of-life decision making. However, very different portraits emerge for each patient. Ms. Guerrera characterizes herself and is described by others as self-reliant and independent, with a strong desire to be involved in the process of decision making about her medical treatment. In contrast, Mr. Hurtado's narrative reveals more "traditional" values concerning the need to protect the patient from information or decisions that might cause emotional pain or discomfort. These two distinct representations of the relationship between cultural background and end-of-life care call attention to the importance of recognizing intracultural variation and the limitations of broad ethnic categories such as "Latino" for predicting response to medical decision making. As the case narratives illustrate, there is considerable diversity in beliefs about end-of-life care among patients who appear to share a similar cultural heritage. The ethnographic approach used in this study made possible the in-depth look at the complex interaction between ethnic background and treatment decisions among cancer patients at the end of life.

Case Two: Clinical Ethics Consultation

Clinical ethics consultation services provided by individual consultants or hospital ethics committees offer an important mechanism for resolving moral dilemmas that occur in medical practice. In the field of medical ethics, there are ongoing debates about the goals and practices of ethics consultation. Investigators have addressed a broad range of issues, including the professional background and training of consultants, patient and family participation, and legal issues that arise in ethics consultations (Baylis 1994; La Puma and Schiedermayer 1994; Fletcher, Quist, and Jonsen 1989). Findings from empirical investigations have been reported (Orr and Moon 1993; Skeel, Self, and Skeel 1993), but few studies have explored the social process of ethics consultation or described contextual factors that encourage or inhibit ethics consults (Marshall 1996; Crigger 1995).

A three-month ethnographic study was conducted at acute-care facilities in a large metropolitan area on the West Coast (Kelly et al. 1997). Data were collected by a medical student working as an ethnographer under the direction and supervision of a medical anthropologist. Ethics consultations and committee proceedings were observed at five facilities: a health maintenance organization, a university hospital, a university-affiliated community hospital, a county hospital, and a Veterans Administration hospital.

Three ethnographic methods of data collection were employed. First, eight ethics committee meetings were observed; field notes were recorded following each observation. Bylaws, mission statements, and committee minutes were reviewed. Additionally, the ethnographer accompanied the ethics consultants and observed the consultation process in order to develop in-depth studies of nine cases where consultations were requested. Second, retrospective chart reviews were conducted for each of the nine consultations. Third, semistructured interviews were completed with all possible individuals involved in the nine cases. Twenty-nine people were interviewed, including fourteen physicians, six nurses, two social workers, two patients, and five family members. Informed consent was obtained from all participants in the study. Field notes and interview transcripts were coded to ensure confidentiality.

Using standard techniques for qualitative analysis of data, four problematic areas were revealed: (1) access to ethics consultation; (2) the contingent and negotiated nature of ethics consults; (3) variable interpretations regarding the key issues involved; and (4) the nature and stability of consensus achieved following the ethics consultation. Results of analysis indicated that local power issues and interpersonal dimensions play an important role in the practice of ethics consultation and the resolution of ethical problems. The investigators found that few of the issues that emerged were ethical in a "formal" sense; issues of communication or problematic power struggles were common. Moreover, findings showed that individuals from outside the hospital milieu were marginalized from the process of the consultation and only rarely given an opportunity to express their concerns.

In this study, important information about the social processes underlying ethics consultation came to light through the systematic application of ethnographic methods. This information would not have been revealed through other empirical methodologies. The use of ethnographic techniques provided opportunities to explore the moral space where difficult ethical problems in patient care are defined, negotiated, and controlled. The discussions and meetings that constitute ethics committee and consultation activities are shown to provide locations for significant ethical "practices" to occur, practices that include the emotional work of grieving in addition to the education of patients, families, and staff about institutional norms and legal requirements. Principle-based discussion of ethical issues was less frequent. As the investigators (Kelly et al. 1997) suggest, this study raises questions about the cultural contexts within which ethics consults are initiated and calls attention to dimensions of ethics committee work.

CONCLUDING COMMENTS

Ethnographic research strategies have enormous potential for the examination of ethical issues that arise in medical practice and in the development and application of scientific technologies. Ethnography and related qualitative methods highlight the phenomenology of moral experience through detailed descriptions of beliefs and behavior in social contexts. Ethnographic research accommodates the complicated social interactions and experiences of everyday life and in this way provides a framework for a deeper and more contextualized understanding of moral challenges in medicine.

Medical ethicists have increasingly recognized the importance of empirical investigations for informing the theoretical basis of moral arguments. Ethnographic accounts of problems in medical ethics offer the possibility of furthering our understanding of the ways in which medical morality is socially constructed and reinvented through cultural practices at particular historical moments.

NOTES ON RESOURCES AND TRAINING

In recent years, the use of ethnographic methods in social science and humanistic research has grown considerably. While this phenomenon has given some scholars reason to celebrate, others are concerned about the appropriation of ethnographic methods by researchers who lack training or experience with ethnographic techniques. The experiential and unstructured aspects of ethnographic fieldwork may invite methodologically naive investigators to pursue an ethnographic research design without the necessary attention to community and institutional issues, protocols for field observation and data analysis, or consideration of ethical dilemmas that may arise in conducting ethnography. Scholars who want to implement ethnographic research but lack experience should familiarize themselves with the literature and enlist the help of others who are trained in conducting ethnography.

In this chapter, we have cited a number of volumes that address a broad range of issues related to ethnographic inquiry. A recent volume edited by Russell Bernard, *Handbook of Methods in Cultural Anthropology* (1998, Thousand Oaks, CA: Altamira Press), provides a strong foundation, including specific information on implementing ethnographic research and analyzing qualitative ethnographic data. Similarly, Norman Denzin and Yvonna Lincoln's edited volume, *Handbook of Qualitative Research* (1994, Thousand Oaks, CA: Sage Publications), offers a thorough treatment of all aspects of qualitative research, including ethnography. Information on computer applications for ethnographic analysis is provided in *Computer Programs for Qualitative Data Analysis* (1995, Thousand Oaks, CA: Sage) by Eben A. Weitzman and Matthew B. Miles.

Two collections of papers address the theoretical dimensions of empirical research in bioethics, with a particular focus on ethnography. A special issue of the journal *Daedalus,* "Bioethics and Beyond" (Vol. 128, No. 4, fall 1999), was edited by Arthur Kleinman, Renee Fox, and Allan Brandt. The *Hastings Center Report* published a series of papers asking, "What can the social scientist contribute to medical ethics?" (Vol. 30, No. 1, Jan./Feb. 2000).

There are a number of websites that provide useful information on books and other resources for ethnographic research design. The following two websites include the extensive list of publications on qualitative and ethnographic methods from Altimira Press and Sage Publications: www.altamirapress.com and www.sagepub.com. The websites for the computer software program called The Ethnograph is found at www.QualisResearch.com.

Individuals interested in training in ethnographic methods have several options in addition to consulting with departments and programs at local universities. For example, the group called Research Talk (e-mail: information@researchtalk.com) offers courses and workshops for individuals with different levels of experience; the training includes an introduction to NUD*IST, a software application for ethnographic analysis. Their Web site address is: www.researchtalk.com. Individuals interested in participating in ethnographic field schools should contact the American Anthropological Association located at 4350 North Fairfax Drive, Suite 640, Arlington, Virginia 22203; phone (703) 528-1902; website: www.aaanet.org.

Research that has incorporated ethnographic methods is published in a wide range of professional journals in the social sciences, education, nursing and, less frequently, medical journals. The following list represents a number of avenues for publication of manuscripts based on qualitative and ethnographic data: (1) *Qualitative Inquiry* (a methods journal); (2) *Qualitative Health Research*, http://www.ualberta.ca/qhr/; (3) *Social Science and Medicine*; (4) *Culture, Medicine and Psychiatry*; (5) *Medical Anthropology Quarterly*; (6) *Sociology of Health and Illness*; (7) *Medical Anthropology*; and (8) *Human Organization*.

Finally, for those interested in learning more about the application of ethnographic techniques, there is an annual conference called "Qualitative Health Research" that is organized by Jan Morse, the editor of the journal of the same name.

REFERENCES

Anspach, R. 1987. "Prognostic Conflict in Life-Death Decisions: The Organization as an Ecology of Knowledge." *Journal of Health and Social Behavior* 28:215–31.

———. 1993. *Deciding Who Lives: Fateful Choices in the Intensive-Care Nursery.* Berkeley: University of California Press.

Atkinson, P. M. 1994. "Ethnography and Participant Observation." In *Handbook of Qualitative Research,* ed. N. Denzin and Y. Lincoln. Thousand Oaks, CA: Sage Publications, pp. 248–61.

Barnes, D. M., A. J. Davis, T. Moran, C. J. Portillo, and B. A. Koenig. 1998. "Informed Consent in a Multi-Cultural Cancer Patient Population: Implications for Nursing Practice." *Nursing Ethics* 5:412–23.

Baylis, F. E., ed. 1994. *The Health Care Ethics Consultant.* Totowa, NJ: Humana Press.

Bernard, H. R. 1994. *Research Methods in Anthropology: Qualitative and Quantitative Approaches.* Thousand Oaks, CA: Sage Publications.

Blackhall, L. J., S. T. Murphy, G. Frank, V. Michel, and S. Azen. 1995. "Ethnicity and Attitudes toward Patient Autonomy." *Journal of the American Medical Association* 274:820–25.

Bosk, C. L. 1979. *Forgive and Remember: Managing Medical Failure.* Chicago: University of Chicago Press.

———. 1992. *All God's Mistakes: Genetic Counseling in a Pediatric Hospital.* Chicago: University of Chicago Press.

Brown, K. 1994. "Outside the Garden of Eden: Rural Values and Health Care Reform." *Cambridge Quarterly of Health Care Ethics* 3:329–37.

Carrese J. A., and L. A. Rhodes. 1995. "Western Bioethics on the Navajo Reservation: Benefit or Harm?" *Journal of the American Medical Association* 274:826–29.

Carson, R. A. 1990. "Interpretive Bioethics: The Way of Discernment." *Theoretical Medicine* 11:51–60.

Churchill, L. 1990. "Hermeneutics in Science and Medicine: A Thesis Understated." *Theoretical Medicine* 11:141–44.

Clifford, J., and G. Marcus, eds. 1986. *Writing Culture: The Poetics and Politics of Ethnography.* Berkeley: University of California Press.

Conrad, P. 1994. "How Ethnography Can Help Bioethics." *Bulletin of Medical Ethics* (May): 13–18.

Crigger, B. J. 1995. "Negotiating the Moral Order: Paradoxes of Ethics Consultation." *Kennedy Institute of Ethics Journal* 5:89–112.

Denzin, N. 1997. *Interpretive Ethnography: Ethnographic Practices in the 21st Century.* Thousand Oaks, CA: Sage Publications.

Denzin, N., and Y. Lincoln. 1994. *Handbook of Qualitative Research.* Thousand Oaks, CA: Sage Publications.

———. 1998. *Collecting and Interpreting Qualitative Materials.* Thousand Oaks, CA: Sage Publications.

Emerson, R., R. Freta, and L. Shaw. 1995. *Writing Ethnographic Fieldnotes.* Chicago: University of Chicago Press.

Fetterman, D. 1998. *Ethnography: Second Edition: Step by Step.* Thousand Oaks, CA: Sage Publications.

Fletcher, J., N. Quist, and A. Jonsen, eds. 1989. *Ethics Consultation in Health Care.* Ann Arbor, MI: Health Administration Press.

Fox, R. 1959. *Experiment Perilous.* New York: Free Press.

Frank, G., L. J. Blackhall, V. Michel, S. T. Murphy, S. P. Azen, and K. Park. 1998. "A Discourse of Relationships in Bioethics: Patient Autonomy and End-of-Life Decision Making among Elderly Korean Americans. *Medical Anthropology Quarterly* 12(4): 403–23.

Geertz, C. 1973. *The Interpretation of Cultures.* New York: Basic Books.

———. 1983. *Local Knowledge: Further Essays in Interpretive Anthropology.* New York: Basic Books.

Guillemin, J. H., and L. L. Holmstrom. 1986. *Mixed Blessings: Intensive Care for Newborns.* New York: Oxford University Press.

Gupta, A., and J. Ferguson, eds. 1997. *Anthropological Locations: Boundaries and Grounds of a Field Science.* Berkeley and Los Angeles: University of California Press.

Hammersley, M., and P. M. Atkinson. 1995. *Ethnography: Principles in Practice.* 2nd ed. New York: Routledge.

Harris, M. 1968. *The Rise of Anthropological Theory: A History of Theories of Culture.* New York: Thomas Y. Crowell.

Hern, H., B. A. Koenig, L. Moore, and P. Marshall. 1998. "The Difference that Culture Can Make in End-of-Life Decision Making." *Cambridge Quarterly of Health Care Ethics* 7:27–40.

Hoffmaster, B. 1992. "Can Ethnography Save the Life of Medical Ethics?" *Social Science and Medicine* 35:1421–32.

Hogle, L. 1999. *Recovering the Nation's Body: Cultural Memory, Medicine, and the Politics of Redemption.* New Brunswick, NJ: Rutgers University Press.

Jennings, B. 1990. "Ethics and Ethnography in Neonatal Intensive Care." In *Social Science Perspectives on Medical Ethics,* ed. G. Weisz. Philadelphia: University of Pennsylvania Press, pp. 261–72.

Kaufert, J. M., and J. D. O'Neil. 1990. "Biomedical Rituals and Informed Consent: Native Canadians and the Negotiation of Clinical Trust." In *Social Science Perspectives on Medical Ethics,* ed. G. Weisz. Philadelphia: University of Pennsylvania Press, pp. 41–63.

Kayser-Jones, J., and B. A. Koenig. 1994. "Ethical Issues in Qualitative Research in Long-Term Care Settings." In *Qualitative Methods in Aging Research,* ed. J. F. Gubrium and A. Sankar. Thousand Oaks, CA: Sage Publications, pp. 15–32.

Kelly, S., P. Marshall, L. Sanders, T. Raffin, and B. A. Koenig. 1997. "Understanding the Practice of Ethics Consultation: Results of an Ethnographic Multi-Site Study." *The Journal of Clinical Ethics* 8:136–49.

Kleinman, A. 1995. "Anthropology of Bioethics." In *Encyclopedia of Bioethics,* ed. W. Reich. New York: Macmillan, pp. 1667–74.

Koenig, B. A. 1988. "The Technological Imperative in Medical Practice: The Social Creation of a Routine Treatment." In *Biomedicine Examined,* ed. M. Lock and D. Gordon. Boston: Kluwer, pp. 351–74.

———. 1997. "Cultural Diversity in Decision Making about Care at the End of Life." In *Approaching Death: Improving Care at the End of Life,* ed. M. J. Field and C. K. Cassel (Institute of Medicine). Washington, D.C.: National Academy Press, pp. 363–82.

Krueger, R. A. 1997. *Analyzing and Reporting Focus Group Results.* Thousand Oaks, CA: Sage Publications.

La Puma, J., and D. Schiedermayer. 1994. *Ethics Consultation: A Practical Guide.* Boston: Jones and Bartlett.

Levin, B. W. 1986. *Caring Choices: Decision Making about Treatment for Catastrophically Ill Newborns.* Unpublished Ph.D. dissertation, Columbia University, New York, New York.

———. 1999. "Adolescents and Medical Decision Making: Observations of a Medical Anthropologist." In *The Adolescent Alone,* ed. J. Bluestein, N. Dubler, and C. Levine. Cambridge: Cambridge University Press, pp. 160–79.

Lock, M. 1995. "Contesting the Natural: Moral Dilemmas and Technologies of Dying." *Culture, Medicine and Psychiatry* 19:1–38.

Lofland, J., and L. Lofland. 1995. *Analyzing Social Settings: A Guide to Qualitative Observation and Analysis.* 3rd ed. Belmont, CA: Wadsworth Publishing Company.

Malinowski, B. 1961. *Argonauts of the Western Pacific.* Reprint. New York: E.P. Dutton.

Marcus G., and M. J Fischer. 1986. *Anthropology as Cultural Critique.* Chicago: University of Chicago Press.

Marshall, P. A. 1992a. "Research Ethics in Applied Anthropology." *IRB: A Review of Human Subjects Research* 14:1–5.

———. 1992b. "Anthropology and Bioethics." *Medical Anthropology Quarterly* 6:49–73.

———. 1996. "Boundary Crossings: Gender and Power in Clinical Ethics Consultations." In *Gender and Health: An International Perspective,* ed. C. Sargent and C. Brettell. Englewood Cliffs, NJ: Prentice Hall, pp. 205–26.

———. January 2000. *Final Report: The Relevance of Culture for Informed Consent in U.S. Funded International Health Services.* The President's National Bioethics Advisory Commission. Available at http://bioethics.gov/pubs.html.

Marshall, P., and A. Daar. 2000. "Ethical Issues in Human Organ Replacement: A Case Study from India." In *Global Health Policy, Local Realities: The Fallacy of the Level Playing Field,* ed. L. M. Whiteford and L. Manderson. Boulder, CO: Lynne Rienner Publishers, Inc., pp. 205–30.

Marshall, P., and B. A. Koenig. 1996. "Bioethics in Anthropology: Perspectives on Culture, Medicine and Morality." In *Medical Anthropology: Contemporary Theory and Method,* ed. C. Sargent and T. Johnson. 2nd ed. Westport. CT: Praeger Publishing Co., pp. 349–73.

Marshall, P., B. A. Koenig, D. Barnes, and A. Davis. 1998a. "Multiculturalism, Bioethics and End-of-Life Care: Case Narratives of Latino Cancer Patients." In *Health Care Ethics: Critical Issues for the 21st Century,* ed. J. Monagle and D. Thomasma. Gaithersburg, MD: Aspen Publishers, pp. 421–31.

———. 1998b. "Ethical Issues in Immigrant Health Care and Clinical Research." In *Handbook of Immigrant Health,* ed. S. Loue. New York: Plenum Press, pp. 203–26.

Muller, J. 1994. "Anthropology, Bioethics and Medicine: A Provocative Trilogy." *Medical Anthropology Quarterly* 8:448–67.

Murphy S. T., J. M. Palmer, S. Azen, G. Frank, V. Michel, and L .J. Blackhall. 1996. "Ethnicity and Advance Directives." *Journal of Law, Medicine and Ethics* 24:89–100.

Orona, C. J., B. A. Koenig, and A. J. Davis. 1994. "Cultural Aspects of Nondisclosure." *Cambridge Quarterly of Health Care Ethics* 3:338–46.

Orr, R., and E. Moon. 1993. "Effectiveness of an Ethics Consultation Service." *Journal of Family Practice* 36:49–53.

Press, N., and C. H. Browner. 1998. "Characteristics of Women Who Refuse an Offer of Prenatal Diagnosis: Data from the California Maternal Serum Alpha Fetoprotein Blood Test Experience." *American Journal of Medical Genetics* 78:433–45.

Rabinow, P. 1999. *French DNA: Trouble in Purgatory.* Chicago: University of Chicago Press.

Rapp, R. 1999. *Testing Women, Testing the Fetus: The Social Impact of Amniocentesis in America.* New York: Routledge.

Scheinfeld, D., P. Marshall, D. Beer, and K. Tyson. 1989. "Knowledge Utilization Structures, Processes and Alliances in a Psychiatric Hospital Study." In *Making Our Research Useful: Case Studies in the Utilization of Anthropological Knowledge*, ed. J. Van-Wiligen, B. Rylko-Bauer, and A. McElroy. Boulder, CO: Westview Press, pp. 201–18.

Sharp, L. 1995. "Organ Transplantation as a Transformative Experience: Anthropological Insights into the Restructuring of the Self." *Medical Anthropological Quarterly* 9: 357–89.

Singer, M., P. Marshall, R. Trotter, and J. Singer. 1999. "Ethics, Ethnography, Drug Use, and AIDS: Dilemmas and Standards in Federally Funded Research." In *Integrating Cultural, Observational, and Epidemiological Approaches in the Prevention of Drug Abuse and HIV/AIDS*, ed. P. Marshall, M. Singer, and M. Clatts. Bethesda, MD: US Department of Health and Human Resources, National Institutes of Health, National Institute on Drug Abuse, pp. 198–222.

Skeel, J. D., D. J. Self, and R. T. Skeel. 1993. "A Description of Humanist Scholars Functioning as Ethicists in the Clinical Setting." *Cambridge Quarterly of Health Care Ethics* 2:485–94.

Strenski, T., P. A. Marshall, J. Gacki, and C. Sanchez. 2000. "The Impact of Emergent Syringe Exchange Programs on Shooting Galleries and Injection Behaviors in Three Ethnically Diverse Chicago Neighborhoods." *Medical Anthropology Quarterly* 18:415–38.

Thomasma, D. C. 1994. "Clinical Ethics as Medical Hermeneutics." *Theoretical Medicine* 15(1994): 93–112.

Tyler, S., ed. 1996. *Cognitive Anthropology.* New York: Rinehart & Winston.

11

Quantitative Surveys[1]

Robert A. Pearlman and Helene E. Starks

Quantitative study of problems in medical ethics can be quite useful. For instance, this approach to studying ethical problems has fostered increased communication and understanding between ethicists and clinicians. Ethicists have also learned about the variability in practice behaviors (e.g., how physicians sometimes provide and sometimes withhold treatment based on their own subjective perceptions of patient benefit), ethical issues that clinicians confront (e.g., requests from patients or their families for treatment perceived to be medically futile), and the difficulties that clinicians face when trying to implement ethics policies (e.g., the difficulties of shared decision making with regard to foregoing cardiopulmonary resuscitation). This approach to ethical analysis and the results of multiple studies helped ethicists reframe old questions and deliberate about new ones (Brody, 1990; Pearlman, Miles, and Arnold 1993; Pearlman, 1994). Over the last two decades, many more clinicians have also started to study ethical problems in medicine in a broader sense, perhaps because quantitative methods and inferential statistics permitted broader interpretations and generalizations. In addition, this area of inquiry gradually became a legitimate career pathway for physician and nurse researchers.

In this chapter, quantitative survey methods are described and critiqued. Examples are presented to demonstrate how these methods have addressed topics of concern in medical ethics.

TECHNIQUE

Planning a Study

Before conducting a study, several issues need to be considered. First and foremost, it is essential to identify and to specify explicitly the goal(s) of the study. After these goals are specified, they should be formulated into answerable study questions. For example, an investigator might have the goal of wanting to characterize how physicians respond to requests for assisted suicide. The answerable study questions, however, might be the following: (1) How do physicians discuss with patients (and their families) the motivation for these requests? (2) How do physicians modify their treatment plans after hearing about patients' interest in assisted suicide? (3) Do physicians obtain other professional opinions for help in managing these requests, and if so, from whom? And (4) How often do physicians respond affirmatively to such requests, and under what circumstances?

After the study questions are formulated, the literature should be reviewed to see whether these questions have been previously investigated. If so, one must then determine if the previous research was done well, if it involved the same population, and if the limitations of the previous study could be overcome. It is also essential to discern whether the study goals are still justified. At this time, research questions should be refined if necessary or appropriate.

After identification of the overall study objectives and resultant study questions, the research design needs to be developed. Although the design is an essential component to any research protocol, for the purposes of this chapter we concentrate on designs employing quantitative surveys including cross-sectional or longitudinal interviews.

Next, the desired target population needs to be identified. The choice of the study population is influenced by the relevance of the study questions to the potential respondents, their ability to participate in the study, and the ability to recruit them. The plan for budgetary support also needs to be ascertained. If there is an available budget, this may shape the scope and format of the research. If government or foundation funding is going to be requested, then budgeting will be assessed after the development of a study proposal in which the details are specified.

The strategy for sampling also needs to be considered. With exploratory investigations, it is usually acceptable to obtain "convenience" samples. Sampling patients who attend a morning clinic in which there is an available room for interviewing, interviewing all patients in a clinic, or sampling ones' professional colleagues are all examples of convenience sampling. If the purpose of the survey is to infer that the results generalize to a larger population, then more representative sampling is required. The most rigorous sampling technique that permits generalization to a larger population, since it is less likely to be biased, is *random sampling*. Random sampling means that each of the respondents chosen for the study has the same chance of being included and that no single respondent has any influence on the selection of another respondent. Random sampling can be achieved by random digit dialing, using a list of random numbers (which are usually available in the appendices of statistics textbooks), or having a computer generate a list of random numbers. Other sampling strategies that promote generalizing, but are not random, include systematic sampling, stratified sampling according to a pertinent set of characteristics, and disproportionate sampling. *Systematic sampling* means that the investigator chooses a selection system and applies it to the entire possible study population. For example, instead of approaching every patient in a clinic, an investigator could decide to approach the fourth and seventh patients on every clinician's roster. *Stratified sampling* is used to ensure that the study sample will have proportional representation of key respondent characteristics. For example, if educational level is thought to be a factor in opinions about completing advance directives, the investigator might stratify the sample to be sure that equal numbers of people with less than a high school education, a high school diploma, some years of college, a bachelor's degree, and postgraduate degrees are included in the study. In *disproportionate sampling*, an investigator may oversample a subpopulation to ensure sufficient responses to be able to analyze this group. Some investigators question whether oversampling or disproportionate sampling truly achieves its goals.

Gordon published an excellent research workbook that outlines how to plan a study (Gordon 1978). In the workbook the author identifies and elaborates on a multistep process to ensure thoughtful quality research. The major steps are presented in Table 11.1. These steps also help investigators pinpoint their needs for support and other resources.

Survey Techniques

Mode of Administration

A central question in designing survey research is to choose an appropriate mode of administration. Whether the survey is conducted in-person, over the telephone, or by mail is determined by many factors. Foremost is whether the study participants can read, write, or hear. In addition, it is important to consider the complexity of the topic, the format of the questionnaire (e.g., vignette-based surveys are difficult to conduct over the telephone), the degree of burden of the survey itself on respondents, the desire or need for respondent anonymity or confidentiality, and the format for how the questions are answered. Lastly, the choice also will be influenced by budgetary and time considerations. Mail and telephone interviews are less expensive than in-person, interviewer-administered surveys, but often result in a lower response rate and incomplete data. The choice of administrative mode may be influenced by the desired sample. Telephone interviews require that the respondents have telephones. Calling during the day will undoubtedly oversample people who are not working or working at home. With mailed surveys, it may be unclear who is responding within a household or whether the respondent has access to any literature that might contaminate the responses. Similarly, it may be unclear what motivates people to respond to mailed surveys, especially when there is no financial or in-kind benefit. Table 11.2 presents advantages and disadvantages of different survey methods.

Survey Format

There are many issues that relate to how the survey itself is organized and formatted on paper. For instance, the order in which questions are asked requires consideration. Questionnaires often use *skip patterns* to guide respondents through the questionnaire. For example, if a respondent answers "yes" to a question, she goes on to the next question, but if she

TABLE 11.1   *Sequential Approach to Planning a Study*

Step	Activity
1.	Select a researchable question.
2.	Search and review related work, and then justify the research question again.
3.	Develop hypotheses.
4.	Identify instruments and data sources.
5.	Develop the research protocol.
6.	Eliminate procedural bias.
7.	Identify the study limitations.
8.	Identify how the results will be reported.
9.	Identify the statistical analyses.
10.	Maintain notes for consideration for the discussion, interpretation, or conclusions.

TABLE 11.2   *Survey Methods: Advantages and Disadvantages*

Survey Types	Advantages	Disadvantages
Mail	• Permits large numbers of respondents. • Geographically unlimited. • Absence of interviewers.	• Limited response rate. • Risk of incomplete data. • Often requires multiple mailings. • Reading and language barriers. • Respondent identity is uncertain.
Telephone	• Permits large numbers of respondents. • Minimal geographic limitations. • Respondent is identified. • Complete data likely. • Quality assurance possible.	• Language and hearing barriers. • Only targets people at home who answer the telephone. • Interviewer costs (training, time, and quality assurance). • Uncertainty about whether respondent is paying attention.
Face-to-Face Interview	• Complete data very likely. • Respondent is identifiable. • Controlled environment. • Complex tasks and visual aids are possible. • Quality assurance possible.	• Smaller number of respondents usually due to the costs. • Often limited by geographic considerations. • Interviewer costs (see above). • Travel costs.

answers "no," she is instructed to skip the next two questions. Moderate use of skip patterns is acceptable, but excessive use can cause increased burden and confusion for the respondent. For example, a respondent should never have to refer to a previous page to answer a question. Nor should a respondent have to endure complicated routing between questions. Lastly, information design experts recommend leaving significant white space on the page, using a printer's font that is large and easy to read, and choosing paper colors that provide good contrast with the type style.

Questionnaires can be designed with or without the use of clinical cases or vignettes. When the survey does not use vignettes, the series of questions are usually grouped by topic and when possible, placed together on the same page. There is usually a heading or introduction of some kind to signal the reader what the questions are about. When the topic changes, the next set of questions begins on a new page with a new header or introduction. When clinical vignettes are used, these are placed at the beginning of the page and then are followed by a series of questions that relate to the particularities of the case.

Regardless of whether the format is a survey questionnaire or vignette, the questions usually provide closed-ended, ordered choices. This works well for eliciting information about well-defined issues or characterizing the dimensions within issues. This format, however, restricts thinking to the dimension being explored by the investigators.

Question Format   The questionnaire format often is used to explore knowledge, beliefs, attitudes, and behaviors. The ideal way to study behaviors is through direct, unobtrusive observation. Questionnaires are used to obtain an approximation or self-report of behaviors since it is often logistically impractical to conduct observational studies. For example, recent surveys have explored physician attitudes, as well as behaviors, regarding physician-assisted suicide. In a 1994 study, Cohen and colleagues used a physician survey to characterize attitudes about physician-assisted suicide, demonstrating that physicians had widely divergent views about these activities and the role of the profession. In a national telephone survey, oncologists were asked whether they had "actually prescribed drugs to a patient knowing the patient intended to use them to end his or her life." The telephone interview also obtained information about each oncologist's behavior in his or her most recent case of being approached about physician-assisted suicide. From the data, the investigators were able to assess the degree to which the oncologists participated in assisted suicide and fulfilled three proposed safeguards (Emanuel et al. 1998). In another study, Meier and colleagues mailed a survey to a national stratified probability sample of physicians (Meier et al. 1998). This research team discovered that approximately 18 percent of the physicians had received a request for assistance with suicide and of those receiving requests, 16 percent had written at least one prescription.

Vignette Format Clinical vignettes are used to present a standardized scenario from which respondents express their attitudes or indicate intended behaviors. They are used when the investigator wants to control for, or modify in a controlled way, many of the variables that could influence a decision or behavior. Using vignettes allows the investigator to present each respondent with the same information to test for the effect of this information on responses.

In one approach to using vignettes, the investigator specifies many of the issues within the case and then tries to characterize the other factors that might influence a behavior or decision. For example, in one study physicians were asked to respond to a standardized vignette regarding whether to withhold mechanical ventilation and allow a patient to die (Pearlman, Inui, and Carter 1982). Physicians were allowed to ask for different details about the case, such as laboratory results, spousal preferences, and the patient's functional abilities. Physicians then were asked to explain their intended behaviors. They also provided demographic information about themselves. In this study, physicians who withheld the mechanical ventilator were more likely to (1) be physicians in training or attending physicians, compared to private physicians, (2) preferentially request social information about the patient, and (3) believe that the hypothetical patient had a very limited life expectancy and poor quality of life.

In another approach, the investigator presents multiple vignettes with carefully modified attributes. When aspects of the case are changed, the investigator can use this variability to study the relative importance and influence of the changing characteristics on the decisions. For example, in one study, physician attitudes about withholding feeding tubes from nursing home patients were characterized (von Preyss-Friedman, Uhlmann, and Cain 1992). The investigators systematically modified information in the vignettes, such as the patient's age, sex, and functional status, to see how these patient attributes affected withholding of this treatment.

A third approach to case-based surveys involves asking respondents to recall a recent clinical case of their own with variables of interest to the investigator and then answer survey questions based on this specific encounter or occurrence. The advantage of using real clinical cases is that respondents are asked to report on actual behaviors as opposed to speculating as to how they might behave given a hypothetical clinical vignette. As an example, investigators conducted a study characterizing the consideration of medical futility as a rationale for writing "do not attempt resuscitation" (DNAR) orders (Curtis et al. 1995). They asked medical residents to identify who amongst their patients in the hospital had DNAR orders. These cases were then characterized by the residents' responses to questions about the patient's likelihood of surviving CPR to hospital discharge and the current and anticipated quality of life for the patient. In another example, investigators wanted to understand how Washington State physicians responded to requests for assisted suicide (Back et al. 1996). In anonymous mailed surveys, the investigators asked physicians to answer a series of questions about their most recent request. These data were analyzed in order to characterize both the patients making the requests (e.g., age, gender, disease, prognosis, symptom burden, perceived rationale for the request) and the physicians' behaviors in response to these requests (e.g., discussion, referral, refusal, psychiatric evaluation, prescriptions for symptom relief and depression, prescription for assisting the suicide).

The use of vignettes in survey research gives rise to an unavoidable tension regarding their composition. While brief, "short-hand" versions of clinical scenarios may be quick and easy to read, they are often unrealistic and do not provide enough information for a well-informed decision regarding an intended behavior. Longer, more specific vignettes permit the elicitation of more informed preferences and intended behaviors and probably have a stronger relationship between intention and true behavior (Ajzen and Fishbein 1977). For example, in recent studies using vignettes concerning circumstances of decisional incapacity and end-of-life decisions, a team of investigators characterized health states by providing information about cognition, mobility and ability to walk, ability to perform activities of daily living, and level of pain (Patrick et al. 1997). Similarly, they described treatments with reference to the acute or chronic condition that created the need for treatment, the nature of the treatment, its side effects, the likelihood of success, and the potential outcomes other than returning to the baseline situation. The benefits of this approach are that study respondents have more specific details to create a mental image of hypothetical scenarios. These can reduce the likelihood of unrealistic or folk beliefs, such as the belief that patients in a coma "could catch up on their rest," or that a mechanical ventilator "was the equivalent of an iron lung." The limitation of these specific scenarios is that the preferences only applied to very specific conditions and treatments. Longer narratives may be used to convey the richer details of a case, thus making the story more complex and realistic. However, the length of these narratives may limit their use in a survey because of the time required for respondents to read and synthesize the details and the risk of cognitively overloading the reader with too much detail. Table 11.3 presents examples of levels of descriptive detail.

Writing Good Questions

Writing good questions is a skill that requires practice. To write a good question, one should (1) use simple words, (2) avoid ambiguous or incomprehensible terms or concepts, (3) be brief, (4) be specific, and (5) be neutral. In addition, questions should avoid using terms that are leading, suggest a "correct" answer, or promote an answer that is socially desirable. If extra information is included that frames the question, one should try to present this information in a balanced way. For example, if the investigator is asking about treatment

TABLE 11.3   *Types of Vignettes*

Clinical "short hand"

Imagine that you have Alzheimer's disease. Would you want CPR if your heart stops?

Functional description

Imagine that you are 82 years old and you:

- Cannot think or talk clearly, are confused, and no longer recognize family members.
- Are not in any pain.
- Are able to walk, but get lost without supervision.
- Need help with getting dressed, bathing, and bowel and bladder functions.

Now imagine that your heart stops beating and you lose consciousness (black out). You could receive cardiopulmonary resuscitation (CPR) which would involve:

- Electric shocks, pumping on your chest, help with breathing, and heart medications through your veins.
- Possible side effects include broken ribs, sore chest, and memory loss.
- Possible outcomes are a 20 percent chance of returning to your baseline, a 5 percent chance of coma, or a 75 percent chance of death.

Would you want CPR in this situation if your heart were to stop beating?

Narrative

   Imagine that you have severe memory loss. You sit in a chair most of the day and do not interact with others. You have full health care coverage that includes the cost of living in a nursing home, which is necessary because you cannot control your bladder or bowels and you must be spoon fed. Your family members come to visit you every two days and you enjoy their visits, although you cannot speak and do not know who they are.
   In addition to your memory loss, you have an irregular heartbeat. Your doctor wants your family to decide if you should receive cardiopulmonary resuscitation (CPR) if your heart suddenly stops beating. He tells them that CPR would include applying electric shocks to your chest to "jump start" your heart. A breathing tube would be placed into your lungs to help you breathe and you would receive medications through a tube placed in your veins. This would go on for 15–30 minutes until your heartbeat was restored and you would probably go to the hospital afterwards for follow-up care in the intensive care unit. You would have a 1–4 percent chance of returning to your previous health condition and going back to the nursing home. What should your family advise the doctors regarding the use of CPR if your heart suddenly stops beating?

preferences, the question should include the likelihood of both success and failure of the treatment. This can be presented as the risk of surviving and the risk of dying. One should avoid "double barrel" questions, or questions that ask about more than one issue at a time. Any question that contains an "and" or an "or" should be reviewed critically. Multiple-choice questions should include the full range of possible responses to avoid leaving out participants whose responses are at the bottom of the range ("floor effects") or the top of the range ("ceiling effects"). When a questionnaire is used multiple times in a longitudinal study, questions that are insensitive to change may have limited value. Table 11.4 presents examples of poorly written questions and shows how they could be modified to make them better.

Scaling Methods

A complementary activity to writing good questions is choosing how the answers will be measured. The investigator must consider the level of specificity of the desired answers and the scaling methods. There are three principal types of measurements: nominal, ordinal, and interval. *Nominal data* categorize information without an ordered relationship. For example, the presence or absence of an advance directive, gender, and ethnic background represent nominal data. *Ordinal data* reflect an ordering of values, such as from small to large, slightly to predominantly, and none to moderate to severe. With ordinal data the size of the intervals between categories cannot be specified. In some surveys a statement is presented and a *Likert scale* is used to facilitate responses. A Likert scale is an ordinal scale that indicates the strength of the response to a statement. Example response categories include "strongly agree," "agree," "disagree," and "strongly disagree." *Interval data* are similar to ordinal data in being ordered, but also represent intervals of known size. Examples of interval data are the number of requests per year to a physician for assisted suicide and the percentage of cases of perceived medical futility (from the physician's perspective) for a particular treatment.

A *Thurstone-type*, or equal-appearing interval, scale presents the respondent with a series of intervals that either are labeled with ordinal descriptions for each interval or labeled only at the end points. An example of a question using a Thurstone-type scale is, "On average, how bad is your pain, where 0 equals no pain and 10 equals pain as bad as it could be?" These scales are ordinal, but have the appearance of being interval. Some investigators will mistakenly assume that statistics that require interval data are appropriate for these data. It is best to assume that the data are ordinal. Repeat statistical analyses can evaluate whether it makes a statistical difference when the intervals are treated as being equal. If statistical tests that assume interval data are employed, the use of such tests should be justified.

Measurement Safeguards

The methodological rigor needed to develop quantitative surveys always argues for a search for questionnaires (also referred to as instruments) that have been shown to be valid and reliable. The expression, "do not re-create the wheel," is always good advice in this context. *Valid instruments* measure what is intended to be measured. Several lines of evidence establish validity. These include *face and content validity* (preliminary lines of evidence that make sense "on the face of it" without external comparative measures), *criterion validity* (showing the relationship between what is measured and other proven measurements of the same or similar phenomena), and *construct validity* (showing the relationship between two hypothetical assumptions or constructs).

Reliable data are reproducible. *Test-retest reliability* assesses the degree to which the same sample of respondents provides the same answers to a questionnaire over a short period of time (usually between two and six weeks). *Interrater reliability* is the degree to which two (or more) investigators ask the same questions or review the same data and obtain the same answers. Reliability is also determined by the *internal consistency* of the questions. This

TABLE 11.4   *The Development of Survey Questions: Draft and Revised Examples*

Original Draft Questions	Problem with the Question	Revised, Improved Questions
• Would you consider hastening your death by physician-assisted suicide? • Do you agree or disagree with the proposed policy that requires a psychiatric evaluation of patients requesting assisted suicide?	• The term "physician-assisted suicide" is undefined. • Assumes that the respondent understands the basis for the proposed policy.	• Have you seriously considered obtaining medications from a physician to hasten your death? • Should all terminally ill patients who request physician-assisted suicide see a psychiatrist to make sure that depression is not the source of the request?
• Have you considered requesting PAS or active euthanasia?	• Double barrel question: Asks two questions in one. Also uses an undefined acronym.	• Have you requested physician-assisted suicide (PAS) for yourself (i.e. obtaining a prescription from your doctor with the intent of hastening your death)? [separate euthanasia question]
• Most experts recommend completion of an advance directive. To what degree do you think this is a good idea? (Responses: very much, a little, very little, not at all.)	• Suggests a "correct" (or socially desirable) answer. The term "advance directive" is undefined. The response categories don't match the question.	• Do you agree or disagree with the idea that older adults should complete an advance directive (e.g., Living Will) to help guide their health care in the event they are too sick to make decisions on their own? (Responses: strongly agree, somewhat agree, neither agree nor disagree, somewhat disagree, strongly disagree.)

is achieved by asking about the same topic in two different but similar ways and then comparing the answers. A related concern, especially for longitudinal studies, is *responsiveness*. This is the degree to which a question is sensitive to change over time.

Pilot Testing

Questions should be evaluated critically before incorporating them into questionnaires. When this step is left out, investigators typically invest enormous resources only to find at the end of the study that their data cannot answer their research questions. The value of pilot testing questions and questionnaires is underappreciated by many trainees. Pilot testing can be done using focus groups or by having a small sample of individuals that is similar to the study population complete the questionnaire. Focus groups allow investigators to get feedback on the "big picture" issues, such as formatting, font size, paper color, sequence of the questions, and any questions that are confusing. Jobe and Mingay (1990) describe a technique known as "cognitive debriefing" that can also be used with individuals. In cognitive debriefing, the investigator sits with the respondent while she is completing the questionnaire and asks her to discuss what the questions mean to her as she is answering them. The cognitive burden of individual questions or the questionnaire as a whole can be assessed during this type of debriefing. Pilot testing (or pretesting) should address the issues identified in Table 11.5.

Sometimes pilot testing provides fascinating, unexpected insights. In a pilot test of vignettes depicting decisional incapacity (e.g. stoke, dementia), we identified that patients were unwilling to imagine some psychological dimensions, such as sadness. They were willing to imagine being cognitively impaired, bed-bound, and unable to care for themselves,

TABLE 11.5   *Issues Addressed in Pilot Testing of Surveys*

Questions	Questionnaire and Administration
• comprehension/understanding • jargon • appropriate reading level • acceptability of cognitive burden • responsiveness of the scales • presence of floor or ceiling effects • repeat items to assess reliability • positive versus negative structure to assess framing effects	• monitor the time to administer • assess reliability: test-retest, interrater, internal consistency • feedback on content, comprehensiveness • assess patterns of responding due to format (e.g., sequencing, ensuring that responses are aligned to a common scale) • check on validity (content measures what it is supposed to) • assess response rate (by question and overall) • observe interviewers: assume neutral roles, use exact wording, record exact responses, use nondirected probes • ensure quality graphic design and simple, easy-to-follow formatting

but not sad for part or most of the time. Without pilot testing we would have never imagined this selective aversion to imagining a psychological state. As a result we identified a structural limitation to the use of vignettes.

Protection of Human Subjects

Prior to initiating any research with human subjects, investigators must establish a protocol. Institutional Review Boards (IRBs) critically review research protocols to ensure that the appropriate standards for conducting research are satisfied. Moreover, IRBs review the informed consent process (including a consent form if appropriate) to ensure that investigators will obtain voluntary, informed consent. Including a few sample questions in consent forms can give potential participants an idea of the kinds of questions they will be asked. With quantitative surveys it is prudent to include at least one example of a difficult question and one example of a sensitive question. For example, one study about advance care planning included the following questions on the consent form as examples of sensitive questions (Patrick et al. 1997). "Imagine that you develop a life-threatening illness and couldn't speak for yourself, would you want kidney dialysis for the rest of your life?" "To what extent do you feel you are a burden on your family and friends?"

CRITIQUE OF SURVEY RESEARCH IN MEDICAL ETHICS

As in the development of any research endeavor, some critical questions to ask at the beginning of the project are: In what ways are the research questions interesting and timely, and who are the intended audiences for the results? In studies that rely on questionnaires, it is also worth ensuring that the results, regardless of the findings, should be important and noteworthy. The reason for this latter caveat is a practical one. Trainees and faculty conduct these investigations, and dissemination of the results is desirable. Thus, it is prudent to frame the research so that the results are of interest to the target audience(s).

Unfortunately, many of the empirical studies in medical ethics that employ questionnaires or vignettes exhibit poor methodological rigor. At the most fundamental level, questionnaires often are developed without consideration of hypotheses, theoretical underpinnings, or conceptual models. A common mistake is to generate one or two study questions and jump straight to a study design without stepping back and considering whether those questions capture the complexity of the problem. For example, consider the case in which an investigator wants to study the influence of uncertainty on how patients make decisions. An inexperienced investigator interested in this topic decides he will design a short questionnaire that asks patients about their general discomfort with uncertainty in decision making and whether they feel that their physicians discuss uncertainty in a balanced way. He provides a definition of uncertainty, but does not provide the context of the discussions and the decisions. While of great interest and relevance, this study, as conceived, fails to address several important issues that would lead to a broader understanding of potential influential factors. For example, the role of uncertainty in clinical decisions may play out differently if the decision refers to a diagnostic test or a clinical decision. Other factors include whether the decision is about a life-saving or elective intervention, the degree of uncertainty or relative likelihood of success or failure (small, moderate, large), the patient's attitudes about risk, the setting and timing of the disclosure, the clinician's comfort level with sharing uncertainty, and how the probability estimate is communicated (verbally, with visual cues, likelihood of success and/or likelihood of failure, etc.).

If the investigator had limited his study to his original design, he would likely discover that his results raise more questions than provide answers. Thinking broadly before getting focused on the study or questionnaire design helps frame the issues and then forces the investigator to select explicitly which aspects of an issue are going to be explored. Thoughtful reflection is enhanced when an interdisciplinary group is incorporated into the planning stages of the research. Interdisciplinary is meant to suggest a broad array of scholars with interests that relate to the question or phenomenon. Many quality research endeavors using quantitative techniques have benefited from collaboration with anthropologists, psychologists, sociologists, philosophers, and health services researchers.

Strengths and Weaknesses of Survey Methodology

Even though there are many threats to the quality of surveys, this research method has many strengths. Surveys are often simple, easy to administer, and present limited risks to the respondent. The greatest risk is usually the discomfort of being asked to consider a sensitive topic. Surveys permit analyses involving large numbers of respondents in a relatively short period of time, can be used to make comparisons between groups, and are usually cost-effective. They can serve multiple purposes, including describing the attitudes, beliefs, and behaviors of populations, patients, and health care providers. They also can be used to test hypotheses and infer generalizable associations through the use of inferential statistics.

However, surveys are limited in the richness of the information that can be obtained. Surveys usually only obtain a limited description of attitudes or behavior. Moreover, they are limited to the approach and resultant questions of the investigator. For richer understanding of issues, qualitative methods need to be employed (see chapter 9).

The other weaknesses of survey methods are mostly those previously described. However, a common problem sometimes occurs with research trainees. In a paradigmatic situation, a trainee in geriatric medicine or general internal medicine embarks on conducting a survey with limited time and budget, a sketchy understanding of the conceptual basis for studying the question(s), imprecise study objectives, and inadequate resources and expertise to ensure that naïve mistakes are avoided. Rather than being an intrinsic weakness in the research method, however, this more accurately reflects a weakness in research training.

CONCLUDING COMMENTS

Quantitative surveys have become a well-appreciated approach to studying problems in clinical ethics. When survey methods are employed in a study, careful attention needs to be directed at the identification of the appropriate target population, the mode in which the survey is administered, and the use of clear language and simple formatting.

Helping to ensure that a quantitative survey provides meaningful and valuable interdisciplinary input in the early stages of planning can help identify the scope of the inquiry and as a consequence the questions to be addressed. Here, critical feedback from other researchers with expertise in survey methods helps ensure scientific rigor. Finally, pilot testing helps assure that the survey results are reliable and valid.

NOTES ON RESOURCES AND TRAINING

In order to conduct survey research with scientific rigor, the investigator needs to have adequate education and training. Education needs to focus on research and survey methods, questionnaire design, cognitive and social psychology, the strengths and weaknesses of scaling techniques, psychometric properties of measurement, and the assumptions and limits of statistical tests. Training requires responsible supervision from trained survey researchers and statisticians to ensure that reliable and valid information is obtained, that appropriate statistical analyses are done, and that the collection of data occurred voluntarily and with informed consent.

One of the more ideal situations involves a multistep process of developing a research study, only one or a few components of which would focus on questionnaire development. In many training programs, such as the Robert Wood Johnson Clinical Scholars Program, research fellows present their early study ideas and obtain feedback and criticism. Subsequent reviews that occur prior to beginning the research focus on the choice of questionnaire design, measurements and scales, goals of pilot testing, and the results and proposed changes due to the pilot. After completion of data collection, supervision of data analyses and reporting is essential. This program has been emulated in many fellowship programs in general internal medicine and to a lesser degree with some geriatric medicine fellowship programs.

Another aspect of training is hands-on experience. Conducting pilot interviews and obtaining feedback is humbling and educational. Another element of hands-on experience is soliciting the impressions and hearing the experiences of the interviewers. With longitudinal studies it is imperative that interviewers be observed for "drift" from the original protocol. Even with closed-ended interview schedules, interviewers can get sloppy over time and skip over instructions or paraphrase questions they consider wordy or confusing. Investigators should participate in this observational review process. If the investigators are collecting primary data, their behavior should be reviewed and critiqued by someone else.

Many of the resources for conducting survey research reside within universities. Universities usually have faculty with expertise in sociology, psychology, statistics, and questionnaire design. Depending on the topic, there also may be experts with interest in the study topic. This can include individuals with expertise in ethics and the related clinical or research entity. Trainees should take advantage of their academic environment and not restrict their search for assistance to their clinical or departmental areas. In addition, textbooks exist that provide excellent overviews and advice about how to conduct survey research (Babbie, 1990; Dillman, 1978; Labaw, 1980; Green and Lewis 1986).

Three other general approaches to identifying resources include (1) contacting academic scholars who have published in the area of interest and requesting their feedback on ideas and questionnaires, (2) accessing resources through the Internet, and (3) communicating with graduate training programs in ethics to see if they have faculty with expertise in empirical research in ethics. A listing of graduate medical ethics programs is available through the Hastings Center in Garrison, New York. Programs that clearly embrace empirical work include the Bioethics Institute (Johns Hopkins University), the Center for Bioethics (University of Pennsylvania), Center for Ethics in Health Care (Oregon Health Sciences University), Center for Medical Ethics (University of Pittsburgh), Center for the Study of Medical Ethics and Humanities (Duke University), Department of Medical History and Ethics (University of Washington), and the MacLean Center for Clinical Medical Ethics (University of Chicago).

It is important to remember that interdisciplinary review often provides useful insights. Moreover, many academic faculty provide consultations and guidance to research trainees from distant sites.

NOTE

1. Work on this chapter was supported in part by the Project on Death in America (Open Society Institute). Dr. Pearlman was supported as a faculty scholar by this program.

REFERENCES

Ajzen, I., and M. Fishbein. 1977. "Attitude-Behavior Relations: A Theoretical Analysis and Review of Empiric Research." *Psychological Bulletin* 84:888–918.

Babbie, E. R. 1990. *Survey Research Methods.* Belmont, CA: Wadsworth Publishing.

Back, A. L., J. I. Wallace, H. E. Starks, and R. A. Pearlman. 1996. "Physician-Assisted Suicide and Euthanasia in Washington State: Patient Requests and Physician Responses." *Journal of the American Medical Association* 275:919–25.

Brody, B. A. 1990. "Quality of Scholarship in Bioethics." *Journal of Medicine and Philosophy* 15:161–78.

Cohen, J. S., S. D. Fihn, E. J. Boyko, A. R. Jonsen, and R. W. Wood. 1994. "Attitudes toward Assisted Suicide and Euthanasia among Physicians in Washington State." *New England Journal of Medicine* 331:89–94.

Curtis J. R., D. R. Parks, M. R. Krone, and R. A. Pearlman. 1995. "Use of Medical Futility Rationale in Do Not Attempt Resuscitation Orders." *Journal of the American Medical Association* 273:124–28.

Dillman, D. A. 1978. *Mail and Telephone Surveys: The Total Design Method.* New York: John Wiley & Sons.

Emanuel, E. J., E. R. Daniels, D. L. Fairclough, and B. R. Clarridge. 1998. "The Practice of Euthanasia and Physician-Assisted Suicide in the United States. Adherence to Proposed Safeguards and Effects on Physicians." *Journal of the American Medical Association* 280:507–13.

Gordon, M. J. 1978. "Research Workbook: A Guide for Initial Planning of Clinical, Social, and Behavioral Research Projects." *Journal of Family Practice* 7:145–60.

Green L.W., and F. M. Lewis. 1986. *Measurement and Evaluation in Health Education and Health Promotion.* Palo Alto, CA: Mayfield Publishing.

Jobe, J. B., and D. J. Mingay. 1990. "Cognitive Laboratory Approach to Designing Questionnaires for Surveys of the Elderly." *Public Health Report* 105:518–24.

Labaw, P. J. 1980. *Advanced Questionnaire Design.* Cambridge, MA: Abt Books.

Meier, D. E., C.A. Emmons, S. Wallenstein, T. Quill, R. S. Morrison, and C. K. Cassel. 1998. "A National Survey of Physician-Assisted Suicide and Euthanasia in the United States." *New England Journal of Medicine* 338:1193–1201.

Patrick, D. L., R. A. Pearlman, H. E. Starks, K. C. Cain, W. G. Cole, and R. F. Uhlmann. 1997. "Validation of Life-Sustaining Treatment Preferences: Implications for Advance Care Planning." *Annals of Internal Medicine* 127:509–17.

Pearlman, R. A. 1994. "Advance Directives: Are We Asking the Right Questions?" *Hastings Center Report* 24:S24–27.

Pearlman, R. A., T. S. Inui, and W. B. Carter. 1982. "Variability in Physician Bioethical Decision Making: A Case Study of Euthanasia." *Annals of Internal Medicine* 97:420–25.

Pearlman, R. A., S. H. Miles, and R. Arnold. 1993. "Empirical Research in Ethics." *Theoretical Medicine* 14:197–210.

von Preyss-Friedman, S. M., R. F. Uhlmann, and K. C. Cain. 1992. "Physicians' Attitudes toward Tube Feeding Chronically Ill Nursing Home Patients." *Journal of General Internal Medicine* 7(1): 46–51.

12

Experimental Methods

Marion Danis, Laura Hanson, and
Joanne M. Garrett

Empirical research in medical ethics is useful to test the effectiveness of interventions deemed valuable on theoretical grounds. When researchers wonder whether ethical reasoning can influence clinical action, or whether ethical guidelines can influence clinical outcomes, they can utilize a range of research methods, from observation and description of interventions to an experimental approach in which an intervention is planned, conducted, and monitored for an expected outcome. In this chapter we focus on the experimental approach. We will emphasize the unique aspects of experimental research that tests whether an intervention is able to affect outcomes with moral significance.

An experimental design should be used when the investigator's goal is to determine whether human knowledge, attitudes, or behaviors can be changed, and whether doing so leads to some valued good. Research questions appropriate for this design might include, for example, the following: Can an educational program improve medical students' knowledge and practice of obtaining informed consent? Does the clinical use of pain scores, in conjunction with vital signs, result in an increased proportion of patients receiving satisfactory pain relief? Or, do programs that teach clinic staff to respect cultural diversity increase access to services for minority patients attending primary care clinics? The investigator who seeks to answer such questions using experimental methods will design an intervention and then evaluate its effect on specified, relevant outcomes. In the course of this chapter, these questions will serve to illustrate issues in the design of experimental research in medical ethics.

While the chapter is meant to help those who are interested in conducting experimental trials do so more effectively, it is also intended to be useful to the non-experimentalist, by making them aware of the important insights that such research yields for the discipline of medical ethics as a whole. The experimental research that demonstrated the limited effectiveness of written advance directives serves as an important example of just how important experimental studies are in testing widely held beliefs in medical ethics (Danis 1991; Schneiderman 1992). Anyone with an interest in medical ethics who wishes to have a well-rounded understanding of the discipline should appreciate what experimental research can contribute and know how to critically evaluate this type of research.

As we planned this chapter, the insights of Weiss about the nature of experimental research were particularly helpful, and we wish to acknowledge that many of our explanations derive from his chapter on randomized controlled trials (Weiss 1996).

DEFINITION

The *experimental method* differs from other research methodologies in that it requires control over a phenomenon under study. The researcher assumes some control over the experience of study subjects so that experimental subjects receive an intervention and are compared to control subjects who do not receive the intervention. To the degree possible, other sources of differences between the intervention and control groups are eliminated. Experimental studies in clinical research are called *clinical trials*—studies that test interventions to improve health or change clinical practices. Such studies have a prospective design and require longitudinal follow-up to measure the effects of the intervention. Investigators may also study the effects of interventions designed and controlled by others, as, for example, when a new educational program or governmental policy influences clinical action. These studies, termed *natural experiments*, are observational rather than experimental in nature, but may still offer insight into purposeful efforts to change clinical practice.

Experimental studies can play a crucial role in ethics research, as we have already suggested, by allowing a re-examination of some of the assumptions derived from observational and theoretical work. At times, results of an experiment may challenge ethicists to re-examine ethical theory. Medical ethicists often develop a systematic approach to clinical dilemmas based on theoretical principle and the reflective analysis of cases. A controlled trial of an intervention may be used to apply the approach and test its impact on desired outcomes. For example, the Study to Understand Prognoses and Preferences for Outcomes and Risks of Treatment (The SUPPORT Principal Investigators 1995) was a randomized, controlled trial to test whether nurses' facilitation of communication about patients' preferences and prognosis would change the treatment experienced by seriously ill patients with short life expectancy. The design of the intervention was based on the ethical principles of autonomy and truth telling and on evidence from descriptive studies that concluded that patients preferred less aggressive life support than the current standard of care. In spite of a careful design that was consonant with current ethical thinking, the SUPPORT intervention had no impact on the treatment experienced by patients. The study results challenged fundamental assumptions in clinical ethics and raised new questions about the meaning of autonomy and the translation of ethical reasoning into clinical practice.

TECHNIQUES

Conducting an experiment to test a hypothesis is a costly and laborious endeavor. It is advisable for the investigator to identify a problem worthy of this effort. Unlike descriptive studies, an experimental study is usually begun after substantial previous observational study and theoretical analysis provide some basis for anticipating a successful outcome. Furthermore, because of their cost, experiments are generally reserved for questions of the greatest merit—interventions that, if successful, would offer significant benefit to large numbers of persons. Once convinced of the need to use experimental design, the investigator must make decisions about overall study design, design of the intervention, selection of subjects and controls, measurement of outcomes, and the plan for interpretation of the results.

Study Design

The overall design of an intervention study may be of three types: a randomized controlled trial, a nonrandomized controlled trial, or an uncontrolled trial. The fundamental distinction between these trial designs is the process of choosing intervention and control groups. In *randomized trials,* subjects enter control or intervention groups by random assignment. *Nonrandomized controlled trials* include studies with historical controls, control subjects who elect not to receive the intervention, or other comparison groups chosen without random assignment. *Uncontrolled trials* study the impact of an intervention by measuring and comparing some key outcome measures for a single group of subjects before and after the intervention. Strictly speaking, the latter two study designs do not adhere to an experimental method. Subjects self-select for the intervention, a process that will introduce bias if those selecting the intervention differ in important ways from those who do not select it. Nonetheless, as described below, these study methods may be useful and feasible in situations in which randomization is logistically or ethically prohibited.

Randomized Controlled Trials

Randomization of subjects to intervention or control groups allows investigators to study the isolated effect of an intervention. Study subjects are informed of the trial's design and purpose, and after informed consent they are assigned randomly to one of the study groups. The control group may receive either no intervention or the usual care, or they may receive a partial or different intervention from the one under study. Chance alone dictates group assignment, creating groups that do not differ (except by chance) in ways other than their experience of the intervention. Randomization creates similar study groups, thus removing known and unforeseen causes of *bias,* which is nonrandom or systematic error, that could lead to false conclusions.

Nonrandomized Controlled Trials and Uncontrolled Trials

While the randomized controlled trial is considered the gold standard for evaluation of the effect of an intervention, there are circumstances that limit the use of this study design. Subjects who can serve as a comparison group for measuring the effect of an intervention can be derived through other approaches. A common strategy is to use *historical controls,* the same or a similar group of patients who received services prior to introduction of the intervention. For example, perceived access to care could be measured before and after implementation of a new program to improve access. Researchers may also choose to use a *convenience sample of control subjects* from a similar population to whom the intervention is not offered, such as patients in a neighboring hospital. A third alternative is to permit subjects to elect or refuse the intervention, and use *self-selected controls.* Nonrandomized trials permit comparison of two study groups, but strictly speaking are truly descriptive rather than experimental in design.

Nonrandomized and uncontrolled trials are useful when (a) a randomized trial would be too costly, (b) randomization is considered ethically unsound, or (c) the proposed intervention is comprehensive or complex. Randomized controlled trials typically require more time and resources than any other study design, and may not be feasible because of cost. More often, an investigator interested in ethical questions will choose a nonrandomized design for ethical reasons. While randomization gives the investigator complete control over one aspect of the patient's experience or therapy, this approach is ethically permissible only when patients are willing to forgo a personal choice, and when there is no clear evidence that subjects assigned to this intervention will face great risk, or that control subjects will give up an effective or important intervention. At the present time, for example, one could not study whether the informed consent process results in a true increase in patient knowledge and satisfaction, since it would be impermissible to withhold informed consent from control subjects. Likewise, while clinically important information could be gained from a randomized controlled trial that compared survival and satisfaction with tube feeding versus manually assisted feeding for seriously ill patients, the trial would abrogate a patient's right to choose whether to have a feeding tube.

Many interventions with ethical implications will never be studied in randomized controlled trials because it is difficult for a team of investigators to offer the intervention to one group of patients without influencing the care of the control group at all. If, for example, a diversity training study involves an educational program for clinicians at a primary care clinic, any clinicians who receive the training must have all their patients assigned to the intervention group, because it would be hard for clinicians to treat some of their patients according to the newly taught approach and other patients according to the older approach. If it is the clinicians who are assigned to intervention and control groups, it might also be difficult to teach a new approach to the clinicians in the intervention group without their influencing those colleagues in the control group in the course of their daily interactions. These difficulties may be avoided in multisite studies, but such studies are extraordinarily complex and expensive and present other problems due to differences among sites.

It may be even more difficult to conduct a randomized trial when the intervention requires systematic changes in the delivery of clinical services. Examples include changes in health care policy or health systems that result in differential access to care, promising new services, or changes in the physician-patient relationship. Investigators must use nonrandomized designs to study the clinical outcomes of new services or policy changes. For example, a university practice may set a goal to increase the use of advance directives and implement a combined program of physician and patient education. Randomization may be impossible within a single system, thus a nonrandomized study design can be used to evaluate impact and improve such a program.

If investigators choose to design a study with intervention and control groups to which study subjects are not randomly assigned, several minimum criteria should be met (Weiss 1996): (1) control and intervention subjects must be clearly defined and enumerated; (2) eligibility criteria should be explicit and identical for intervention and control subjects; (3) in planning the study the two groups should be selected to be as similar as possible to minimize factors other than the intervention that would influence the outcome of interest; and (4) the tools for monitoring the outcome of interest should be identical for both study groups. In nonrandomized studies, intervention and control subjects might be matched on important variables, such as gender or educational attainment, or selected from similar geographic or service settings. The investigator must recognize that when historical controls are used in a study with prolonged follow-up, other *secular trends* or changes in health care delivery may impact the outcome. For example, the use of advance directives is steadily increasing over time in the United States, as a result of general media coverage and implementation of the Patient Self-determination Act. Therefore, a study comparing rates of advance directive use before and after an institution-wide educational program will be strengthened if the investigators include information on advance directive use in a larger geographic area that can show the impact of these secular trends over the time frame of their study.

Designing the Intervention

Once a study design has been selected, the design of the intervention becomes the focus. In designing the intervention, the investigator should consider (a) existing evidence for the effect of the proposed intervention, (b) practical concerns about generalizability, (c) selection of control or comparison groups, and (d) whether to conduct an efficacy or effectiveness trial.

In designing an intervention, the investigator needs to decide how much to subsume under the label of one intervention. As an example, consider an educational intervention to teach medical students about informed consent. Review of educational literature might suggest many possible educational methods: discussion groups, presentation of panels of patients or research subjects who discuss their perceptions of the value of informed consent, role plays in which students take on the roles of clinicians and patients, or modeling of informed consent by senior physicians working with the students. If the primary research question is whether one can improve medical students' knowledge of the principles and practice of informed consent, the investigators might wish to use several approaches in an effort to make the intervention as potent as possible. Their intervention might include as many of these strategies as possible as a combination of curricular materials presented in all four years of medical education. Alternatively, the investigators' review of the educational literature might suggest that two strategies—role playing and modeling by senior physicians—are the most effective educational methods. They might then combine these two techniques as the study intervention in the belief that a more defined intervention would be more practically incorporated into any medical school's curriculum. Alternatively, if prior successful trials had used varied methods to improve knowledge, the investigators might design a study to test one educational method against another, or to test whether educational efforts could be concentrated in preclinical courses. For this study, investigators would use existing studies to select a single teaching method with the best evidence of success.

If an intervention is to benefit patients in general (i.e., outside of a research setting), it needs to be designed so that it can be feasibly reproduced in practice. Consider, for example, a randomized controlled trial of a multidisciplinary team to promote the autonomy of stroke patients with speech deficits. If the intervention requires intensive hours of speech and physical therapy but yields only modest benefit for patients, it is likely that the intervention will be considered too cumbersome and costly and not sufficiently portable or useful for other clinicians and patients. Thus, in designing an intervention that one hopes will be generally useful it ought to be as simple, inexpensive, and easy to export to other settings as possible.

The investigators must also design the control or comparison group's experience. Should the comparison group receive the contemporaneous standard approach or should the intervention be compared to doing nothing? Alternatively, should a placebo, an intervention that is expected to be of no benefit, be given to the control group? The latter approach would be analogous to using a placebo in a clinical trial of a drug (Freedman 1990).

The ethical acceptability of having a control group that receives no intervention or a placebo can be quite controversial. In clinical trials, opponents of placebos consider their use unethical when a standard, proven treatment exists (Freedman, Glass, and Weijer 1996; Rothman and Michels 1994). Those who endorse placebos suggest that placebo-controlled trials may be ethical when deferral of therapy will not harm a patient (Temple and Ellenberg 2000). Safeguards that are recommended to make the use of placebos ethically acceptable involve the adherence to certain standards for their use, including minimization of risk, informed consent for study subjects, and optimization of treatment at the conclusion of a study (Miller 2000). The possibility of a control group that receives no intervention, or less than the standard of care, becomes even more complex when international research involves communities with differing standards of care. Which community standard to follow is a matter of intensive debate (Angell 1997; Varmus and Satcher 1998).

In standard clinical trials two groups are being compared, but if the investigator chooses to study two interventions, then subjects may be randomized to one of two possible interventions groups with a third group serving as a control. One must consider the impact of this choice on the power of the study to detect differences between groups. Study *power*, the probability of detecting an intervention's effect in the study sample, if it exists in the population at large, is determined by the number of subjects in each group and the magnitude and variability of the difference in outcome between intervention and control groups. If a fixed number of potential subjects are divided into three groups, it will diminish the power of the study to detect differences between groups. Similarly, if a limited intervention is compared to a more potent one, the two groups may differ less than if a true control group without intervention was studied.

Intervention studies may be designed either as efficacy or effectiveness trials. In an *efficacy trial*, investigators wish to know whether an intervention has impact on the outcome of interest under optimal circumstances. Efficacy trials are generally used when an intervention is relatively unproven and are designed to maximize the impact of the intervention. They examine the outcome of an intervention under idealized circumstances. Efficacy trials may exclude patients who are less likely to benefit. The intervention is designed to be as powerful as possible.

Once efficacy has been demonstrated, investigators may then design an *effectiveness trial* in which they set out to examine whether the benefits endure under nonideal conditions. Thus, if one has completed an efficacy trial that demonstrates that an educational intervention to promote cultural sensitivity improves minority access to medical services, one might design an effectiveness trial to determine whether the intervention can work in a pressured work environment where clinic employees see patients in brief visits and where there is rapid staff turnover.

Defining Outcome Measures

Each intervention is designed with a goal in mind—a plan to influence some *outcome* of interest because it reflects an aspect of ethical reasoning or behavior. Thus, the outcome is as important as the intervention itself. Why else conduct the study? Defining the outcome of interest and deciding how to measure it is crucial. It may be difficult to find tangible measures of morally relevant outcomes because complex human beliefs and behaviors are not easily captured by quantitative measures. Investigators will begin with a broad concept of benefit, such as patient satisfaction with pain management. In the design of a study, they must consider whether, for example, family surrogates' satisfaction can substitute as an outcome measure for patients incapable of response (Sulmasy et al. 1998) and how to adjust for the strongly positive bias in most satisfaction scales (Hays and Ware 1986).

Clinical outcome measures may be usefully divided into process measures and patient-centered outcomes (Donaldson and Field 1998). *Process measures* are intermediate steps or easily identified components of care that may be used as proxies for the true outcomes of interest. *Patient-centered outcomes* are the best measures of successful clinical interventions, since the primary aim of most clinical research is to improve patient care. However, researchers may choose process measures when they lack the resources for extensive follow-up or interviews with patients. For example, in a study of medical student education on informed consent, the investigators might hope these students will do a better job with informed consent once they enter into practice. Since it would be impractical to conduct the study long enough to measure this endpoint, the investigator must measure other more proximate endpoints. Any process measure should be selected based on some evidence that it is a good predictor of the ultimate outcome of interest. Thus, one might observe medical students obtaining informed consent during an Objective Structured Clinical Examination (OSCE), a standardized assessment tool used to evaluate examination skills (Roberts and Norman 1990). Other process measures, such as the students' knowledge and attitudes about informed consent and patient autonomy, might be measured to evaluate the short-term effects of the educational intervention.

As medical practice has become more costly, intervention trials have begun to examine the economic cost of offering an intervention. Thus Torgerson et al. argue that cost should be considered one of the outcome variables of interest in any trial (Torgerson, Ryan, and Ratcliffe 1995).

Given the longitudinal nature of an intervention study, the investigator exercises control over the timing between the intervention and measurement of the outcome. The longer the period of follow-up, the more costly the study becomes. Also, the longer the interval, the more likely it is that the effect of the intervention will decay over time and fail to influence the outcome. On the other hand, short-term studies may be of very little realistic use. For example, a study testing the merits of a weekend retreat to teach medical students about ethics, which measured the difference in the students' knowledge before and after the weekend, may show a substantial gain from Friday to Sunday, but one wouldn't want to rely on these results if one was hoping for retained knowledge in the long term.

In all intervention studies it is important to measure and account for other factors that might influence the study outcome of interest. Thus, once the outcome measure is defined, data collection will need to include variables that could concurrently influence that outcome. In the example of the informed consent study, a survey might assess cultural background and demographic information of students that might influence their attitudes toward autonomy or communication with patients.

Part of the definition of outcome measures entails the selection of study instruments. In conducting a trial related to an ethical issue, it is quite likely, for instance, that the attitudes of research participants will be an important outcome measure. Questionnaires therefore will be necessary to measure these attitudes. The selection of the instrument to use for this purpose raises issues that are addressed elsewhere in this volume (see chapter 11). When possible, investigators benefit from the use of survey instruments that have been previously developed and validated so that the investigator need not devote energies to instrument design, which entails a study in itself (Pequegnat and Stover 1995).

Selection of Study Subjects

In order to conclude that the results of an experiment are *generalizable* to other populations, the participants who form the *study sample* must be similar to a larger population, or *target population,* for whom the intervention might be useful. While it is rarely possible to derive the study sample as an exact subset of the proposed clinical population, it is important to have the study sample be as similar to the population of interest as possible. If, for example, one wishes to learn about the effect of written advance directive materials on elderly individuals with low literacy, then studying the materials' impact on college students is not helpful. Further, it might be prohibitively expensive or impractical to identify a random sample of chronically ill, older adults with limited education. However, a sample of visitors to a senior center in an impoverished neighborhood might be reasonably similar to the target population. Even after selecting such an appropriate study sample, it remains important to collect information from participants about their age, chronic disease experience, and education, so that others then may compare their situation to the study sample when they are considering whether the study results might be applicable to them.

In selecting study subjects the investigator should define inclusion and exclusion criteria. It is important to appreciate that doing so can have opposing effects on the efficacy and generalizability of the study. If, for example, one is trying to teach cultural sensitivity to clinic staff to improve access to care for minority patients, one might specify in the inclusion criteria that these patients be able to read and write so that one can prepare written materials to offer them in clinic and survey them at the completion of the study by use of a written questionnaire. But patients who can read and write may be the easiest patients to help gain access, since health literacy has a substantial impact on health outcomes (Baker et al. 1998). By including only such patients one has a higher likelihood of demonstrating that the intervention is effective. However, if the vast majority of clinics serving minority populations have patients that are not literate, then the exclusion of illiterate patients reduces the generalizability of the study results. The majority of clinics will not find the intervention useful, or they will find it useful for only a segment of their clinic population.

Determination of the Sample Size

Aside from defining the characteristics of the study subjects, the number of study subjects must be determined. To set the *sample size*, the investigator must identify the hypothesis to be tested; select a statistical test that will be used to test whether the hypothesis has been proven; choose an *effect size*, indicating how much of a difference between the treatment and control group will be considered clinically important; and decide how much one is willing to tolerate making an error about the results (how acceptable it would be to have either a falsely positive study result, referred to as a type I error, or to have a falsely negative result, referred to as a type II error) (Hulley and Cummings 1988; Cohen 1988). The larger the sample size the greater the statistical power will be to detect a significant difference between the groups. One strategy for guaranteeing an adequate number of study subjects while minimizing the cost of conducting a study is to alter the sampling ratio so that the number of subjects in the control group exceeds the number of subjects in the intervention group (Morgenstern and Winn 1983).

Selection of the Study Site

A variety of other decisions are involved in the design of an experimental trial. Should the trial be multicentered or located at one study site? One study site will suffice if that site can provide an adequate number of research subjects that represent the target population and if the study site has sufficient space, resources, and supporting staff. If one is interested in an ethnically diverse population, then one study site may not suffice unless it is a site with many cultural groups. If one is studying a fairly complex intervention, such as a whole course or various additions to the curriculum, it may be difficult to reproduce the intervention in more than one site. One advantage of a single site is that it can provide more reliably consistent data collection because the same staff collects all the data (Chow and Liu 1998). An advantage of a multisite study, when one is examining ethically charged issues, is that individual study sites can remain unidentified during reporting, leaving institutions less susceptible to being labeled "ethically deficient" as a result of their participation in a study. Use of multiple study sites permits the inclusion of urban and rural sites, geographically dispersed sites, or sites that include ethnically and religiously diverse populations. Given the relationship of moral values to culture and religion, this can be an important consideration in a study of an intervention intended to have an ethically meaningful outcome.

In selecting a study site, an important decision involves whether to conduct the study in an academic or nonacademic setting. While it is often easier to conduct a study in the academic setting where an investigator may be located, or because other resources are easily accessible there, the generalizability to the nonacademic setting cannot be assumed. Here again is a reason for a multisite study, so that the results can be generalized.

As the global economy becomes more interdependent and dynamic, and as research is conducted across international boundaries, the possibility of conducting ethics research internationally arises. Here researchers are faced with a particularly complicated task of being attentive to the reality that ethical norms vary in different societies. One must be very cautious and wary about studying ethical interventions across cultures that have different ethical beliefs and practices.

Developing and Writing the Experimental Protocol

The *protocol* is a written mechanism that describes how the trial will be conducted. The protocol will include the criteria for inclusion of research subjects, the recruitment method, the method for recording data, the consent form, procedures for handling individuals who refuse to participate or drop out, and instructions for research subjects, investigators, and trial personnel (Spilker 1991).

Obtaining Institutional Review Board (IRB) Approval

Since the interventional studies discussed here involve the participation of human subjects, they require the preparation of informed consent forms and approval by an IRB (U.S. Department of Health and Human Services 1991).

Subject Recruitment

Spilker and Cramer have developed some rules to follow during the design of a protocol and during the initiation of the trial itself, in order to promote subject recruitment (Spilker and Cramer 1992). These include identifying the actual and potential pool of subjects, developing a recruitment strategy, devising methods to optimize this strategy, developing alternative strategies, and writing the trial protocol with some sensitivity to its impact on recruitment. Following their recommended rules can facilitate maximal recruitment.

The Conduct of the Trial

Given the complicated nature of many clinical trials, detailed procedures are required to ensure correct conduct of the trial. A thorough description of the conduct of a clinical trial has been particularly well outlined by Spilker (1991).

Analysis

Data Interpretation

The interpretation of the results of a trial includes three types of evaluation: data analysis, interpretation, and extrapolation (Spilker 1991). *Data analysis* involves a determination of the statistical significance of the study results and involves the use of statistical procedures and evaluations. Statistical significance does not automatically imply that the results are clinically important. *Interpretation* involves a determination of the clinical significance of the results based on clinical judgment. If, for example, a large trial across the country testing the impact of a class in medical ethics on first-year medical students shows a difference of ten points in test scores measuring understanding of the reasons for informed consent (scores of 75 percent in the control group and 85 percent in the intervention group), this difference may be statistically significant, but it may not lead an ethicist to consider adopting this teaching strategy in a first-year medical school class. To determine that the results of a trial are clinically significant, it is best to establish criteria for significance before the trial begins. One must decide how large a response in the most important outcome measured in the study would be necessary to convince the relevant audience to use the intervention. One might decide beforehand that first-year students should demonstrate a 25 percent difference in scores in order to consider the intervention an educational success. *Extrapolation* requires the use of judgment and logic to determine relevance of the study results for practice settings or circumstances beyond the precise circumstances created in the trial.

Statistical Analysis

The ability to analyze study results is a crucial ingredient in conducting and understanding experimental research. For the interested reader, we venture here to explain the strategy for selecting a statistical approach to experimental research because it is difficult to locate a logical and concise strategy for statistical analysis anywhere in the literature.

The responses of research subjects to the intervention provide the clinical endpoints or data that will require analysis before the investigator can assess the effectiveness of the study intervention. The data may be either *qualitative* (nonnumeric data) or *quantitative* (numerical data). Qualitative data can be classified in categories and hence are labeled *categorical data*. If the categories can be ordered then they may be called *ranked* or *ordered categorical data*. For example, in our hypothetical study of medical student training to obtain informed consent, we may use as our endpoint patients' satisfaction with the consent discussion as determined by interview following the consent process. These interviews may be analyzed with qualitative analytic techniques. Patients' responses may be placed in categories—such as unsatisfied, somewhat satisfied, and very satisfied—depending upon their comments about the student's ability to discuss the consent with them. Alternatively, we may ask patients to rank the interview on a numerical scale. The resulting data will be *numerical data*. If there are numbers with gaps between them, then the variables are *discrete variables*. If there are no such gaps, then the data are considered *continuous*.

To aid in our discussion of data analysis, we refer the reader to three diagrams, developed by Garrett, which provide a guide to the use of the most common statistical tests for data analysis. Figs. 12.1, 12.2, and 12.3 provide decision strategies for selecting tests when performing an analysis with one (*univariate*), two (*bivariate*), or many variables (*multivariable analysis*), respectively. In general, the strategy for selecting a statistical test is based on the characteristics of the variables, whether the variables are categorical or continuous. As indicated above, categorical means that the data collected for the variable can be classified into categories (such as gender, race, type of disease, or location of death) but cannot be quantified in the standard way that quantifiable variables (such as age, temperature, amount of pain, or degree of satisfaction) can be. By contrast, continuous data are measured on a continuum that contains no gaps. In general, the analytic approach one takes should be justified based on the character of the data and is best selected before the data is in hand to be certain that the analytic approach is not chosen to yield some desired result.

Before using statistical tests it is important to examine the values of each variable in order to assess for inaccurate, missing, or extreme data values, and to determine what is the most appropriate form in which to use these variables in further analysis. Since one is dealing here with one variable at a time, it is appropriate to use univariate methods (Fig. 12.1).

If the independent variable, X, is designated to represent whether or not the study subject received the intervention, then X is a categorical variable. If the dependent variable, Y, is the outcome of the study, it may be categorical or continuous. If it is continuous, it further may be classified as normally or not normally distributed. By *normally distributed*, we mean, technically, that the values are distributed in a fashion (called a *probability distribution function*) that looks like a bell shaped curve, with the area under the curve equaling 1, and values ranging from -∞ to ∞. To analyze the effectiveness of the study intervention, one would use the test statistic that is appropriate for the particular type of variable with which one is dealing.

If the study is uncontrolled and the major variable of interest is the study outcome, then it is appropriate to conduct a bivariate analysis. In this case, the baseline and follow-up measurements of the outcome variable are considered separate variables, or repeated measures on the same sample of study subjects. Here the investigator would choose a paired t-test or McNemar's test to compare the baseline and follow-up measurements, depending upon whether the dependent variable is continuous and normally distributed, or categorical (Fig. 12.2).

If the study is a controlled trial, then it is appropriate to carry out a bivariate analysis, with X representing the independent variable (whether the subject was in the control or intervention group) and Y representing the outcome. Take, for example, a hypothetical study to determine whether a pain assessment as a "vital sign" (i.e., asking patients whether and how much pain they have every time their usual vital signs of blood pressure, pulse, respiratory rate, and temperature are checked) leads to improved pain management. The in-

FIGURE 12.1   *Analysis Plan for Univariate Data*

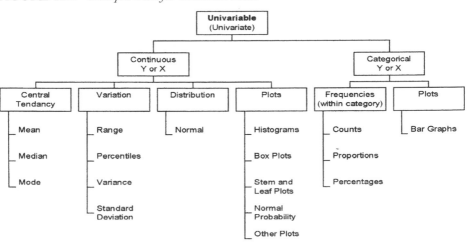

FIGURE 12.2   *Analysis Plan for Bivariate Data*

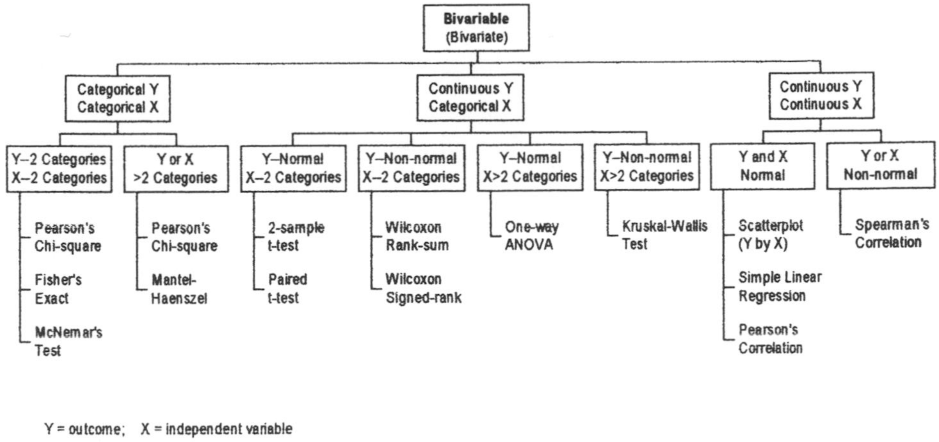

```
                              ┌──────────────┐
                              │  Bivariable  │
                              │ (Bivariate)  │
                              └──────────────┘
         ┌──────────────────────────┼──────────────────────────┐
  ┌───────────────┐         ┌───────────────┐          ┌───────────────┐
  │ Categorical Y │         │ Continuous Y  │          │ Continuous Y  │
  │ Categorical X │         │ Categorical X │          │ Continuous X  │
  └───────────────┘         └───────────────┘          └───────────────┘
```

Y–2 Categories X–2 Categories	Y or X >2 Categories	Y–Normal X–2 Categories	Y–Non-normal X–2 Categories	Y–Normal X>2 Categories	Y–Non-normal X>2 Categories	Y and X Normal	Y or X Non-normal
Pearson's Chi-square	Pearson's Chi-square	2-sample t-test	Wilcoxon Rank-sum	One-way ANOVA	Kruskal-Wallis Test	Scatterplot (Y by X)	Spearman's Correlation
Fisher's Exact	Mantel-Haenszel	Paired t-test	Wilcoxon Signed-rank			Simple Linear Regression	
McNemar's Test						Pearson's Correlation	

Y = outcome;   X = independent variable

dependent variable, X, represents whether or not the patient received the pain assessment. Thus, X is a categorical variable with two categories. Our dependent variable, Y, is a pain score. If the patients' responses to the pain score seem to divide cleanly into two groups—those patients whose pain is satisfactorily relieved and those whose pain is not satisfactorily relieved—then we can consider our outcome measure a categorical variable. Alternatively, we may choose to group the responses into several categories—very unsatisfactory, somewhat unsatisfactory, somewhat satisfactory, and very satisfactory. Yet another option, if the responses to the summary pain score seem to range along a continuum, would be to consider our outcome as a continuous variable. If one modifies an analytic approach after the data is available, the data should be analyzed using several strategies to be certain whether the analytic approach itself influences the significance or interpretation of the findings. Ultimately, the selected analytic approach must be justified to the reader. Alternatively, if the interpretation of the results differs with use of different analytic approaches, the investigator can include these differing interpretations in publication of the results.

We choose a test statistic that is appropriate when X is categorical. If we choose to handle the outcome data as categorical and the scores are divided into two categories, we use Pearson's Chi-square or alternatively Fisher's exact test if the sample is quite small (Fig. 12.2). If we choose to divide the pain scores into more than two categories, we use Pearson's Chi-square or the Mantel-Haenzel test for trend. If the pain scores are continuous and have a normal distribution, we would select a two-sample t-test. If the pain scores are continuous but not normally distributed, we pick the Wilcoxon rank-sum test. Had we designed our study to have more than two treatment arms, it would be appropriate to use one-way analysis of variance (if Y is normally distributed) or the Kruskal-Wallis test (if Y is non-normal).

If we wish to examine the joint contribution of sets of variables, to see the independent contribution of each variable, then we would use multivariable analysis (Fig. 12.3). The X variable in any of the models depicted in Fig. 12.3 can be categorical or continuous. The analysis we choose is determined by the distribution of the outcome variable, Y.

FIGURE 12.3   *Analysis Plan for Multivariate Data*

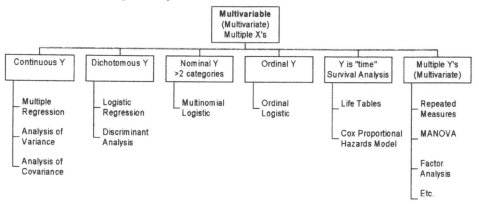

Y = outcome;   X = independent variable

Evaluating Treatment Efficacy in Subgroups of the Study

Study subjects are not all the same and may respond to a study intervention differently. We may wonder if their responses are a function of some particular characteristic. In our pain assessment study the overall results may be negative, but we may notice that children participating in the study tend to show different outcomes in the control and intervention groups. We may therefore choose to perform a subgroup analysis, separating out and analyzing results exclusively for children.

Alternatively, we may be disappointed with the overall negative results and wish to look for patient characteristics that would be associated with greater efficacy of the intervention but not have any one characteristic in mind. Thus, we may choose to perform a multivariable analysis.

Interpretation of Clinical Significance

One judges the clinical significance of the study results according to the expectations one sets out at the beginning of the trial. A statistically significant difference in outcomes between the intervention and control groups may not necessarily be clinically meaningful. Using the example of our hypothetical study of the use of a pain assessment item along with the usual vital signs, if the patients in the intervention group had statistically significantly more pain relief than the control group, as judged by responses to pain scores measured two hours after checking vital signs, but were no more comfortable by midday or evening and reported being no more satisfied with their care, one might judge that the intervention was not effective from the clinical standpoint, despite the statistical results.

Extrapolation

Another important outcome is the influence of the study results upon ethical theory. While SUPPORT was a negative study, as mentioned above, one might argue that it had a profound effect upon medical ethicists' thinking about life-sustaining treatment decision making. The study provided an impetus to find other approaches to improve care at the end of life. Thus, while the study intervention did not have its intended effect, the study certainly served to advance understanding of the ethical aspects of end-of-life care (Schroeder 1999).

Additional Analytical Issues

Whether in a randomized controlled trial or a nonrandomized trial, study subjects may fail to receive the intervention, and the investigator must decide, when analyzing the data, how to handle subjects who failed to receive the intervention. This may happen because the execution of the intervention may not have occurred as intended during its design; the intervention may have been withheld or withdrawn because of some anticipated or actual adverse consequence of the intervention for a particular study subject; or the subject may have chosen not to undergo the intervention after agreeing to participate in the study. In analyzing a randomized control trial, the investigator chooses among three options: to include the subject in the intervention arm, to include the subject in the control group, or to exclude the subject from the analysis altogether. It is generally preferable to take the first approach, called *intention to treat analysis,* since it avoids the possibility of bias or distortion of the results that may occur because of subjects with certain characteristics shifting from one group to another. One might imagine, for example, that medical students who are uncomfortable discussing difficult topics with patients might be less enthusiastic about training in the informed consent process and thus avoid the training intervention. If they were analyzed with the control group, the participants in the intervention group would appear to demonstrate more capability in offering informed consent than they would have had these reluctant students been included among them. The intervention thus will look more effective than it would have had the data been analyzed by intention to treat. If the investigator chooses to include the subject in the control group, this undermines the randomized nature of the study design, but reduces misclassification, which would underestimate the effect of the intervention (Fisher, Dixon, and Herson 1990). If the investigator removes a subject from analysis because the subject was placed in the intervention arm but did not receive the intervention, the benefit of randomization diminishes, since the subjects remaining in the two arms are no longer similar.

Finally, an experimental study is a longitudinal study in which the occurrence of outcome events may be studied over time. In our hypothetical study of the impact of teaching about cultural sensitivity on access to care among minority patients, these patients may be at risk for illness that requires care and be followed over a two-year time period. We might choose to follow patients with regular phone calls and chart reviews and compare the duration of time until the occurrence of some undesirable outcome, such as an illness during which some needed care was not provided. We could compare the length of time until the occurrence of such adverse events in the intervention and control groups using a technique called *survival analysis* (Peto et al. 1977).

Reporting Results

If the investigator conducts an excellent trial but does not report it well, the quality of the study will not be appreciated. Balas and colleagues have developed a tool for evaluating the quality of RCTs (Balas et al. 1995). It is worth utilizing their criteria as one prepares to report the study results.

CRITIQUE OF EXPERIMENTAL METHODS

Appropriate Questions

Experimental research methods can provide answers to empirical questions—questions that are amenable to measurable answers. Normative questions will never be answered by empirical examination. Thus, a philosopher who asks whether it is acceptable ethically to make health care decisions for comatose patients by relying on those patients' previously written instructions for care will answer this question by examining the theoretical arguments about whether or not the conscious individual who is writing the directive is still the same person when he is in a coma, and whether it is best to have such a written advance directive speak for the comatose individual or whether it is ethically preferable for someone else to make treatment decisions on that person's behalf. The philosopher establishes such an argument on theoretical grounds.

Not all empirical questions that one might be interested in asking are amenable to investigation by an experimental trial. Given the enormous effort needed to conduct such a trial, the intervention that the investigator wishes to test ought to be at a certain stage in its evolution to warrant its examination in a clinical trial. The decision to test an intervention should be based not simply on sound theoretical arguments but also on some prior empirical evidence. Such an intervention would be one that is based on a matured idea for which some preliminary empirical evidence exists. At the same time, one ought to still have sufficient doubt about the efficacy of an intervention to warrant conducting the study. Thus, it might be an idea that ethicists have begun to debate and about which there are coherent opposing arguments. The scholarly community ought to be in a position of equipoise in which one is in genuine doubt about the likely outcome of the study in order to proceed with a randomized trial (Freedman 1987).

Strengths and Weaknesses

The experimental method has the potential to provide definitive evidence of the effectiveness of an intervention. While one may have anecdotal experiences, or a series of observations that influence one's belief in the efficacy of an ethical practice, such unsystematic observations are notoriously susceptible to biases. Interventional studies, therefore, provide an invaluable check upon one's beliefs. While this is true for experimental studies in general, some research methodologists consider randomized controlled trials to provide a uniquely impeccable demonstration of effectiveness. Those who promote the use of evidence-based medical practice—recommending that practice be based on effectiveness that has been demonstrated in scientific studies—often argue that randomized controlled trials are the *sine qua non* of definitive evidence. By controlling differences between the intervention and control groups, the likelihood of finding differences that are not truly due to the intervention can be eliminated.

There are, however, significant drawbacks to conducting intervention trials. They are expensive. Aside from monetary expense, they require the expenditure of untold hours of personnel time. At the conclusion of a study, the results may be negative for a variety of reasons unrelated to the merit or the veracity of the hypothesis itself. The intervention as designed by the investigators may not have been as effective as it possibly could be; the design might have been excellent but the execution of the intervention during the conduct of the study might not have been successful; the sample size might not have been large enough to demonstrate a significant difference between the intervention and control group. These and other reasons may lead to the false conclusion that the tested intervention is not effective.

At the other extreme, study findings may be positive and yet the intervention may not have any practical value by the time the study is done (Dupont 1985, Fletcher 1989). This may be because the subjects selected for the trial may differ from typical persons seen in clinical practice; the end points measured in the trial may be of minimal clinical importance; or the intervention tested in the trial may be obsolete by the time the trial is over.

CONCLUDING COMMENTS

Experimental research has not been a part of the traditional armamentarium of the scholar in medical ethics. Yet an increasing number of experiments examining questions of ethical import demonstrate how valuable testing one's assumptions can be. While arguments about how we should conduct ourselves may not always be settled by demonstration of empirical evidence of consequences, for those who wish to make consequentialist arguments, it is important to demonstrate that the outcomes one expects to see from a recommended course of action really do occur. Beyond this, experiments at times provide new and surprising insights into human attitudes and behavior that are relevant to anyone with an interest in ethics. Ethicists do well to pay attention to such empirical findings as they conduct conceptual work.

NOTES ON RESOURCES AND TRAINING

The many skills that contribute to the conduct of a well-done clinical trial are not the domain of any single discipline. Rather, a multidisciplinary team with individuals trained in several fields is appropriate. An indispensable ingredient is an understanding of ethics with sufficient understanding of theory to generate a plausible hypothesis. Additional skills include: study design, grant writing, questionnaire design, project management, interviewing, chart review, data editing, data entry, computer programming, data analysis, and manuscript preparation.

While we have emphasized the need for multidisciplinary collaboration for the conduct of experimental studies in ethics, it is worth considering what sort of training and experience is warranted for those individuals who hope to lead this research effort. Principal investigators are likely to be familiar with the medical ethics research literature and will also require research training for a substantial duration of time, such as a two- or three-year fellowship. They may combine an interest in ethics with skills in health services research or epidemiology.

An excellent text for acquiring a general understanding of the design of experimental research is the textbook, *Designing Clinical Research* (Hulley and Cummings 1988). Several textbooks provide valuable resources for the investigator engaged in the conduct of clinical trials (Pequegnat and Stover 1995; Weiss 1996; Spilker 1991; Spilker and Cramer 1992; Chow and Liu 1998), although these last three texts provide advice for clinical trials of pharmacologic agents. The investigator who wishes to test an intervention to alter an ethically important outcome is testing something far more complex than a medication or most other clinical interventions and should therefore be cautious in extrapolating from these texts to her own work.

Aside from useful texts, there is no substitute for seeking the advice of experienced investigators to learn about the conduct of experimental trials. Respected investigators are likely to be available in most major medical centers and in a growing number of independent clinical research organizations and survey research firms.

While much scholarly research in medical ethics requires modest financial resources, this is not the case for experimental studies. Therefore, attention to such resource requirements is essential. The conduct of a well-designed, well-conducted, and carefully analyzed experimental study is a costly endeavor that requires designated funds that are not likely to be available in an institution's usual operating budget. To seek funds from outside of their institution or to carefully justify the expenditure of their own organizational funds requires investigators to prepare a grant proposal. Pequegnat and Stover have written a useful guide for doing so (Pequegnat and Stover 1995). The development and justification of a budget should parallel the development of the research plan. Part of this process involves the outline of a detailed timeline. Without this, it is impossible to know in which year to budget key items.

The key categories for expenditures should include: personnel, equipment, supplies, travel, patient care costs, other expenses such as publication costs, and consortium or contractual costs. Compensation should be requested for personnel, including the principal investigator and possibly coinvestigators; a project manager; research personnel who will perform a myriad of tasks, including recruiting research subjects, conducting interviews, performing chart reviews, logging in and checking accuracy of data, performing computer data entry, cleaning data postentry; data programmers; statistician; and administrative assistants who handle correspondence, telephone calls, management of funds, and ordering supplies.

REFERENCES

Angell, M. 1997. "The Ethics of Clinical Research in the Third World." *New England Journal of Medicine* 342:967–69.

Baker, D. W., R. M. Parker, M. V. Williams, and W. S. Clark. 1998. "Health Literacy and the Risk of Hospital Admission." *Journal of General Internal Medicine* 13:791–98.

Balas, E. A., S. M. Austin, B. G. Ewigman, G. D. Brown, and J. A. Mitchell. 1995. "Methods of Randomized Controlled Trials in Human Services Research." *Medical Care* 33:687–99.

Chow, S.-C., and J. Liu. 1998. *Design and Analysis of Clinical Trials: Concepts and Methodologies.* New York: John Wiley and Sons, Inc.

Cohen, J. 1988. *Statistical Power Analysis for the Behavioral Sciences.* 2nd ed. Hillsdale, NJ: Lawrence Erlbaum Associates, Publishers.

Danis, M., L. I. Southerland, J. M. Garrett, J. L. Smith, F. Hielema, G. Pickard, D. M. Egner, and D. L. Patrick. 1991. "A Prospective Study of Advance Directives for Life-Sustaining Care." *New England Journal of Medicine* 324:882–88.

Dupont, W. D. 1985. "Randomized vs. Historical Clinical Trials." *American Journal of Epidemiology* 122:940–46.

Donaldson, M. S., and M. J. Field. 1998. "Measuring Quality of Care at the End of Life." *Archives of Internal Medicine* 158:121–28.

Fisher, L. D., D. O. Dixon, and J. Herson. 1990. "Intention to Treat in Clinical Trials." In *Statistical Issues in Drug Research and Development,* ed. K. E. Peace. New York: Marcel Dekker.

Fletcher, R. H. 1989. "The Cost of Clinical Trials." *Journal of the American Medical Association* 262:1842.

Freedman, B. 1987. "Equipoise and the Ethics of Clinical Research." *New England Journal of Medicine* 317:141–45.

———. 1990. "Placebo-Controlled Trials and the Logic of Clinical Purpose." *IRB* 12:1–6.

Freedman, B., K. C. Glass, and C. Weijer. 1996. "Placebo Orthodoxy in Clinical Research: II: Ethical, Legal, and Regulatory Myths." *Journal of Law, Medicine, and Ethics* 24:252–59.

Hays, R. D., and J. E. Ware Jr. 1986. "My Medical Care Is Better than Yours: Social Desirability and Patient Satisfaction Ratings." *Medical Care* 6: 519–24.

Hulley, S. B., and S. R. Cummings. 1988. *Designing Clinical Research.* Baltimore: Williams and Wilkins.

Miller, F. G. 2000. "Placebo-Controlled Trials in Psychiatric Research: An Ethical Perspective." *Biological Psychiatry* 47:707–16.

Morgenstern, H., and D. M. Winn. 1983. "A Method for Determining the Sampling Ratio in Epidemiologic Studies." *Statistics in Medicine* 2:387–96.

Pequegnat, W., and E. Stover. 1995. *How to Write a Successful Research Grant Application: A Guide for Social and Behavioral Scientists.* New York: Plenum Press.

Peto, R., M. C. Pike, P. Armitage, N. E. Breslow, D. R. Cox, S. V. Howard, N. Mantel, K. McPherson, J. Peto, and P. G. Smith. 1977. "Design and Analysis of Randomized Clinical Trials Requiring Prolonged Observation of Each Patient II: Analysis and Examples." *The British Journal of Cancer* 35:1–39.

Roberts, J., and G. Norman. 1990. "Reliability and Learning from the Objective Structured Clinical Examination." *Medical Education* 24:219–23.

Rothman, K. J., and K. B. Michels. 1994. "The Continuing Unethical Use of Placebo Controls." *New England Journal of Medicine* 331:394–98.

Schneiderman, L. J., R. A. Pearlman, R. M. Kaplan, J. P. Anderson, and E. M. Rosenberg. 1992. "Relationship of General Advance Directive Instructions to Specific Life-Sustaining Treatment Preferences in Patients with Serious Illness." *Archives of Internal Medicine* 152:2114–22.

Schroeder, S. A. 1999. "The Legacy of SUPPORT: Study to Understand Prognoses and Preferences for Outcomes and Risks of Treatment." *Annals of Internal Medicine* 131:780–82.

Spilker, B. 1991. *Guide to Clinical Trials.* New York: Raven Press.

Spilker, B., and J. A. Cramer. 1992. *Patient Recruitment and Clinical Trials.* New York: Raven Press.

Sulmasy, D. P., P. B. Terry, C. S. Weisman, D. J. Miller, R. Y. Stallings, M. A. Vettese, and K. B. Haller. 1998. "The Accuracy of Substituted Judgments in Patients with Terminal Diagnoses." *Annals of Internal Medicine* 128:621–29.

The SUPPORT Principal Investigators. 1995. "A Controlled Trial to Improve Care for Seriously Ill Hospitalized Patients: The Study to Understand Prognoses and Preferences for Outcomes and Risks of Treatments (SUPPORT)." *Journal of the American Medical Association* 274:1591–98.

Temple, R., and S. S. Ellenberg. 2000. "Placebo-Controlled Trials and Active-Controlled Trials in the Evaluation of New Treatments." *Annals of Internal Medicine* 133:455–63.

Torgerson, D. J., M. Ryan, and J. Ratcliffe. 1995. "Economics in Sample Size Determination for Clinical Trails." *Quarterly Journal of Medicine* 88:517–21.

U.S. Department of Health and Human Services. 1991. *Rules and Regulations.* 45 CFR 46.

Varmus, H., and D. Satcher. 1998. "Ethical Complexities in Conducting Research in Developing Countries." *New England Journal of Medicine* 18:1331–32.

Weiss, N. S. 1996. *Clinical Epidemiology: The Study of the Outcome of Illness.* 2nd ed. Oxford: Oxford University Press.

13

Economics and Decision Science

David A. Asch

I doubt that many health economists or medical decision scientists believe they are making contributions to the fields of medical ethics in the course of their everyday work. The methods used by scholars in these fields are attractive in part because they appear highly quantitative and value free. Those characteristics might make these approaches seem out of place within a list of tools to address problems in ethics, since ethical problems are so often seen as conflicts of value. Some economists and decision scientists probably take refuge in the view that their methods are ostensibly silent on the issue of values. But even if these fields really are value free at the level of their methodology, their contribution to the manipulation and analysis of values provided from other sources still offers much to empirical work in medical ethics. However, at a very fundamental level, these fields take an implicit value-laden stance—one based largely on some form of utilitarianism. Sometimes that stance is obscured by the methodology that overlies it, but understanding what values may lurk underneath these seemingly sterile approaches will help scholars and policy makers understand both the potentially profound applications and the limitations of these methods.

In this chapter, I focus on certain popular and normatively appealing techniques, such as decision analysis, broadly; cost-effectiveness analysis; and related forms of clinical economics, more specifically. However, there is much more to decision sciences than just decision analysis. For example, decision analysis is a technique for choosing among alternatives in the face of uncertainty. It is a *normative* approach. But many who consider themselves decision scientists focus on *descriptive* observational or experimental studies of decision processes in an attempt to understand how clinicians and patients actually make medical decisions, to uncover biases in those processes (against some normative standard), and, more *prescriptively*, to de-bias, or in other ways improve them.

Similarly, there is much more to health economics than cost-effectiveness analysis or cost-benefit analysis. Health economists also address the social and clinical implications of changes in health care financing, such as the introduction of new insurance products or modifications in the incentive structure for health systems or clinicians. Similarly, they may study the implication of changes in clinician labor force (size, specialty, or geographic distribution) or related changes in projected patient demand, given changing demographics or the introduction of new medical technologies. These fields are broad, and much that health economists or medical decision scientists do is beyond the scope of this chapter.

This chapter focuses on those techniques of economics and decision science designed to evaluate alternative clinical approaches and, in other ways, determine best practices when the best choice is not already known. I first describe how these approaches might be used to evaluate a clinical decision and then provide an example of how it might be adapted for the ethically charged area of carrier screening for cystic fibrosis.

THE TECHNIQUE OF DECISION ANALYSIS

An Abbreviated Primer on Decision Analysis

Imagine a physician who has just begun to set up her office but does not yet have the ability to perform diagnostic tests. With some frequency, she sees patients who complain of urinary symptoms (burning on urination, a sense of urgency, and the like) that might signal a urinary tract infection (UTI) that could be treated with antibiotics. Since the physician does not yet have the ability to perform any diagnostic tests, such as an examination or culture of the urine that might help her make the diagnosis, she recognizes that she must decide on her own how likely it is that each patient with such symptoms has a urinary tract infection. Although much judgment is involved, the task is not too difficult: young women are much more likely to have urinary tract infections than young men; people who have had them before are more likely to get them again; some symptoms are particularly representative of urinary tract infections. Given her experience and judgment, she can assign a probability to each patient she sees that reflects her judgment about whether or not the patient has a urinary tract infection.

However, this physician now faces the question of deciding what probability of urinary tract infection is high enough to justify treatment with an antibiotic or, conversely, what probability is too low to justify such treatment. She reasons that this decision must reflect some combination of factors, including the risks or costs of treating patients with antibiotics when they do not have an infection, the risk or costs of not treating patients when they do, and, if she had been able to use a test to help her with the diagnosis, the risks, costs, and accuracy of the test.

Decision analysis is a structured approach designed to help incorporate these different kinds of information and so identify the best choice when the best choice is otherwise uncertain. Fig. 13.1 displays one way in which a decision analyst might represent the clinical problem of the UTI. As the tree is read left to right, the square node on the left indicates a *choice* the physician makes between treating the symptoms with antibiotics or not. The circular nodes represent *chance* events over which the physician has no control. In this case, the chance event is whether or not the patient indeed has a UTI, represented here with a probability, p; this chance event and its associated probability are the same regardless of the choice the physician makes. At the end of each branch is some reflection of the outcome, for example, a treated UTI.

More thorough descriptions of the techniques and methods of decision modeling are available elsewhere, including techniques based on trees, like the UTI example, or those based on Markov models or other simulations (Detsky et al. 1997a, 1997b; Naglie et al.

FIGURE 13.1. *Sample Decision Tree for the Management of Suspected Urinary Tract Infection. The square node represents a choice to be made. Circular nodes represent chance events, in this case at probability,* p. UTI = urinary tract infection.

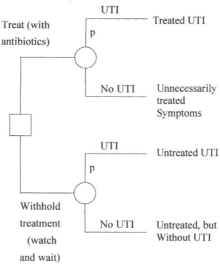

1997; Krahn et al. 1997; Naimark et al. 1997; Weinstein and Fineberg, 1980; Sox et al. 1988). Even so, the simple structure of the UTI example follows many of the steps and contains many of the elements essential to all of these models:

1. Imagine the model and draw the tree.
2. Identify the probabilities.
3. Identify the outcome variables.
4. Calculate the expected values.
5. Perform sensitivity analyses.

The first step is to structure the clinical problem and represent it in a tree format so that the consequences of alternative choice and chance events can be understood. Both science and art are necessary to structure trees well. Real clinical problems are complex, but useful clinical *models* simplify and constrain circumstances and choices. In the UTI example, only the choices to treat or withhold treatment are presented. However, real clinicians might see other options. For example, they might wait a day or two to see if the symptoms resolve on their own and then treat only if they do not. Individual branches on a tree must be mutually exclusive, so that there is no overlap or confusion. Moreover, they must be exhaustive—meaning that together they encompass all of the important possibilities. However, how many "twigs" ought to be included on each branch, or how finely detailed the model ought to be, is a matter of judgment, which is to say that the choices often reflect the values of the decision analyst. Skilled decision analysts find themselves "pruning" the trees of their students, who tend to include too much detail. Those who miss the big picture are often said to have "missed the forest for the trees"; in decision analysis, the risk is missing the tree because of the branches.

The second step is to identify the probabilities of various chance events occurring. In Fig. 13.1, a circular chance node reflects the mutually exclusive and exhaustive possibilities that a UTI is either present or not. In this example, the source of that probability could be the physician's judgment. For example, the physician might estimate that there is a 40 percent chance that a twenty-two-year-old woman has a UTI, given that she complains of new urinary frequency and burning on urination, but she is sexually inactive and has no prior history of UTI. Accurate or not, that estimate of probability, if it really is the physician's best estimate, ought to influence her management of the patient—whether or not it is incorporated into a formal decision analysis. In more legitimate analyses the best sources of this information are well-conducted studies published in the medical literature. Such studies are often unavailable for some or many parts of a model, and so investigators often rely on practical, but less credible sources, such as expert opinions.

The third step is to identify the outcomes and assign values to them. The UTI example expressed in Fig. 13.1 includes only four outcomes, reflecting that the patient either does or does not have a UTI and is either treated with antibiotics or not. Many of the ethically relevant issues in a decision analysis are concentrated in choices about how these outcomes are valued. Because of their importance, these issues will be discussed more extensively in a later section. In the meantime, these outcomes might be ranked, from best to worst, in the following order:

1. The patient does not have a UTI and is not treated [0]
2. The patient does not have a UTI and is treated with antibiotics [–10]
3. The patient has a UTI and is treated with antibiotics [–20]
4. The patient has a UTI and is not treated [–50]

This order reflects that some outcomes are clearly better than others. For example, if we consider only the outcomes in which the patient does not have a UTI (1 and 2), it is better to be untreated than treated, so 1 > 2. Similarly, if we consider only the outcomes in which the patient has a UTI (3 and 4), it is better to be treated than untreated, and so 3 > 4. Finally, if we consider only the outcomes in which the patient receives antibiotics (2 and 3), it is better not to have a UTI than to have one, and so 2 > 3.

For a decision analysis, these outcomes must be given some relative values, not just a rank ordering, and some potential relative values are included in brackets in the list. These values might be considered as "utilities," which are abstract representations of some amount of good. Or, they could be expressed in dollars or some other value metric. In this example, the first outcome was given a value of 0, to reflect that the patient neither has the disease nor receives any treatment. The last was given a value of –50, reflecting that sometimes an untreated UTI can get worse and cause other problems, and that symptoms might persist longer than with treatment. These values, and the ones in between, were assigned somewhat arbitrarily. More formal, rigorous, and methodologically defensible techniques for assigning values to outcomes are described in a variety of sources, but are conceptually and procedurally complex (Torrance 1986; Redelmeier and Detsky1995; Froberg and Kane 1989). Some sources catalog utility measures for many different health states (Fryback et al. 1993).

The fourth step is to calculate the expected values. This step is a mathematical exercise in which the values of the outcomes (from step 3) are weighted by the probabilities that they will occur (from step 2). In the UTI example, given a 40 percent chance of a UTI (which means there is a 60 percent chance of no UTI), the "expected value" (EV) of following the upper branch of Fig. 13.1 and providing treatment is:

EV(Treatment) = 0.4 × (−20) + 0.6 × (−10) = −14.

The expected value of following the lower branch of Fig. 13.1 and withholding treatment is:

EV(Withhold Treatment) = 0.4 × (−50) + 0.6 × (0) = −20.

Because the expected value of treating this patient (−14) exceeds the expected value of withholding treatment (−20), this decision analysis suggests that treatment is the preferred option. The calculation of expected value is a mathematical approach with *consequentialist* goals, which are to achieve the highest expected value.

The final step is to perform a *sensitivity analysis*. In this example, the values assigned to the outcomes were not well justified and might plausibly be quite different. A decision analyst might ask whether the conclusion to prescribe antibiotics would be sustained under alternative plausible assumptions about these values. Similarly, in this example the probability of a UTI was estimated at 40 percent. However, this physician might want to know whether antibiotics are appropriate if the probability of a UTI falls to 10 percent or, more generally, what level of probability represents the threshold between prescribing antibiotics or not. A sensitivity analysis tests the stability of the conclusions across alternative assumptions about one or more variables in the model; it determines how sensitive the conclusions are to certain model assumptions, alone or in combination. For example, Fig. 13.2 reveals a sensitivity analysis for the UTI example and shows the expected value of the Treat and Withhold strategies over all probabilities of UTI, from 0 to 1. The two lines intersect at a probability of 0.25, meaning that, given the structure of the tree and the assumptions about the value of the outcomes, patients whose likelihood of UTI is less than 25 percent should not be treated with antibiotics, and patients whose likelihood of UTI exceeds 25 percent should be treated.

The UTI example is simplistic in many ways, but it illustrates decision analysis' main purpose of structuring choices and analyzing them systematically. Indeed, a central advantage of decision analysis is that through its formal process, one can avoid many of the emotional pitfalls that accompany conventional decision making. Nevertheless, decision analysis is not value free. Not only are the choices one makes in creating a decision analysis often questions of value, but decision analysis can also be used to structure ethical questions. The next section discusses the question of valuing outcomes, followed by an example of using decision analysis to explore carrier screening for cystic fibrosis.

A Closer Look at the Issue of Valuing Outcomes

In the previous section, the valuations of the outcomes in the UTI example were presented without much explanation, merely to move the example forward. However, the

FIGURE 13.2.   *One-way Sensitivity Analysis for Suspected Urinary Tract Infection. The expected value (EV) of the Treat and Withhold strategies is shown. For any probability of disease indicated on the horizontal axis, the best strategy can be found by identifying which strategy provides the highest expected utility. At probabilities less than .25, withholding treatment provides the greatest expected value. At probabilities exceeding .25, treating provides the greatest expected value.*

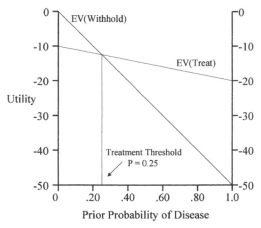

choices made in valuing these outcomes reflect underlying beliefs about what issues are important. To the extent that decision analyses are sensitive to these valuations—as they often are—these beliefs determine the results of the analysis and, in turn, what advice is given to patients or policy makers. For this reason, the methods used in valuing outcomes need some special attention.

For example, decision analysts are nearly always interested in clinical outcomes, such as serious illness or death. However, some clinical outcomes do not reflect serious illness or death, but nevertheless are associated with pain or anxiety. Although these symptoms are often very important to patients, they are included only in some decision analyses—largely because they are so difficult to measure. In deciding what aspects of each outcome to account for, decision analysts, in effect, determine what considerations are seen as important; i.e., effects on mortality will be included, but effects on anxiety or patient worry will not. For example, one potential advantage of chorionic villus sampling over amniocentesis, for prenatal diagnosis, is that the former can be performed earlier during a pregnancy, and therefore the results can be available sooner. A decision analysis comparing amniocentesis with chorionic villus sampling that looks only at how accurately the test performs or how well it identifies abnormalities in the fetus may fail to reflect the concerns of women and couples if diagnostic delay is something to be avoided.

Decision analysts also must decide whether to include economic costs in addition to clinical outcomes when they evaluate alternatives. Cost-effectiveness analyses and cost-benefit analyses, for example, are decision analyses that include as measured outcomes not just the clinical outcomes, but also the economic outcomes of alternative clinical strategies. Incorporating costs into a decision analysis is as ethically value laden as incorporating considerations of costs into real-time clinical decisions. First, some people are uncomfortable incorporating costs into a clinical decision because they believe, rightly, that this approach implicitly puts a monetary value on human life. The only reason to compare the cost-effectiveness of two clinical approaches, for example, is to help one later decide whether the increased costs of the more expensive approach are justified by any increased health benefits. However, they might not be, either because the more expensive approach does not convey any additional benefits (which makes decision making easy: use the cheaper approach because it is at least no worse), or because the additional benefits provided by the more expensive approach just are not worth the additional cost. Those who feel that no price can be put on life are implicitly supporting an impossible position. If one fails to put a finite price on the value of saving a life, then one effectively commits unlimited resources to saving lives and goes bankrupt. If, instead, one puts a finite price on saving a life, then there will be some costs that will exceed that limit (Asch 1995).

A second fundamental ethical challenge to clinical economics is that the answer to the question, How much does it cost? depends critically on who is asked. A patient with full, first dollar insurance coverage bears no additional charge when a more expensive option is chosen over a cheaper one. The insurance company may see greater charges, or may not if it has previously negotiated an arrangement with the physician or health system to provide either option at the same rate. But in the latter case, the health system may face greater costs if, indeed, the more expensive option consumes more resources (staff time, equipment) that could be put to other use. Costs and charges are different (Finkler 1982). Charges measure the cost only to those who pay those charges.

Most economists now argue that costs should be viewed from the "societal" perspective when performing economic assessments, in which the societal perspective reflects the consumption of resources regardless of who pays the bill (Gold et al. 1996). There are advantages to this approach, in that it is less susceptible to manipulation and because most of these analyses are designed to take societal perspectives into consideration in the first place. Nevertheless, the results of a cost-effectiveness analysis that measures costs from the societal perspective will misrepresent the interests of individual patients who may view costs very differently than society as a whole. Clinicians who choose a less-costly, less-effective alternative because the additional benefit of the more expensive alternative is not worth it need to recognize that they may not be saving their patient's money, but someone else's. How comfortable we feel about those decisions is inherently a question of values.

Several resources provide more thorough descriptions of the techniques of clinical economics (Gold et al. 1996; Drummond, Stoddard, and Torrance 1987; Sox et al. 1988; Eisenberg 1989). The next section provides an illustration of how these techniques can be used in an ethically charged clinical area.

Carrier Screening for Cystic Fibrosis[1]

Asch and colleagues used cost-effectiveness analysis to evaluate several alternative strategies for screening couples for the genetic mutations responsible for cystic fibrosis (CF). Approximately one in twenty-five Caucasians in the United States carries the gene for cystic fibrosis, and approximately one in 2,500 babies born is affected. Cystic fibrosis is an autosomal recessive disease, which means that if both reproductive partners are carriers, one in four of their children will have CF. Most children with CF are born to couples without a family history who learn they are carriers only through the birth of an affected child. However, even though the CF gene has been identified, the hundreds of distinct mutations of this gene make it impractical to screen for all of them. For this reason, most DNA-based screening tests for only five or ten of the most common mutations, representing, in aggregate, about 85 percent of carriers (U.S. Congress 1992).

Population-based CF carrier screening is controversial, in part because genetic screening, in the setting of reproductive planning, raises important ethical issues, and also because even very good tests perform poorly when applied to low-prevalence conditions.

The application of CF carrier screening is further complicated because many different screening strategies may be constructed using different decision rules for proceeding to further testing or deciding whether to continue a pregnancy (Asch et al. 1996). For example, one screening strategy might screen both partners in a couple for the presence of the gene. Those couples for whom both partners are found to carry the gene (which causes no problems in those who merely carry one copy) might then proceed to prenatal diagnosis using amniocentesis or chorionic villus sampling to determine if the fetus has inherited both mutations and therefore might be affected. Alternatively, partners within a couple might be screened in sequence: the second partner is screened only if the first partner is found to carry the mutation, and the fetus is tested only if both partners in the couple are carriers. Many other permutations of tests are possible, varying the breadth of the screen used, or using combinations of tests. Altogether, Asch and colleagues examined sixteen different strategies, each likely to lead to different clinical and economic outcomes. Thus, the clinical and economic questions are not only whether widespread CF carrier screening should be done but how it should be done.

Several representative branches of the overall decision tree are shown in Fig. 13.3. All branches end with a clinical outcome reflecting a pregnancy that either is delivered, miscarried, or terminated. In addition, each pregnancy represents a fetus that is affected with CF or not.

These outcomes under consideration distinguish this kind of cost-effectiveness analysis from many others. Most analyses target few and relatively uncontroversial goals. For example, policies toward childhood immunization, prostate cancer screening, or dietary fat reduction have as explicit goals the reduction of disease and disability, the promotion of health, or related goals easy to share. Typically, these policies become controversial only when these clinical goals conflict with other goals to reduce costs.

In contrast, genetic carrier screening, for the purposes of reproductive planning, leads to clinical outcomes that are more controversial. These strategies often raise issues concerning abortion, eugenics, contraception, and reproductive choice—issues that can incite or challenge strong feelings (Wilfond and Fost 1992). More important, the kinds of economic evaluations these analyses address can seem unusual.

Table 13.1 displays the distribution of a hypothetical cohort of 500,000 pregnancies over these six clinical outcomes (delivery, miscarriage, or termination × CF or not CF) for selected strategies from the original analysis. Strategy A reflects the no screening option and is used for comparison. A description of the other strategies is not essential for this illustration, but can be found elsewhere (Asch and Hershey 1998).

FIGURE 13.3 *Selected Branches of the Decision Tree and Subtree for Cystic Fibrosis Carrier Screening Problem.*[a] *Each pregnancy can either be terminated (subtree A) or continued (subtree B). If it is terminated, it might have led to the birth of a child with CF or without CF. If it is continued, it might lead to a miscarriage or to delivery, and in either case might be affected with CF or not. MIE—microvillar intestinal enzyme analysis—is a biochemical test that could be used to improve diagnosis of CF but is now no longer used.*

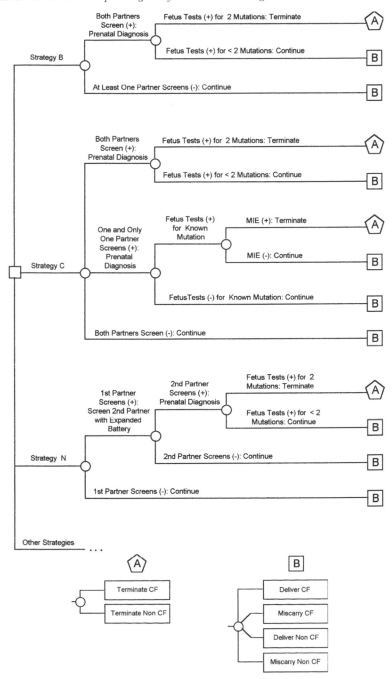

[a]Adapted from Asch et al. 1998.

TABLE 13.1   *Base-Case Analysis for Selected Alternative Cystic Fibrosis Carrier Screening Strategies*[a]

Strategy	CF			Non-CF			CF Births Avoided (rel. to A)	Total Cost	Cost Per CF Birth Avoided (rel. to A)
	Births	Abortions	Miscarriages	Births	Abortions	Miscarriages			
A	195	0	5	487,305	0	12,495	0	$1,530,313,000	—
B	57	142	1	487,302	0	12,498	138	$1,623,710,000	$676,000
C	8	191	0	486,787	340	12,673	187	$1,641,185,000	$594,000
E	6	194	0	486,737	358	12,705	189	$1,694,522,000	$867,000
F	39	160	1	487,300	0	12,499	156	$1,627,544,000	$625,000
N	49	150	1	487,301	0	12,499	146	$1,583,972,000	$367,000
O	49	150	1	487,301	0	12,499	146	$1,607,352,000	$527,000
P	32	167	1	487,045	169	12,586	163	$1,593,807,000	$391,000

[a]Selected from Asch et al. 1998. The figures represent the results of a strategy applied to a cohort of 500,000 pregnancies that have survived through 16 weeks gestation. Birth outcomes are rounded to the nearest 1 and costs to the nearest $1,000 in 1995 dollars.

These results reveal much about the consequences and tradeoffs of different policies. Fewer children are born with CF with Strategy C than Strategy A (no screening), but one of the nonfinancial costs of achieving this goal is that more total abortions are performed, and these tend to be terminations of pregnancies that would have resulted in the delivery of unaffected children had the pregnancies been continued. The reason for the large number of abortions in Strategy C is that the identification of each additional affected pregnancy requires tests of lower and lower specificity used on pregnancies of only intermediate risk. The result is an increasing rate of false positive tests. The rate of miscarriages increases in this strategy as well because more couples undergo prenatal diagnosis, and this procedure induces a small but tangible risk of miscarriage. Costs also differ considerably among the strategies—whether these costs are considered either as a whole or as a ratio of the cost per CF birth avoided.

If one were interested only in avoiding as many CF births as possible, one would choose Strategy E. However, this strategy comes with many abortions of pregnancies that would not result in the delivery of a child affected with CF, a higher rate of miscarriages attributable to the risks of prenatal diagnoses, the highest total costs, and second highest cost per CF birth avoided. If, in addition, one wanted to avoid abortions of unaffected pregnancies, Strategy F might seem attractive, but it is much costlier than Strategy N. More generally, even if the goal of CF carrier screening is to reduce the number of children born with this condition, many would want to balance that goal with the outcomes reflected in other cells of the table.

Table 13.1 illustrates the genuine tradeoffs that exist in this clinical situation. The economic and decision-analytic approach that produces this table helps make these tradeoffs explicit, but it does not clearly point to a best strategy, or, in general, a way to resolve these tradeoffs. Moreover, the reporting of the results in Table 13.1 itself reflects a series of value-laden choices about what outcomes are useful to measure and track. Some might believe that costs or abortions ought not to matter. Others might believe that certain outcomes currently not reflected in this table (such as the amount of anxiety couples face while they are awaiting the news of prenatal diagnosis) ought to be included or featured prominently.

Problems with Values[2]

Table 13.1 also introduces a different set of concerns related to the economic evaluation of these clinical strategies. In a *cost-benefit* analysis, all outcomes are evaluated in monetary terms and compared to the additional costs incurred. Strategies producing an excess of benefits over costs are desirable. In a *cost-effectiveness* analysis, clinical outcomes are measured and related to a measure of costs. Often, the analysis is expressed as a ratio of the cost incurred while achieving these clinical goals—for example, dollars per year of life saved. Even in a cost-effectiveness analysis, however, one must eventually have some sense of how many dollars saving a year of life is worth or strategies in the end are unevaluable.

Nevertheless, many clinicians are uncomfortable with economic analyses, because they do not believe the measures of value are valid, because they find difficult or offensive the requirement that clinical outcomes be evaluable in monetary terms, or because they think costs ought not to matter. Even those comfortable with economic analysis in the main may have special problems evaluating outcomes in the case of genetic screening. In a conventional screening strategy for breast cancer, for example, one evaluates strategies that help individuals present at earlier and more easily treated stages. With genetic carrier screening, one evaluates strategies that prevent the *births* of individuals with the disease, rather than the disease in people already born. From a population perspective, the two approaches can yield identical results, but from an individual perspective, conventional screening strategies work by preventing or treating disease, and reproductive genetic screening strategies work by preventing the births of persons who might develop the disease. Absent specific therapy, genetic screening in the reproductive setting at best replaces individuals with genetic conditions with those without them. It does nothing positive for the individuals who are affected, or those who would be.

How does one measure the value of avoiding a delivery that would have resulted in the birth of a child with CF? Presumably, if the parents attach a positive value to the birth, they would not terminate a pregnancy, even at high risk. Conversely, a couple that chooses to terminate such a pregnancy reveals a set of values for which the birth of an affected child would be worse than an abortion. Such a decision would not imply, however, that should a child with CF be born to these parents, having that child survive is worse than having that child die. Most children with CF are deeply loved by their families. More likely the decision to terminate a pregnancy is based on an expectation that the abortion will be followed by a new pregnancy and a second chance at delivering an unaffected child.

In theory, for a specific couple or a specific individual, one could engage in an exercise to assess the value, in monetary or nonmonetary terms, of each of the six clinical outcomes represented in Table 13.1, in the context of an overall reproductive plan, spanning several pregnancies. Such an exercise might help individuals make choices, which is the purpose of policy analysis applied to the individual case. But in this case, great individual variation in values is likely, so it is virtually certain that no general policy could be ideal for everyone. In the case of conventional screening for breast cancer, all are likely to agree that more years of health are better than fewer, though they probably do not agree on how much better they are, and at how much cost in money, pain, or disfigurement. But as hard as it is to set a national policy for breast cancer screening, it is probably impossible and not very useful to set a uniform policy for genetic screening where values are likely to be even more varied.

A CRITIQUE OF DECISION ANALYSIS

Appropriate Questions

This chapter began with the estimate that most health economists or medical decision scientists probably do not believe they are making contributions to the fields of medical ethics in the course of their everyday work. For what questions in medical ethics, then, might these approaches be useful?

These techniques have their greatest application to medical ethics when understanding the *consequences* of alternative choices is likely to define the most appropriate path. Many ethical questions surround the use of CF carrier screening in the reproductive setting. Some of these center around ethical principles of reproductive choice, or concerns about eugenics, or the social construction of disease. Others are based on a legitimate desire to understand the likely clinical and economic consequences of screening, to help understand what tradeoffs are involved, and whether those tradeoffs are worth it.

The next two sections outline the strengths and weaknesses of these approaches in more detail, but the basic focus of these approaches is on understanding the consequences of choices, when the best choice is not otherwise clear.

Strengths

The fundamental power of decision-analytic and economic approaches to clinical or medical ethics problems is that these approaches are explicit, formal, and systematic. The tradition in these fields, and the nature of the work, demands that individual assumptions are specified and, in the best case, open to view. Similarly, the results can be presented following the same explicit rules. For example, the CF analysis reported in Table 13.1 provides an organized view of the consequences of several alternative ethically charged choices. Sometimes these consequences are unanticipated or make sense only in retrospect.

The second strength of these approaches is that the process used to construct a model may be a useful end in itself. Scholars willing to go through the exercise of structuring a decision tree may find that the process helps clarify their own thinking because of the regimented steps that are required. Formalizing a problem in this way enforces discipline and helps to distance scholars from their visceral reactions to a medical ethics problem. That distance can be useful if those visceral reactions do not help illuminate an issue and are not defensible by clearer heads.

A third strength of these approaches is that the need to assign values to the outcomes encourages careful attention to how patients feel about clinical outcomes. People generally want to avoid a miscarriage, but making good decisions often requires a more detailed sense of exactly how that outcome is valued. As with other elements, the process of decision analysis enforces disciplined thinking in essential areas.

Finally, modeling provides tremendous power in its opportunity to support sensitivity analyses. Sensitivity analyses allow scholars to test the impact of alternative plausible assumptions about all aspects of the problem. What if the risk of miscarriage following amniocentesis was higher? What if the test had a higher rate of false positives? What if we decided that we needed to understand the impact of couples' anxiety? These analyses are useful in two ways. First, they can indicate what assumptions, when changed, critically alter the results, so that one would choose a different approach after viewing those results. When a sensitivity analysis shows this, and the alternative assumptions are plausible, then it is time to return to the literature, the laboratory, the clinic, or wherever necessary to get more precise information about those particular assumptions. Or, as in the CF case, perhaps it means that if different values lead to vastly different management strategies, then developing an appealing uniform policy across individuals would be impossible. Second, sensitivity analyses can indicate what assumptions, even when changed substantially, leave the overall conclusions unaffected. Such a finding indicates that those assumptions are simply not important to the situation, and certainly that no more work should go into increasing the precision of their estimates.

Weaknesses

There is a vast and growing literature on the weaknesses of economic approaches to evaluating health care programs. The aim of much of this literature is to refine methods to address problems and thereby move the field forward. Much of the literature also addresses ways to standardize approaches across investigators, to make studies comparable, and to increase the confidence that results are not subject to manipulation by idiosyncratic accounting procedures. For example, critical issues in the use of these methods include ways to incorporate life expectancy and quality of life into economic models; whether public or patient values are most appropriate in evaluating health states; distinguishing between fixed and variable costs and allocating the costs of infrastructure; appropriate techniques in the temporal discounting of costs or health benefits; and clear ways to reflect uncertainty in model results.

These specific challenges to the field reflect technical advances or choices and are summarized well in a published guide (Gold et al. 1996). However, there are weaknesses in these methods that are more specific to applications in medical ethics. Underlying these weaknesses is the fundamental issue that decision-analytic reasoning is inherently utilitarian. Although one can think of modifications to decision analyses that might incorporate notions of individual rights (for example, one simply might not structure decision trees with branches that violate important individual rights), decision analyses evaluate strategies only by the outcomes they produce, and not how they get there. This consequentialist approach may thereby conflict with the approach of many theoretical medical ethicists.

Asch and Hershey have examined one particular tension that can arise in the conduct of these analyses (Asch and Hershey 1995; 1998). Most decision analyses, when they take a population perspective, inherently aggregate the outcomes of individuals across the population. In this way, although some individuals may realize bad outcomes, these may appear to be offset by the good outcomes realized by other individuals. More generally, these analyses often present the central tendency of the analysis, or the average result, without giving much attention to the distribution of outcomes across individuals in the population. If programs are evaluated only on the basis of the average outcome, they may be misevaluated—because most individuals will not bear the average outcome, but some other outcome that will be like the average only when viewed in combination with what happens to everyone else.

Tsevat and colleagues calculated the gains in life expectancy attributable to reducing various coronary heart disease risk factors. They found that reducing serum cholesterol to 200 mg/dl for thirty-five-year-old men would result in a population-wide increase in individual life expectancy of 0.7 years. The authors were careful and correct to note that individual gains could be much more substantial (Tsevat et al. 1991). If everyone bore the average burden of a health intervention and received the average benefit, many might jump at the chance to give up 0.7 years of life in exchange for the comfort of eating high-fat foods with abandon. Of course, many of these patients would give up nothing, and some would suffer very early mortality. The population-based perspectives of the boardroom often miss the point that clinicians and patients care about the full distribution of outcomes, as well as the central tendency (Asch 1999).

Some forms of utilitarianism shy away from interpersonal comparisons, but other forms are premised on the idea that the good outcomes achieved by some individuals offset the bad outcomes achieved by others. In contrast, rights-based or deontological theories of justice get their support, in part, from the view that by averaging outcomes across individuals, utilitarian perspectives elide important distinctions between persons (Rawls 1971). Those who want to use the techniques of clinical economics or decision analysis to help them address problems in medical ethics need to be keenly aware of the implicit philosophical assumptions that underlie these methods.

CONCLUDING COMMENTS

Ethical values are inherently represented in the conduct of cost-effectiveness analyses and other forms of quantitative decision analysis, despite the seeming objectivity and value neutrality of these techniques. These techniques embody a form of utilitarianism that can contrast with other systems of justice based on rights, for example. For these reasons, the decision to adopt the results of a decision analysis in addressing a question of health policy is, in part, the adoption of that moral framework.

Indeed, the utilitarian framework is one of the virtues of decision analysis in that the utiles or other units of these analyses can be summed and compared—at least mathematically. Arguments based on rights, for example, often lose their heuristic appeal when different rights compete—or at least the solution to such conflicts is often not clear. Decision analyses provide a structured approach to examining such conflicts, and the insistence on common metrics of value makes it easier to resolve what otherwise might become shouting matches.

NOTES ON RESOURCES AND TRAINING

Because of the breadth of these methods, training is available from many different sources and comes in many forms. At one extreme, those aiming to pursue original scholarship in these fields can enter doctoral programs in economics, public policy, operations research, epidemiology, and the like. Some specialized programs focus on health economics.

Masters-level training in these areas is often available in schools of public health and related programs. Some universities offer joint degrees, pairing clinical training with methodologic training in medical decision making or clinical economics. Popular combinations are M.D. or R.N. programs paired with a Ph.D in economics, M.P.H, or M.B.A. programs.

Many scholars who are interested in these areas, but not sufficiently interested to justify long, degree-granting programs, might do well to investigate the short courses offered by The Society for Medical Decision Making (http://www.gwu.edu/~smdm/index.html) during its annual national meeting, held in the fall. Half-day and full-day courses are typically offered in basic and advanced decision analysis, Markov modeling, clinical economics, decision psychology, and the like. Attending the remainder of the scientific meeting, and reading through the journal, *Medical Decision Making*, can provide additional insights.

Many of the papers and books cited in the bibliography were chosen because they represent useful tutorials or guides for those interested in these methods. As mentioned above, the journal *Medical Decision Making* often contains technical notes and other review articles that can help scholars use these methods.

Because these fields are so quantitative, a variety of software programs exist to perform decision analyses. One of the most popular and easy to use programs is DATA, available for Windows or Macintosh platforms (TreeAge Software, Inc.; Williamstown, MA; http://www.treeage.com/).

NOTES

1. Much of the material in this section has been taken from two sources, Asch et al. 1996 and Asch et al. 1998.
2. Much of the material in this section has been taken from Asch et al. 1996.

REFERENCES

Asch, D. A. 1995. "Basic Lessons in Resource Allocation: Sharing, Setting Limits, and Being Fair." *Pharos of Alpha Omega Alpha Honor Medical Society* 58:33–34.

———. 1999. "From Boardroom to Bedside: Bioethical Implications of Policy Research for Clinical Practice." *Journal of Investigative Medicine* 47:273–77.

Asch, D. A, and J. C. Hershey. 1995. "Why Some Health Policies Don't Make Sense at the Bedside." *Annals of Internal Medicine* 122:846–50.

———. 1998. "Avoidable Errors in Health Policy Analysis." *Journal of General Internal Medicine* 13:762–67.

Asch, D. A., J. C. Hershey, M. V. Pauly, J. P. Patton, M. K. Jedrziewski, and M. T. Mennuti. 1996. "Genetic Screening for Reproductive Planning: Methodological and Conceptual Issues in Policy Analysis." *American Journal of Public Health* 86:684–90.

Asch, D. A., J. C. Hershey , M. L. DeKay , M. V. Pauly , J. P. Patton, M. K. Jedrziewski, F. X. Frei, R. Giardine, J. A. Kant, and M. T. Mennuti. 1998. "Carrier Screening for Cystic Fibrosis: Costs and Clinical Outcomes." *Medical Decision Making* 18:202–12.

Detsky, A. S., G. Naglie, M. D. Krahn, D. Naimark, and D. A. Redelmeier. 1997a. "Primer on Medical Decision Analysis: Part 1—Getting Started." *Medical Decision Making* 17:123–25.

Detsky, A. S, G. Naglie, M. D. Krahn, D. A. Redelmeier, and D. Naimark. 1997b. "Primer on Medical Decision Analysis: Part 2—Building a Tree." *Medical Decision Making* 17:126–35.

Drummond, M. F., G. L. Stoddard, and G. W. Torrance. 1987. *Methods for the Economic Evaluation of Health Care Programmes.* New York: Oxford University Press.

Eisenberg, J. M. 1989. "Clinical Economics: A Guide to the Economic Analysis of Clinical Practices." *Journal of the American Medical Association* 262:2879–86.

Finkler, S. A. 1982. "The Distinction between Costs and Charges." *Annals of Internal Medicine* 96:306–10.

Froberg, D. G., and R. L. Kane. 1989. "Methodology for Measuring Health-State Preferences—I. Measurement Strategies." *Journal of Clinical Epidemiology* 42:345–54.

Fryback, D. G., E. J. Dasbach, R. Klein, B. E. Klein, N. Dorn, K. Peterson, and P. A. Martin 1993. "The Beaver Dam Health Outcomes Study: Initial Catalog of Health-State Quality Factors." *Medical Decision Making* 13:89–102.

Gold, M. R., J. E. Siegel, L. B. Russel, and M. C. Weinstein. 1996. *Cost-Effectiveness in Health and Medicine.* New York: Oxford University Press.

Krahn, M. D., G. Naglie, D. Naimark, D. A. Redelmeier, and A. S. Detsky. 1997. "Primer on Medical Decision Analysis: Part 4—Analyzing the Model and Interpreting the Results." *Medical Decision Making* 17:142–51.

Naglie, G, M. D. Krahn, D. Naimark, D. A. Redelmeier, and A. S. Detsky. 1997. "Primer on Medical Decision Analysis: Part 3—Estimating Probabilities and Utilities." *Medical Decision Making* 17:136–41.

Naimark, D., M. D. Krahn, G. Naglie, D. A. Redelmeier, and A. S. Detsky. 1997. "Primer on Medical Decision Analysis: Part 5—Working with Markov Processes." *Medical Decision Making* 17:152–59.

Rawls, J. 1971. *A Theory of Justice.* Cambridge: Harvard University Press.

Redelmeier, D. A., and A. S. Detsky. 1995. "A Clinician's Guide to Utility Measurement." *Primary Care* 22:271–80.

Sox, H., M. A. Blatt, M. C. Higgins, and K. I. Marton. 1988. *Medical Decision Making.* London: Butterworth.

Torrance, G. W. 1986. "Measurement of Health State Utilities for Economic Appraisal: A Review." *Journal of Health Economics* 5 (1986): 1–30.

Tsevat, J., M. C. Weinstein, L. W. Williams, A. N. Tosteson, and L. Goldman. 1991. "Expected Gains in Life-Expectancy from Various Coronary Heart Disease Risk Factor Modifications." *Circulation* 83:1194–1201.

U.S. Congress, Office of Technology Assessment. 1992. *Cystic Fibrosis and DNA Tests: Implications of Carrier Screening.* OTA-BA-532 (August). Washington, D. C.: U.S. Government Printing Office, ch. 2.

Weinstein, M. C., and H. V. Fineberg. 1980. *Clinical Decision Analysis.* Philadelphia: Saunders.

Wilfond, B. S., and N. Fost. 1992. "The Introduction of Cystic Fibrosis Carrier Screening into Clinical Practice: Policy Considerations." *Milbank Quarterly* 70:629–59.

PART III

Relationships and Applications

14

Research in Medical Ethics: Physician-Assisted Suicide and Euthanasia

Daniel P. Sulmasy

The issue of physician-assisted dying, including both physician-assisted suicide and euthanasia, provides an excellent example with which to demonstrate how many methods of medical ethics have contributed to the examination of a single (but particularly vexing) set of questions. This chapter is not a comprehensive review of the literature, but rather a survey of some of the highlights of this vast array of scholarship. My aim is to mention enough of the work to give the reader a feel for the breadth of the investigation and the interactions between a variety of contributing disciplines and their methods, and to point out some of the failures of medical ethicists to take up important aspects of this question or to pursue interdisciplinary dialogue to its greatest potential. While the morality of suicide and euthanasia has been argued for many centuries, I will largely confine my discussion to the literature of the 1980s and 1990s, discussing some of the most recent work in the field.

In this chapter, I use the term *physician-assisted suicide* (PAS) to refer to situations in which physicians enable patients to take their own lives, typically by prescribing medicines that are intended to bring about death. *Euthanasia* refers to situations in which a physician (or another person) acts to create a new, lethal pathophysiological state in a patient with the specific intention that the patient should die by way of that action.

RESEARCH CONTRIBUTIONS OF THE MANY METHODS

Philosophical Methods

Although it has not always been so obvious that philosophers should be doing medical ethics, twenty-five years ago, when questions about the morality of PAS and euthanasia were being raised stridently in the United States, philosophers were already deeply enmeshed in the field. They readily took up these controversial questions.

Perhaps the first major strong, proeuthanasia paper in the modern medical ethics literature was written by James Rachels and published in the *New England Journal of Medicine* in the 1970s. Rachels attacked the distinction between killing patients and allowing them to die (Rachels 1975). He later expanded these arguments into a book (Rachels 1986). Tom Beauchamp, initially challenging Rachels (Beauchamp 1982), later evolved to a position of agreement that the traditional distinction between killing patients and allowing them to die is mistaken (Beauchamp 1996), and now believes that physician-assisted suicide is justified and ought to be legalized. Dan Brock (1989; 1992; 1993) and Peggy Battin (1994; 1998a) have also mounted vigorous attacks on the traditional prohibition on these actions. The latter two authors differ with Beauchamp in that they fail to see a relevant moral distinction between PAS and euthanasia and argue in favor of the legalization of both. All these authors have employed rigorous analytic philosophical methods. Their arguments can be characterized as taking three approaches that have not changed fundamentally since Rachels—the argument from liberty, the argument from dignity, and the argument from mercy.

As can be expected, however, the philosophical camp has not been uniformly in favor of PAS and euthanasia. The most prominent medical ethicist arguing against the morality of PAS and euthanasia has been Dan Callahan (1992; 1993). Joining him, with a very different style of argumentation, has been Leon Kass (1989; 1990). They have argued that autonomy is not self-justifying (Callahan 1992), that there are natural limits to life (Callahan 1993), and that professional integrity disallows these actions (Kass 1989; 1990). Deontological arguments based upon rules prohibiting killing have also been advanced (Gert 1988). An important component of the argument against PAS has been a defense of the distinction between killing and allowing to die (Gert 1988; Sulmasy 1998). Slippery slope arguments have also had a prominent place in the philosophical literature against PAS and euthanasia (Sulmasy 1995; Bok 1998).

These philosophical arguments have interacted heavily with the legal system. For example, in the 1997 U.S. Supreme Court cases regarding assisted suicide, a pro-PAS "Philosopher's Brief" was written by prominent moral philosophers who had not previously had a great deal to say about the subject (Dworkin et al. 1997). On the other side, an *amicus curiae* brief was submitted to the U.S. Supreme Court in opposition to PAS, popularly known as the "Bioethicist's Brief" (Brief for Bioethics Professors 1997). What impact either of these briefs had on the Court's decision is hard to tell.

Theology and Religious Studies

Religious voices have had plenty to say about PAS and euthanasia. The Roman Catholic Church, in particular, has forcefully reiterated its long-standing view that both euthanasia and suicide, whether physician assisted or not, are immoral (Sacred Congregation 1980; John Paul II 1995). Catholic theologians have been almost uniform in their rejection of PAS and euthanasia (McCormick 1991; Paris 1992; Kaveny 1997). In contrast to other ethical issues in medicine, such as contraception, there has been almost no dissent from official Church teaching on this issue, with only a few exceptions (e.g., Küng and Jens 1995). Other religions generally have also been opposed, although with varying degrees of vigor (Campbell 1992). For example, Protestant theologians have expressed a wider variety of views, although the majority has argued against the morality of PAS (Campbell 1992; Hamel and DuBose 1996). Verhey (1996) has been among the more visible Protestant authors arguing against PAS. By contrast, Vaux (1989) has argued that it should be considered morally permissible in certain circumstances.

The Episcopal Church has not voted to approve PAS, but the Episcopal bishop of Newark has been a staunch advocate of legalizing the practice (Spong 1996), and a Washington, D.C., Episcopal committee released a paper that outlined arguments for and against PAS without taking a definitive stand (Episcopal Diocese of Washington 1997). Of course, the Episcopal theologian Joseph Fletcher (1954) had argued in favor of euthanasia decades before.

Jewish opinion has also been largely (but not uniformly) opposed. As one might expect, Orthodox (Bleich 1998; Rosner 1979) and Conservative (Dorff 1998) authors have written in opposition, yet there have been some Reform rabbis who have written in favor of the morality of PAS under certain conditions (Reines 1990; McDaniel et al. 1990).

In reviewing this literature, the arguments that theologians have employed in opposition to euthanasia and PAS have generally been quite similar to those of philosophers. Clearly they have read and taken seriously these philosophical arguments. Theologians have also used some unique arguments. Some have been based on traditional scriptural prohibitions on killing derived from the Decalogue. Others have cited the writings of the Church Fathers. Still others are based on a conception of human dignity that differs radically from that of the philosophers, one founded upon the creation of human beings in the image and likeness of God (Campbell 1992; Sulmasy 1994). Arguments from theologians in favor of PAS generally have been, as they were for Fletcher (1954), based on the duty to relieve suffering. More unique theological arguments have been founded upon conceptions of freedom as an essential, God-given human attribute that must be respected in these circumstances (Vaux 1989).

Casuistry

It is rather unique in the recent history of medical ethics that some of the most famous cases regarding PAS and euthanasia were not decided in the courts. Euthanasia was really not a topic much discussed in any circles, let alone in medicine, when in 1988, an anonymous case appeared in the *Journal of the American Medical Association* (*JAMA*) under the title, "It's Over, Debbie." The case described the actions of a house officer who euthanized a terminally ill patient whose decision-making capacity was even questioned by proponents of PAS and euthanasia (Anonymous 1988). The publication set off a flurry of response, including questions about the advisability of *JAMA*'s decision to publish an anonymous paper describing actions that were clearly illegal (Vanderpool et al. 1988). Most observers considered the case of "Debbie" an aberration. Few could have predicted the rapidity with which PAS emerged as a major matter of public policy and debate.

Soon thereafter, a pathologist named Jack Kevorkian thrust himself into the headlines, assisting a woman named Janet Adkins, who suffered from early signs of Alzheimer's disease, in committing suicide inside his van in Oakland County, Michigan, using a machine he called "The Mercitron" (Altman 1990). Kevorkian then embarked on a long series of assisted suicides that ended with his conviction and imprisonment in 1999 (Murphy and Swickard 1999).

Soon after the death of Janet Adkins, the *New England Journal of Medicine* decided to publish an account of PAS by an internist from Rochester, New York, named Timothy Quill (1991). The case of the woman he assisted with suicide, "Diane," brought the topic of assisted suicide to the forefront of medical debate. In contrast to the irascible Kevorkian, Quill was mild mannered and wrote and spoke movingly of his experiences in helping patients to die (Quill 1996). He was a hero around whom a movement could galvanize its forces, and he was willing to accept the role.

These three cases, "Debbie," Janet, and "Diane," launched an intense decade of research and debate. And the intensity persists.

Case-based reasoning in medical ethics has also been employed to examine particular questions related to this debate. For example, Brody (1993) presented a "line of cases" to argue, casuistically, that PAS was woven from the same fabric as cases in which physicians made deliberate decisions to withhold or withdraw life-sustaining therapies. On the other side of the debate, Miles (1994) used case-based arguments to suggest that PAS presented a moral paradox—it could only be justified in cases in which physician and patient were extremely close. But in precisely those cases, PAS could not be permitted because the physician's closeness to the patient would impair his or her objectivity.

Professional Codes

The initial response to the "Debbie" case was a forceful restatement of traditional Hippocratic principles by some of the nation's leading physician-ethicists in an article entitled, "Doctors Must Not Kill" (Gaylin et al. 1988). This manifesto did not go unchallenged, but it seemed to represent physician opinion until more voices in favor of PAS began to appear in the medical literature. Quill and Cassel (1995), for example, invoked a principle of "nonabandonment" of patients as a traditional medico-moral basis for justifying PAS. Pellegrino (1995) responded, in an editorial entitled, "Non-Abandonment—An Old Obligation Revisited." He argued that the principle Quill and Cassel invoked needed to be placed within a pantheon of professional principles and virtues, and could not be used as the sole justification for PAS.

Legal Scholarship and Legal Developments

Legal scholars, the courts, and legislative bodies all weighed in on the euthanasia and PAS debate of the 1980s and 1990s. Each of the legal mechanisms for addressing a contentious issue in medical ethics discussed by Hodge and Gostin in chapter 6 came into play.

Legal scholars such as Orentlicher (1996) and Baron (1997), who argued in favor of legalizing PAS, enunciated arguments that were later used by the courts. They made arguments on the basis of PAS as a protected liberty interest and as a privacy right, and argued that equal protection under the U.S. Constitution should entail that if patients on life support have a right to die by termination of that life support, then patients not dependent upon life support should have the same right to terminate their lives through pharmacological means supplied by a physician. In making their arguments, they relied heavily upon the work of philosophers.

Legal arguments against legalizing PAS were advanced by Annas (1996), Capron (1996), Kamisar (1993), and Wolf (1996). They invoked philosophical work on the meaning of professionalism, expositions of the meaning of codes of medical ethics, and policy cautions about the potential for abuse and the danger of a slippery slope, especially with respect to the care of the vulnerable and disadvantaged. In these arguments, they relied upon the writings of health care professionals more than philosophers. However, they advanced legal arguments based on the distinction between positive rights to goods and services and negative rights not to be interfered with or touched without consent, a distinction itself based upon philosophical distinctions between requests and refusals (Boyle 1977; Gert 1988; Gert, Bernat, and Mogielnicki 1994).

In the United States, where so many debates regarding issues in medical ethics are conducted in the courts, it should come as no surprise that many court cases were heard in the 1980s and 1990s regarding euthanasia and assisted suicide. Both state and federal courts heard important cases.

Jack Kevorkian, as mentioned above, made a public display of his assistance in many of the 130 suicides in which he admitted participating, directly challenging the law and daring authorities to attempt prosecution (Belluck 1998). On the few occasions when charges were brought against him for assisted suicide, he and his attorney, Geoffrey Feiger, successfully used the courtroom as a stage for publicizing the issue of assisted suicide. Charges were brought against Kevorkian for assisted suicide in Michigan four times, but he was exonerated on three occasions and a mistrial was declared in the other (Belluck 1998). His defense invoked the philosophical principle of "double effect" (*New York Times* 1996), although its applicability to these cases seems suspect (Sulmasy and Pellegrino 1999). Perhaps reflecting public opinion in the matter of PAS, the district attorney in Oakland County was defeated in a reelection campaign by a candidate who promised not to bring charges against Kevorkian for PAS again (Associated Press 1996). In curious twists of fate, however, Kevorkian's lawyer, Mr. Feiger, was roundly defeated when he ran for governor of Michigan (*USA Today* 1998). And when Kevorkian crossed the line from assisted suicide to euthanasia, he was once again prosecuted. This time, he was convicted and imprisoned (Johnson 1999).

While Kevorkian occupied the spotlight, other significant cases also took place in state courts. For example, in the case of *Krisher v. McIver* (1997), it was argued that the Florida State law prohibiting assisted suicide violated that state's constitution. Nevertheless, the state Supreme Court found no violation of the state constitution.

Roughly in parallel, two cases were brought in federal courts challenging the federal constitutionality of state statutes prohibiting assisted suicide in Washington (*Compassion in Dying v. Washington* 1994) and in New York (*Quill v. Koppel* 1994). On first appeal, a three-judge panel of the 9th Circuit overturned the decision of the district court that the law violated the U.S. Constitution (*Compassion in Dying v. Washington* 1995). However, the full 9th Circuit Court heard the case *en banc*, and reversed the 9th Circuit panel's judgment, ruling that the law in Washington State *did* violate the U.S. Constitution (*Compassion in Dying v. Washington* 1996). The 9th Circuit Court's *en banc* ruling relied heavily on an argument that the plaintiffs had a protected liberty interest in having access to assisted suicide, echoing the philosophical argument from liberty, and following the thinking of several legal scholars.

In the New York case, Dr. Timothy Quill, who propelled the issue of PAS into the spotlight by his publication of the case of "Diane" discussed above (Quill 1991), challenged the constitutionality of New York's anti-assisted-suicide legislation with legal action (*Quill v. Koppel* 1994). The 2nd Circuit Court found for Dr. Quill and his fellow plaintiff, Dr. Klagsbrun (*Quill v. Vacco* 1996). In this decision, the court accepted an argument based upon the legal principle of equal protection. This argument, in turn, was based upon the philosophical argument that killing and allowing to die are not morally distinguishable. The legal equal protection argument claimed that it was discriminatory to allow persons who were on life-support to have access to the death they desired by terminating that support while patients who were not dependent upon life-support could not have access to a similarly desired death through the ingestion of pills. As above, several legal scholars had made this line of argument before the court came to its decision.

In 1997, the U.S. Supreme Court upon appeal by the two states decided both of these cases (*Vacco v. Quill* 1997; *Washington v. Glucksberg* 1997). The majority opinion of the Court dismissed the equal protection argument out of hand, relying heavily on clinical tradition and practice and on an appeal to common sense. The Court did not engage the argument philosophically. The majority opinion took the liberty argument a bit more seriously, but decided that states had compelling obligations to preserve life and to defend the vulnerable and that it was within the competence of the states to decide whether to ban or legalize assisted suicide. Although the reasons given in the many concurring opinions varied substantially, the justices ruled unanimously that the U.S. Constitution does not guarantee a right to assisted suicide. However, states were freed up to experiment with liberalized assisted-suicide laws if they chose to do so. Various legal interpretations followed this ruling (Burt 1997; Orentlicher 1997).

Currently, then, the legal action is at the level of the state. Oregon passed its liberal assisted-suicide law by a narrow margin in a referendum in 1994 (Colburn 1994; Oregon Death with Dignity Act 1995), but was restrained from enactment by court challenges and a subsequent legislative decision to bring the question back to the people by a repeat referendum. The repeat referendum (this time to repeal the law) was voted down soundly (Egan 1997). After the U.S. Supreme Court refused to hear a final appeal from opponents of the Oregon law, the assisted-suicide law finally took effect (Booth 1998).

At present, euthanasia is still illegal everywhere else in the United States. Referenda to legalize assisted suicide have been defeated in Washington State (Gross 1991), California (Boschert 1992), Michigan (Cain and Kiska 1998), and Maine (Adams 2000). Several bills introduced in the state legislatures of a number of states were also defeated in the 1990s, and fifteen states newly criminalized the practice from 1986 to 1999 (Pratt 1999). While suicide has been universally decriminalized, the law regarding *assisted* suicide is considered ambiguous in only five states (Pratt 1999), and the latest to explicitly criminalize assisted suicide was Maryland (Md. Ann. Code 1999).

The federal government has enacted legislation denying any states that choose to legalize assisted suicide the right to use federal dollars to support the practice, for example through Medicare or Medicaid (Assisted Suicide Funding Restriction Act of 1997). There have been no federal bills introduced to try to ban the practice, partly because this would raise constitutional concerns about federal vs. state jurisdiction. However, a bill has been introduced that would prohibit the use of substances that are controlled by the federal government's Drug Enforcement Agency (such as barbiturates) from being used to carry out assisted suicide (HR 2260). This very controversial bill was passed by the House in 1999, but has yet to be voted upon by the U.S. Senate (Pear 1999).

Historical Research

Contemporary discussions of suicide, euthanasia, and assisted suicide gave rise to renewed interest in history of these practices. van Hooff (1990) and Droge and Tabor (1992), for example, published major historical studies of these practices in antiquity. Philosophers such as Rachels (1986) and even federal court judges (*Compassion in Dying v. Washington* 1996) refer extensively to classical historical examples in their reasoning. Much of this work has been sharply criticized (see chapter 8), and more carefully conducted historical research leads to very different interpretations (Amundsen 1986; 1989).

This interest also gave rise to the publication of an anthology of studies in the intellectual history of philosophical and theological discussions of these practices throughout Western history (Brody 1989). In addition, a new edition of John Donne's obscure and posthumously published defense of suicide, *Biathanatos*, was also published under the editorship of a leading philosophical proponent of PAS (Battin and Rudick 1982).

Finally, there was a renewed interest in the history of the euthanasia movements of the late nineteenth and early twentieth centuries. There had been historical interest in these issues before the 1980s (Fye 1978), but by the 1990s this history had become part of the debate. For example, a leading opponent of PAS, Ezekiel Emanuel, published work that led him to conclude that the movement was born of a spirit of utilitarianism and social Darwinism in the late nineteenth century ("Euthanasia" 1994; "History of Euthanasia Debates" 1994).

And despite the fact that the history has been very recent, one major history of bioethics has included an extensive discussion of the history of the twentieth-century debates regarding euthanasia up to about 1992 (Jonsen 1998).

Qualitative Research and Ethnography

While philosophers, theologians, physicians, historians, lawyers, legislators, and judges have all been arguing intensely about assisted suicide and euthanasia for the last fifteen years, those who engage in descriptive research in medical ethics have not been idle.

Qualitative researchers have begun to make some important contributions. Gomez, for example, conducted interviews in the Netherlands regarding twenty-six cases to gain firsthand knowledge of the practice there (Gomez 1991). Morrow (1997), a lawyer, conducted nine focus groups of women from minority and other disadvantaged communities regarding whether legalized PAS would be abused, leaving, however, many of the centrally important issues unaddressed. Formally trained anthropologists have studied the reasons why several ethnic groups resist the idea of discontinuing life support as well as differences with respect to telling patients the truth about fatal diagnoses (Koenig and Gates-Williams 1995), but have not reported studies regarding PAS per se.

Despite these reports, the paucity of serious qualitative research about PAS and euthanasia is surprising. This seems an important gap in knowledge and a rich field of research waiting to be explored. It seems important to understand what motivates patients to explore this option or to reject it, and to investigate the complex patterns of relationship between patients and families and health care professionals and cultures that help to shape attitudes, beliefs, and practices.

Surveys

Surveys have been the primary means of conducting empirical research about this important issue in medical ethics. Dozens have been conducted. Most explore opinions and attitudes. Some have attempted to answer more narrowly defined research questions surrounding PAS and euthanasia.

Surveys of the general public have been conducted for decades by Gallup regarding this issue. By 1999, 61 percent of the general public agreed that it should be legal for a physician to assist a patient with suicide in the setting of severe pain and incurable disease (Gillespie 1999). Public health researchers (Blendon, Szalay, and Knox 1992) have also conducted similar surveys. There has been steady growth in public support since the end of World War II. In 1950, only 36 percent of the public supported the statement that "doctors should be allowed by law to end a patient's life," but the figure had already reached 60 percent by 1977, remaining more or less stable since then (Blendon, Szalay, and Knox 1992). Support is lower among the elderly, Catholics, and minorities (Gillespie 1999; Blendon, Szalay, and Knox 1992)

Surveys of health care professionals have been more numerous. Cohen et al. (1994), found 48 percent of physicians in Washington State thought that euthanasia was never justified, and 54 percent thought it should remain illegal. Interestingly, they found that those most in favor of legalization were those in specialties least likely to perform PAS, such as psychiatry. Back and colleagues (1996) found that 12 percent of Washington State physicians reported having had a request for PAS in the previous year. In Oregon, Lee and colleagues (1996) found that 68 percent of physicians thought that PAS should be legal in some cases, and 46 percent might be willing to prescribe for PAS if it were legal. Bachman and colleagues (1996) found that 40 percent of physicians in Michigan supported legalizing PAS. In states where the issue had not become so politically contentious, such as Wisconsin (Shapiro et al. 1994) and Rhode Island (Fried et al. 1993), investigators found substantially less willingness to actively cause death through euthanasia or PAS. Emanuel and colleagues (1996) surveyed oncologists nationally, and found that 46 percent would agree with physician-assisted suicide for unremitting pain and 18 percent would agree with assisted suicide for patients who found life "meaningless." However, 57 percent of these oncologists reported that they would vote against a referendum to make PAS legal. Asch (1996) surveyed nurses in intensive care units and reported that 16 percent had performed "euthanasia" or "assisted suicide." This survey was vigorously criticized for the ambiguity of its definitions (Scanlon 1996). Meier and colleagues (1998) used a much more careful definition in a national survey of physicians and found that 3 percent reported having given a patient a lethal prescription at least once, and 5 percent reported having given a patient a lethal injection at least once.

These surveys have all been subjected to criticisms. Questions have arisen about the definitions used in their surveys, their tendency either to "lump" or "split" in reporting their results, and worries that the researchers may have been overly influenced by their own beliefs in designing the surveys and interpreting the results. Yet, these are the best data available, and they help to understand how the general population and health care professionals think about these issues.

In addition to opinion surveys, some have attempted to answer questions about potential abuse of legalized PAS and about slippery slope considerations. For example, Chochinov and his colleagues have surveyed terminally ill patients' desire for death, showing both how this is highly correlated with depression (Chochinov et al. 1995) and how patients' desire for death fluctuates over time (Chochinov et al. 1999). Sulmasy and colleagues (1998) used survey instruments to show an association between physicians' cost-conserving practice styles and their willingness to assist patients with suicide.

None of these surveys answers any normative questions definitively, but they do illuminate the issues in constructive ways.

Experiments

There have been no randomized controlled trials of assisted suicide or euthanasia, but many have described the legal conditions in the Netherlands and Oregon as "experiments." Empirical researchers, eager to understand what actions have been taken and how these practices are carried out in real life, have treated the jurisdictions where PAS is legally tolerated as "natural" experiments. Of course, interpretation of these studies is limited by the lack of randomization, as explained in chapter 12.

In the Netherlands, the government appointed a commission to examine the practices of Dutch physicians. It released the results of surveys of physicians and death certificate examination in 1991 (van der Maas et al. 1991; van der Maas, van Delden, and Pijnenborg 1992) and published a follow-up physician survey in 1996 (van der Maas et al. 1996). The commission reported that about 2–3 percent of Dutch deaths are due to euthanasia, and that few physicians prescribe assisted suicide. Through these studies it also came to light that about 1 percent of deaths are due to nonvoluntary euthanasia of decisionally incapacitated patients who are construed to be desirous of such a death. Further, another 2 percent of deaths are also not classified as euthanasia, but result from deaths due to rapid increases in opioids at least in part with the intention of hastening death. The total number of such actions appears to have increased slightly between surveys, but no single category increased at a statistically significant rate, and some categories stayed virtually the same as a percentage of all deaths. The Dutch authors interpreted these data as evidence against a slippery slope. However, their presentation of their practices and their interpretation of their own data have been sharply criticized as an attempt to minimize serious deficiencies and problems (Capron 1992; Hendin, Rutenfrans, and Zylicz 1997; Jochemsen and Keown 1999). In turn, the Dutch and their proponents have defended their descriptions of the practice (Battin 1998b; van Delden 1999). Recently, the Dutch have published data on the reasons for the request and on the rate of complications of assisted suicide and euthanasia, such as prolonged time to death or myoclonus (Groenewoud et al. 2000).

Interestingly, throughout the last two decades of this experiment in public policy, the practices of euthanasia and assisted suicide remained technically illegal in the Netherlands. Physicians were immune from prosecution as long as they followed certain guidelines. However, the Dutch now have regularized these practices. On November 28, 2000, Parliament officially made euthanasia and assisted suicide legal, a move that simultaneously was hailed as social progress and decried as further evidence of the slippery slope (Simons 2000).

The Oregon "experiment" has also been intensely studied, and two reports have been published in the *New England Journal of Medicine* detailing the scant information available from monitoring of reported cases in the short time that the practice has been legal (Chin et al. 1999; Sullivan, Hedberg, and Fleming 2000). In addition, a survey of physicians' experiences with the new law has been published (Ganzini et al. 2000). It seems fair to say that because of the small number of cases studied and because these reports relied exclusively upon the descriptions of the physicians themselves, the validity of these data is suspect (Foley and Hendin 1999). Thus, the "experiment" continues.

Economics and Decision Science

Some empirical work has been done in the field of economics and decision analysis regarding end-of-life care, but I am unaware of any formal studies using these methods that directly touches upon the questions of PAS and euthanasia. One published paper has detailed the financial savings that accrue if one denies "potentially ineffective treatments" (Cher and Lenert 1997). However, this study has been criticized because although the treatments were allegedly "ineffective," the survival rate was lower for those who did not receive such treatments than for those who did (Lynn 1998). Another paper was written by two authors, neither trained as economists, suggesting that cost savings would be minimal if assisted suicide were legalized (Emanuel and Battin 1998). In addition, glossing over some significant metaphysical and conceptual questions, one group has actually explored the "utilities" that patients place on dying, comparing the relative advantage of death over "states worse than death" (Patrick et al. 1994).

WHAT HAS BEEN LEARNED?

It should be clear that questions about euthanasia and assisted suicide have attracted enormous research attention in medical ethics in the last fifteen years, and that almost every method described in this book has been used to address directly or indirectly some of these issues. How did this all unfold?

As Jonsen would have predicted (see chapter 7), it seems that *cases* pushed the question to the forefront. The cases of "Debbie," Janet, and "Diane" seemed to come out of nowhere, taking the medical profession by surprise. These cases pushed the issue forward from the 1980s into an intense decade of academic scholarship in the 1990s. Simultaneously, the additional cases associated with Jack Kevorkian kept the issue before the public on a regular basis. Public interest also was sustained by the Hemlock Society, particularly by the publication of its president's controversial book on how to commit suicide, *Final Exit* (Humphry

1991). This public interest, in turn, served as a launching station for scholars' research into these questions.

The first wave of physician response to these cases relied heavily upon arguments from the authority of medical oaths, codes, and traditions, as well as the meaning of professionalism. Social interest led to a series of surveys documenting public and professional views. Philosophers and theologians who had thought that these questions were dormant revived their interest in them. And historians, conscious that this was not the first time that anyone in the West had thought about the morality of suicide, took a look back at some of the roots of the question. Because some of these first cases led to further cases, and because of apparently broadening social support for legalization, legal scholars began to explore arguments for or against the constitutionality of laws prohibiting assisted suicide and drafting model legislation. Some empirical scholarship next began to move beyond opinion polls to look at a few of the psychosocial aspects of the question. Simultaneously, several well-organized movements tried unsuccessfully to legalize assisted suicide in several states before ultimately achieving success in Oregon. After the U.S. Supreme Court decision, a third wave of philosophical, theological, historical, and legal scholarship reacted to that decision. And now that the courts have cleared the Oregon law, a new wave of empirical scholarship has begun to explore the impact of this uncontrolled experiment.

There have been good and bad studies in all this work. But much has been learned. It is clear that there is widespread popular support for PAS, but much less so among Catholics, minority groups, and the elderly. Physicians are about evenly divided over whether they would like to see it legalized. Psychiatrists seem most in favor. A minority of physicians say they would engage in PAS, even if it were legalized. Yet a substantial minority already admit that they have done so, even though it is illegal. Patients who ask for PAS do so largely for reasons having to do with loss of control or perceived loss of dignity, and rarely for uncontrolled pain. It has currently been settled that there is no U.S. Constitutional right to assisted suicide, but that states are free to pass legislation legalizing the practice. No philosopher or theologian argues for suicide on demand, although there is considerable disagreement among both philosophers and theologians about when, if ever, PAS might be a morally right action. Historians have pointed out that the practice is not new, and have corrected views that there has ever been widespread tolerance for the practice at any time in Western history since late antiquity.

HAS MEDICAL ETHICS RESEARCH BEEN GENUINELY INTERDISCIPLINARY IN THE CASE OF PAS?

How have these various research methods and disciplines interacted over the past two decades of investigation of this question by medical ethicists? One way to assess this is to observe the sources that the scholars have cited. While I have not done this quantitatively, clear patterns emerge for any careful reader of this literature.

It is probably fair to say that legal scholars investigating the issues of PAS and euthanasia have cited the widest variety of methods and disciplines. It is clear that they have read history, philosophy, arguments based on professionalism and codes, discussions of cases that never went to trial, and a fair amount of the empirical literature. One cannot be confident, however, that these scholars have critically read work using nonlegal methods. Theologians have read the philosophical arguments thoroughly, as well as the arguments based upon professional codes, and history. They have read ecumenically: Catholics, Protestants, and Jews cite each other's work. They have tended not to read empirical work. And while they occasionally have discussed casuistic literature about cases that never went to trial, they have tended not to read legal scholarship. Philosophers, by and large, have tended to cite more legal scholarship than theologians have, as well as the oft-cited cases that did not go to court. They have tended to ignore the work of theologians and those making arguments on the basis of codes and professionalism. They have read historical selections in philosophy, but often not as comprehensively as historians would hope. And philosophers have generally ignored empirical work. With a few exceptions, empirical researchers in medical ethics have read only the smattering of philosophy and history that finds its way onto the editorial pages of medical journals. Occasionally, a philosopher or theologian will appear as a coauthor on an empirical paper. But by and large, empirical researchers have made little effort to grasp or try to engage the other disciplines. Theology, for example, has been almost completely ignored, even when exploring "religious differences" in beliefs. Codes and arguments from professionalism have been cited, but generally without rigor (see chapter 5).

I conclude that, in the case of the PAS/euthanasia debate, medical ethics research has been extremely *multi*disciplinary. But I also conclude that it has been only moderately *inter*disciplinary. While I cannot say so with certitude, I suspect that this assessment of research about PAS is characteristic of research in the field of medical ethics as a whole. While more genuinely interdisciplinary than most fields, medical ethics still has a lot more work to do in its struggle to become truly interdisciplinary.

PAS AND MEDICAL ETHICS RESEARCH: AN AGENDA FOR THE FUTURE

Besides trying to become more genuinely interdisciplinary, what else might medical ethics take up as a research agenda regarding PAS and euthanasia?

First, it seems that the tracking of the "experiments" in Oregon and the Netherlands will continue to be a subject for empirical research for the next several years. There is intense interest on both sides of the question regarding whether concerns about abuse or the slippery slope are being realized. Equally important, however, will be an examination of the extent to which the debate about PAS and euthanasia has had an effect upon the quality of end-of-life care in general, even in places where it is not used or has not been legalized (Lee and Tolle 1996).

As detailed above, good qualitative research regarding PAS and euthanasia is sorely lacking. It seems important to get behind the numbers of quantitative research to understand more fully what goes on in the minds of persons who seek PAS, as well as those who perform PAS. What are the social and cultural contexts? What are the nonrational sources of this movement? And what does PAS say about Western culture?

Similarly, quantitative empirical research about PAS needs to move beyond opinion surveys to explorations of the psychology of PAS. The future holds a move beyond the simple counting of heads to asking *why*—the testing of hypotheses and the search for explanation. There are few data about the health care professionals who perform PAS, about the patients who seek it, or about their families. Similarly, little is really known about those who oppose it. Motives, moods, and other beliefs and attitudes almost certainly are associated with these practices. This is a major research agenda for those who conduct empirical research about PAS and euthanasia.

The role of humanities research regarding these issues certainly will be to continue to provide a forum for the debate and to continue to refine the moral questions. Very fundamental questions about the nature of morality lie just beneath the surface of the debate about PAS and euthanasia. These unsettled moral questions include those surrounding the scope of autonomy, the scope of privacy, and the meaning of harm. The shape and validity of slippery slope arguments will be a task shared by humanities researchers with those who conduct empirical work. While some consider it an already settled question, I believe debates about the meaningfulness of the distinction between killing and allowing to die will continue, as well as the role of intention in the moral evaluation of PAS and euthanasia. Finally, fundamental questions such as the meaning of dignity and the relationship between dignity and autonomy in human moral affairs must be addressed as part of this debate. These questions will not be settled by empirical means. The PAS and euthanasia debate has opened a crack in the moral crust of Western society, and the task ahead is for historians, lawyers, casuists, physicians, theologians, and philosophers to peer down into this chasm and to deepen our collective understanding of the tectonics of human morality.

CONCLUDING COMMENTS

If PAS is any example, then it should be abundantly clear that all of the methods described in this book can make important contributions in the field of medical ethics. PAS has arisen as a question of enormous normative significance and controversy at the end of the twentieth century. Scholars from many disciplines have jumped into the fray, employing a variety of research methods. All are properly called "medical ethicists," and their research is properly called "medical ethics." This brief excursion through this research, conducted largely in the last ten years and around a single issue, demonstrates that medical ethics is an impressively multidisciplinary field. It holds great promise for becoming perhaps the most profoundly interdisciplinary field of study human intellectual history has known.

REFERENCES

Adams, G. 2000. "Doctor-Assisted Suicide, Gay Rights, Lose in Main Balloting." Associated Press, 8 November.

Altman, L. K. 1990. "The Doctor's World: Use of Suicide Device Sets in Motion Debate on a Disturbing Issue." *The New York Times,* 12 June, sec. C3.

Amundsen, D. W. 1986. "Medicine and the Birth of Defective Children: Approaches of the Ancient World." In *Euthanasia and the Newborn,* ed. C. Richard, H. McMillan Jr., Tristram Engelhardt Jr., and Stuart F. Spicker. Dordrecht, The Netherlands: D. Reidel Publishing Company, pp. 3–22.

———. 1989. "Suicide and Early Christian Values." In *Suicide and Euthanasia: Historical and Contemporary Themes*, ed. Baruch Brody. Dordrecht, The Netherlands: Kluwer Academic Publishers, pp. 77–153.

Annas, G. J. 1996. "The Promised End—Constitutional Aspects of Physician-Assisted Suicide." *New England Journal of Medicine* 335:683–87.

Anonymous. 1988. "It's Over, Debbie." *Journal of the American Medical Association* 259:272.

Asch, D. A. 1996. "The Role of Critical Care Nurses in Euthanasia and Assisted Suicide." *New England Journal of Medicine* 334:1374–79.

Assisted Suicide Funding Restriction Act of 1997. Public Law 105-12 [H.R. 1003] Apr. 30, 1997 (105 P.L. 12; § 3, 111 Stat. 23; 1997).

Associated Press. 1996. "Departing Prosecutor Charges Dr. Kevorkian in 10 Deaths." *American Medical News*, 18 November, p. 71.

Bachman, J. G., K. H. Alcser, D. J. Doukas, R. L. Lichtenstein, A. D. Corning, and H. Brody. 1996. "Attitudes of Michigan Physicians and the Public toward Legalizing Physician-Assisted Suicide and Voluntary Euthanasia." *New England Journal of Medicine* 334:303–09.

Back, A. L., J. I. Wallace, H. E. Starks, and R. A. Pearlman. 1996. "Physician-Assisted Suicide and Euthanasia in Washington State: Patient Requests and Physician Responses." *Journal of the American Medical Association* 275:919–25.

Baron, C. H. 1997. "Pleading for Physician-Assisted Suicide in the Courts." *Western New England Law Review* 19:371.

Battin, M. P. 1994. *The Least Worst Death: Essays in Bioethics on the End of Life*. New York: Oxford University Press.

———. 1998a. "Is a Physician Ever Obligated to Help a Patient Die?" In *Regulating How We Die: The Ethical, Medical, and Legal Issues Surrounding Physician-Assisted Suicide*, ed. Linda L. Emanuel. Cambridge, MA: Harvard University Press, pp. 21–47, 264–67.

———. 1998b. "Euthanasia: The Way We Do It, The Way They Do It." In *Health Care Ethics: Critical Issues for the 21st Century*, ed. John F. Monagle and David C. Thomasma. Rev. ed. Gaithersburg, MD: Aspen Publishers, pp. 311–22.

Battin, M. P., and M. Rudick, eds. 1982. *John Donne's Biathanatos: A Modern-Spelling Edition*. Garland English Texts, 1. New York: Garland.

Beauchamp, T. L. 1982. "A Reply to Rachels on Active and Passive Euthanasia." In *Contemporary Issues in Bioethics*, ed. Tom L. Beauchamp and LeRoy Walters. 2nd ed. Belmont, CA: Wadsworth.

———. 1996. "Refusals of Treatment and Requests for Death." *Kennedy Institute of Ethics Journal* 6:371–74.

Belluck, P. 1998. "Prosecutor to Weigh Possibility of Charging Kevorkian." *The New York Times*, 23 November, sec. A12.

Bleich, J. D. 1998. *Bioethical Dilemmas: A Jewish Perspective*. Hoboken, NJ: KTAV, pp. 61–129.

Blendon, R. J., U. S. Szalay, and R. A. Knox. 1992. "Should Physicians Aid Their Patients in Dying? The Public Perspective." *Journal of the American Medical Association* 267:2658–62.

Bok, S. 1998. "Euthanasia." In *Euthanasia and Physician-Assisted Suicide: For and Against*, ed. Gerald Dworkin, R. G. Frey, and Sissela Bok. New York: Cambridge University Press, pp. 107–27.

Booth, W, 1998. "Oregon Suicide Is Called the First under Law Legalizing Doctor Role." *The Washington Post*, 26 March, sec. A7.

Boschert, S. 1992. "California Narrowly Rejects MD-Assisted Dying." *Internal Medicine News and Cardiology News*, 1 December 1, pp. 3, 20.

Boyle, J. M. 1977. "On Killing and Letting Die." *New Scholasticism* 51: 433–52.

Brief for Bioethics Professors Amicus Curiae Supporting Petitioners, *Vacco v. Quill*, 521 US 793 (1997) (No. 95-1858); *Washington v. Glucksberg*, 521 US 702 (1997) (No. 96-110).

Brock, D. 1989. "Death and Dying." In *Medical Ethics*, ed. Robert M. Veatch. Boston: Jones and Bartlett, pp. 329–56.

———. 1992. "Voluntary Active Euthanasia." *Hastings Center Report* 22 (March–April): 10–22.

———. 1993. *Life and Death: Philosophical Essays in Biomedical Ethics*. New York: Cambridge University Press.

Brody, B., ed. 1989. *Suicide and Euthanasia: Historical and Contemporary Themes*. Dordrecht, The Netherlands: Kluwer Academic Publishers, pp. 77–153.

Brody, H. 1993. "Causing, Intending, and Assisting Death." *Journal of Clinical Ethics* 4.112–17.

Burt, R. 1997. "The Supreme Court Speaks: Not Assisted Suicide but a Constitutional Right to Palliative Care." *New England Journal of Medicine* 337:1234–36.

Cain, C., and T. Kiska. 1998. "Voters Overwhelmingly Reject Assisted Suicide." *The Detroit News*, 4 November, sec. A1.

Callahan, D. 1992. "When Self-Determination Runs Amok." *Hastings Center Report* 22 (March–April): 52–55.

———. 1993. *The Troubled Dream of Life: Living with Mortality*. New York: Simon and Schuster.

Campbell, C. S. 1992. "Religious Ethics and Active Euthanasia in a Pluralistic Society." *Kennedy Institute of Ethics Journal* 2: 253–77.

Capron, A. M. 1992. "Euthanasia in the Netherlands: American Observations." *Hastings Center Report* 22 (March–April): 30–33.

———. 1996. "Liberty, Equality, Death!" *Hastings Center Report* 26 (May–June): 23–24.

Cher, D. J., and L. A. Lenert. 1997. "Method of Medicare Reimbursement and the Rate of Potentially Ineffective Care of the Critically Ill." *Journal of the American Medical Association* 278:1001–07.

Chin, A. E., K. Hedberg, G. K. Higginson, and D. W. Fleming. 1999. "Legalized Physician-Assisted Suicide in Oregon—The First Year's Experience." *New England Journal of Medicine* 340:577–83.

Chochinov, H. M., K. G. Wilson, M. Enns, N. Mowchun, S. Lander, M. Levitt, and J. J. Clinch. 1995. "Desire for Death in the Terminally Ill." *American Journal of Psychiatry* 152:1185–91.

Chochinov, H. M., D. Tataryn, J. J. Clinch, and D. Dudgeon. 1999. "Will to Live in the Terminally Ill." *Lancet* 354:816–19.

Cohen, J. S., S. D. Fihn, E. J. Boyko, A. R. Jonsen, and R. W. Wood. 1994. "Attitudes toward Assisted Suicide and Euthanasia among Physicians in Washington State." *New England Journal of Medicine* 331:89–94.

Colburn, D. 1994. "Assisted Suicide Bill Passes." *Washington Post*, 15 November, Health section, p. 9.

Compassion in Dying v. Washington, 850 F. Supp. 1454, 1461 (W.D. Wash. 1994).

Compassion in Dying v. Washington, 49 F.3d 586 (9th Cir. 1995).

Compassion in Dying v. Washington, 79 F.3d 790 (9th Cir. 1996) (*en banc*).

Dorff, E. N. 1998. *Matters of Life and Death: A Jewish Approach to Modern Medical Ethics*. Philadelphia: Jewish Publication Society.

Droge, A. J., and J. D. Tabor. 1992. *A Noble Death: Suicide and Martyrdom among Christians and Jews in Antiquity*. San Francisco, CA: Harper Collins.

Dworkin, R., T. Nagel, R. Nozick, J. Rawls, T. Scanlon, and J. J. Thompson. 1997. "Assisted Suicide: The Philosopher's Brief." *New York Review of Books*, 27 March, pp. 41–47.

Egan, T. 1997. "In Oregon, Opening a New Front in the World of Medicine." *The New York Times*, 6 November, sec. A26.

Emanuel, E. J. 1994. "Euthanasia: Historical, Ethical, and Empirical Aspects." *Archives of Internal Medicine* 154:1890–1901.

———. 1994. "The History of the Euthanasia Debates in the United States and Britain." *Annals of Internal Medicine* 121:793–802.

Emanuel, E. J., D. L. Fairclough, E. R. Daniels, and B. R. Clarridge. 1996. "Euthanasia and Physician-Assisted Suicide: Attitudes and Experiences of Oncology Patients, Oncologists, and the Public." *Lancet* 347:1805–10.

Emanuel, E. J., and M. P. Battin. 1998. "What Are the Potential Cost Savings from Legalizing Physician-Assisted Suicide?" *New England Journal of Medicine* 339:167–72.

Episcopal Diocese of Washington, D.C., Committee on Medical Ethics (Chair: C.B. Cohen). 1997. *Assisted Suicide and Euthanasia: Christian Moral Perspectives* (The Washington Report). Harrisburg, PA: Morehouse Publishing.

Fletcher, J. 1954. *Morals and Medicine*. Princeton: Princeton University Press, pp. 172–210.

Foley, K., and H. Hendin. 1999. "The Oregon Report: Don't Ask, Don't Tell." *Hastings Center Report* 29 (May–June): 37–42.

Fried, T. R., M. D. Stein, P. S. O'Sullivan, D. W. Brock, and D. H. Novack. 1993. "Limits of Patient Autonomy: Physician Attitudes and Practices Regarding Life-Sustaining Treatments and Euthanasia." *Archives of Internal Medicine* 153 (1993): 722–28.

Fye, W. B. 1978. "Active Euthanasia: An Historical Survey of Its Conceptual Origins and Introduction into Medical Thought." *Bulletin of the History of Medicine* 52:492–502.

Ganzini, L., H. D. Nelson, T. Schmidt, D. F. Kraemer, M. A. Delroit, and M. A. Lee. 2000. "Physicians' Experiences with the Oregon Death with Dignity Act." *New England Journal of Medicine* 342:557–63.

Gaylin, W., L. R. Kass, E. D. Pellegrino, and M. Siegler. 1988. "Doctors Must Not Kill." *Journal of the American Medical Association* 259: 2139–40.

Gert, B. 1988. *Morality: A New Justification of the Moral Rules.* New York: Oxford University Press, pp. 295–300.

Gert, B., J. L. Bernat, and R. P. Mogielnicki. 1994. "Distinguishing between Patients' Refusals and Requests." *Hastings Center Report* 24 (July–August): 13–15.

Gillespie, M. 1999. "Kevorkian to Face Murder Charges." Gallup News Service, March 19, (www.gallup.com/poll/releases/pr990319.asp).

Gomez, C. F. 1991. *Regulating Death: Euthanasia and the Case of the Netherlands.* New York: The Free Press.

Groenewoud, J. H., A. van der Heide, B. D. Onwuteaka-Philipsen, D. L. Williams, P. J. van der Maas, and G. van der Wal. 2000. "Clinical Problems with the Performance of Euthanasia and Physician-Assisted Suicide in the Netherlands." *New England Journal of Medicine* 342:551–56.

Gross, J. 1991. "Voters Turn Down Mercy Killing Idea." *The New York Times*, 7 November, sec. B16.

Hamel, R. P., and E. R. DuBose. 1996. *Must We Suffer Our Way to Death? Cultural and Theological Perspectives on Death by Choice.* Dallas: Southern Methodist University Press.

Hendin H. 1996. *Seduced by Death: Doctors, Patients, and the Dutch Cure.* New York: W. W. Norton, p. 53.

Hendin, H., C. Rutenfrans, and Z. Zylicz. 1997. "Physician-Assisted Suicide and Euthanasia in the Netherlands: Lessons from the Dutch." *Journal of the American Medical Association* 277:1720–22.

Humphry, D. 1991. *Final Exit: The Practicalities of Self-Deliverance and Assisted Death.* Eugene, OR: Hemlock Society.

Jochemsen, H., and J. Keown. 1999. "Voluntary Euthanasia under Control? Further Empirical Evidence from the Netherlands." *Journal of Medical Ethics* 25:16–21.

John Paul II. 1995. "*Evangelium Vitae.*" *Origins* 24: 691–727.

Johnson, D. 1999. "Kevorkian Sentenced to 10 to 25 Years in Prison." *The New York Times*, 14 April , secs. A1, A23.

Jonsen, A. R. 1998. *The Birth of Bioethics.* New York: Oxford University Press, p. 265.

Kamisar, Y. 1993. "Are Laws against Assisted Suicide Unconstitutional?' *Hastings Center Report* 23 (May–June): 32–41.

Kass, L. R. 1989. "Neither for Love nor Money: Why Doctors Must Not Kill." *Public Interest* 94 (Winter): 24–46.

————. 1990. "Death with Dignity and the Sanctity of Life." *Commentary* 89 (March): 33–43.

Kaveny, M. C. 1997. "Assisted Suicide, Euthanasia, and the Law." *Theological Studies* 58:124–48.

Koenig, B. A., and J. Gates-Williams. 1995. "Understanding Cultural Differences in Caring for Dying Patients." *Western Journal of Medicine* 163:244–49.

Krisher v. McIver, 697 So. 2d 97 (Fla. 1997).

Küng, H., and W. Jens. 1995. *A Dignified Dying.* London: SCM Press.

Lee, M. A., H. D. Nelson, V. P. Tilden, L. Ganzini, T. A. Schmidt, and S. W. Tolle. 1996. "Legalizing Assisted Suicide—Views of Physicians in Oregon." *New England Journal of Medicine* 334:310–15.

Lee, M. A., and S. W. Tolle. 1996. "Oregon's Assisted Suicide Vote: The Silver Lining." *Annals of Internal Medicine* 124:267–69.

Lynn, J. 1998. "Potentially Ineffective Care in Intensive Care" [letter]. *Journal of the American Medical Association* 279: 652.

McCormick, R. A. 1991. "Physician-Assisted Suicide: Flight from Compassion." *The Christian Century* 108:1132–34.

McDaniel, Y., S. B. Saulson, M. Datz, and A. J. Reines. 1990. "Dialogue on Suicide and Abortion." *Journal of Reform Judaism* 37 (Fall): 49–58.

Md. Ann. Code art. 27, §416 (1999).

Meier, D. E., C. A. Emmons, S. Wallenstein, T. Quill, R. S. Morrison, and C. K. Cassel. 1998. "A National Survey of Physician-Assisted Suicide and Euthanasia in the United States." *New England Journal of Medicine* 338:1193–1201.

Miles, S. H. 1994. "Physicians and Their Patients' Suicides." *Journal of the American Medical Association* 271:1786–88.

Morrow, E. 1997. "Attitudes of Women from Vulnerable Populations toward Physician-Assisted Death: A Qualitative Approach." *Journal of Clinical Ethics* 8:279–89.

Murphy, B., and J. Swickard. 1999. "Convicted of Murder." *Detroit Free Press,* 27 March, p. 1A.

The New York Times. 1996. "Kevorkian Says Wish Is to Ease Suffering, Not to Hasten Death," 6 March, sec. A19.

Oregon Death with Dignity Act. *Oregon Revised Statute* 127.800–127.995 (1995).

Orentlicher, D. 1996. "The Legalization of Physician-Assisted Suicide." *New England Journal of Medicine* 335:663–67.

————. 1997. "The Supreme Court and Physician-Assisted Suicide: Rejecting Assisted Suicide but Embracing Euthanasia." *New England Journal of Medicine* 337:1236–40.

Paris, J. 1992. "Active Euthanasia." *Theological Studies* 53:113–26.

Patrick, D. L., H. E. Starks, K. C. Cain, R. F. Uhlmann, and R. A. Pearlman. 1994. "Measuring Preferences for Health States Worse than Death." *Medical Decision Making* 14:9–18.

Pear, R. 1999. "House Backs Ban on Using Medicine to Aid Suicide." *The New York Times,* 28 October, secs. A1, A29.

Pellegrino, E. D. 1995. "Nonabandonment: An Old Obligation Revisited." *Annals of Internal Medicine* 122:377–78.

Pratt, D. A. 1999. "Too Many Physicians: Physician-Assisted Suicide after Glucksberg/Quill." *Albany Law Journal of Science and Technology* 9:161.

Quill, T. E. 1991. "Death and Dignity: A Case of Individualized Decision Making." *New England Journal of Medicine* 324:691–94.

———. 1996. *A Midwife through the Dying Process: Stories of Healing and Hard Choices at the End of Life.* Baltimore, MD: Johns Hopkins University Press.

Quill, T. E., and C. K. Cassell. 1995. "Non-Abandonment: A Central Obligation for Physicians." *Annals of Internal Medicine* 122:368–74.

Quill v. Koppel, 870 F. Supp. 78 (S.D.N.Y. 1994).

Quill v. Vacco, 80 F.3d 716 (2nd Cir. 1996).

Rachels, J. 1975. "Active and Passive Euthanasia." *New England Journal of Medicine* 292:78–80.

———. 1986. *The End of Life: Euthanasia and Morality.* New York: Oxford University Press.

Reines, A. J. 1990. "Reform Judaism, Bioethics, and Abortion." *Journal of Reform Judaism* 7 (Winter): 43–59.

Rosner, F. 1979. "Suicide in Jewish Law." In *Jewish Bioethics,* ed. Fred Rosner and J. David Bleich. New York: Sanhedrin Press, pp. 317–30.

Sacred Congregation for the Doctrine of the Faith. 1980. "Declaration on Euthanasia." *Origins* 10:154–57.

Scanlon, C. 1996. "Euthanasia and Nursing Practice—Right Question, Wrong Answer." *New England Journal of Medicine* 334:1401–02.

Shapiro, R. S., A. R. Derse, M. Gottlieb, D. Schneiderman, and M. Olson. 1994. "Willingness to Perform Euthanasia: A Survey of Physician Attitudes." *Archives of Internal Medicine* 154:575–87.

Simons, M. 2000. "Dutch Becoming First Nation to Legalize Assisted Suicide." *The New York Times,* 29 November, sec. A3.

Spong, Bishop John S. 1996. "Statement of Bishop John S. Spong, Newark, NJ." *Assisted Suicide in the United States.* Hearing before the Subcommittee on the Constitution of the Committee on the Judiciary, House of Representatives. 104th Congress, Second Session, April 29, 1996, Serial No. 78. Washington, D.C.: U.S. Government Printing Office, pp. 340–48.

Sullivan, A. D., K. Hedberg, and D.W. Fleming. 2000. "Legalized Physician-Assisted Suicide in Oregon—The Second Year." *New England Journal of Medicine* 342:598–604.

Sulmasy, D. P. 1994. "Death and Human Dignity." *Linacre Quarterly* 61 (Winter): 27–36.

———. 1995. "Managed Care and Managed Death." *Archives of Internal Medicine* 155:133–36.

———. 1998. "Killing and Allowing to Die: Another Look." *Journal of Law, Medicine, and Ethics* 26:55–64.

Sulmasy, D. P., B. P. Linas, K. Gold, and K. Shulman. 1998. "Physician Resource Use and Willingness to Participate in Assisted Suicide." *Archives of Internal Medicine* 158:974–78.

Sulmasy, D. P., and E. D. Pellegrino. 1999. "The Rule of Double Effect: Clearing Up the Double Talk." *Archives of Internal Medicine* 159:545–50.

USA Today. 1998. "Final Election Results: Indiana through Mississippi," 5 November, p. 7.

Vacco v. Quill, 117 S. Ct. 2293 (1997).

van Delden, J. J. M. 1999. "Slippery Slopes in Flat Countries—A Response." *Journal of Medical Ethics* 25:22–24.

van der Maas, P. J., J. J. M. van Delden, L. Pijnenborg, and C. W. N. Looman. 1991. "Euthanasia and Other Medical Decisions Concerning the End of Life." *Lancet* 338:669–74.

van der Maas P. J., J. J. M. van Delden, and L. Pijnenborg. 1992. *Euthanasia and Other Medical Decisions Concerning the End of Life.* New York: Elsevier.

van der Maas, P. J., G. van der Wal, I. Haverkate, C. L. de Graaff, J. G. Kester, B. D. Onwuteaka-Phillipsen, A. van der Heide, J. M. Bosma, and D. L. Willems. 1996. "Euthanasia, Physician-Assisted Suicide, and Other Medical Practices Involving the End of Life, 1990-1995." *New England Journal of Medicine* 335:1699–1705.

Vanderpool, H. Y., B. Z. Paulshock, P. Storey, F. H. Miller, G. J. Annas, C. B. Clark, J. G. Manesis, D. C. Shaw, D. Humphry, P. A. Singer, M. G. Lamb, W. Kime, S. D. Wilson, D. Davis, D. A. Hyman, G. B. DiRusso, J. S. Driben, M. R. Druffner, R. Lauricella, S. Sarma, W. D. Fiorini, D. C. Thomasma, and E. Moran. 1988. "It's Over, Debbie" [letters]. *Journal of the American Medical Association* 259:2094–98.

van Hooff, A. J. L. 1990. *From Autothanasia to Suicide: Self-Killing in Classical Antiquity.* London: Routledge.

Vaux, K. L. 1989. "The Theologic Ethics of Euthanasia." *Hastings Center Report* 19 (Jan.–Feb.): 19–22.

Verhey, A. 1996. "Choosing Death: The Ethics of Assisted Suicide." *The Christian Century* 113:716–19.

Washington v. Glucksberg, 117 S. Ct. 2258 (1997).

Wolf, S. 1996. "Physician-Assisted Suicide in the Context of Managed Care." *Duquesne Law Review* 35:455–79.

15

Research in Medical Ethics: Genetic Diagnosis[1]

Gail E. Henderson

Genetic screening is defined in the *Encyclopedia of Bioethics* as "programs designed to canvass populations of healthy individuals to identify those with genotypes that place them or their offspring at high risk for disease or defect." *Genetic testing* is offered to individuals or families who are identified as being at increased risk for developing disorders or passing these defects on to their children (McEwen and Reilly 1995, 1000).[2] The moral features of genetic screening and testing have been noted in the medical ethics literature (summarized in Murray and Botkin 1995, 1005–07), the popular press (Nelkin and Lindee 1995), and a wide number of social science and clinical disciplines (e.g., Conrad and Gabe 1999).

What are the main moral and ethical aspects of genetic diagnosis? First, in many cases, genetic information itself is seen as intellectually, morally, and socially problematic. Data on genetic risk is difficult to understand and interpret, even for physicians. It can also be inherently ambiguous, leading to further difficulty in understanding what a particular diagnosis means. Second, in contrast to some other diagnoses, a genetic diagnosis may herald a future event that may or may not be preventable. Third, a genetic diagnosis is at once both personal and social. It involves information about an individual's genetic identity that is also of direct concern to other, related people, including family members, and also racial and ethnic group members. Finally, a disproportionate share of the burden of prenatal genetic diagnosis and carrier screening falls on women. While most of these features are not unique to genetic testing and screening, in combination they pose a set of impressive ethical challenges to informed consent, confidentiality/privacy, and justice.

These challenges have set the stage for empirical research that has moral and ethical implications.[3] Such research might address any of the following questions: Are people provided adequate information to make decisions regarding genetic screening and testing? If not, how can this be improved? How is the information provided by genetic diagnosis understood? What is the impact of genetic information on a person's life? Does access to information and services vary by ethnic group membership or social class? Are individual interests in conflict with those of family, ethnic group, or medical care providers, and if so, how can those interests best be reconciled? Is confidentiality of genetic information protected?

Do people, families, or groups experience stigmatization or discrimination after genetic diagnosis? If so, how can this be prevented? Are current laws and regulatory policies adequate to protect against infringement of individual rights?

This rich and varied set of questions has produced a great number of empirical studies. In this chapter, I review the social science research that addresses questions about informed consent, privacy/confidentiality, and justice in the application of genetic screening and testing. Three themes dominate the published reports and serve as the organizing framework for this analysis. The first addresses the meaning of genetic information, and how people make sense of genetic diagnoses. The second concerns the process of informed consent for screening and testing, how it is being done, and how it can be improved. The third concerns broader economic and social implications of genetic diagnosis, namely discrimination and eugenics. For each of these topics, I describe the articulation of specific research questions, the methods that are employed to investigate these questions, and a summary of findings.

This chapter provides an opportunity to survey a collection of research projects that have been generated by a revolutionary new medical technology. In addition, it provides examples of many of the descriptive research methods that are featured in this volume. The range of qualitative and quantitative methods includes observation, in-depth interviews, survey research, and longitudinal and experimental studies. As in all empirical research, the type of research question often dictates the method of data collection. Thus, while the chapter is organized thematically, there are links between topics and methods. For example, research on the meaning of genetic information is mainly qualitative, while studies of knowledge and behavior (e.g., Does a patient understand the information that a test might reveal and does he or she decide to be tested?) are more quantitative. This dichotomy is overly simplistic, however. Research on the multifaceted issues raised by informed consent in genetic screening and testing, for example, includes a spectrum of methodological approaches, from focus groups to textual analyses to quantitative survey research.

The studies reviewed include works by anthropologists, sociologists, physician-researchers, and public health and policy scholars. They were selected through electronic searches (using keywords and subject indexes) of the medical, bioethics, and social science literatures, as well as through more traditional bibliographic explorations.

As it turns out, empirical research on the ethical implications of genetic diagnosis is a fragmented set of literatures, and the analytic organization of this essay imposes my own interpretive framework on the research. Some investigations are intended to advance understanding of a particular problem, such as failure to understand genetic information, and the ways to resolve it. Others are less applied, speaking to a set of theoretical concerns. At the same time, it should be acknowledged that many questions about genetic diagnosis raise ethical issues that are not easy to investigate empirically (e.g., Should we offer a choice for predictive information about a disease for which prevention or treatment is uncertain?).

Despite these caveats, when the body of research related to genetic diagnosis is reviewed, a different kind of ethical dimension becomes visible. This dimension involves the moral implications inherent in the empirical research agendas themselves. Why have some issues received more attention than others? Why are some "at-risk" populations studied less than others? It is evident that research does not exist apart from the social world. When we choose to define research questions in particular ways, we are reflecting, consciously or unconsciously, the values of society as well as its research funding sources. Thus, not only are the methods and findings described below of interest, but, in a broader view, the framing of the research itself offers another kind of assessment.

MAKING SENSE OF GENETIC INFORMATION

Genetic information is increasingly prevalent in the news media, medical and scientific journals, medical care and even fashion advertisements. Dorothy Nelkin (1990; Nelkin and Lindee 1995) and others (e.g., Conrad 1997; Henderson and Kitzinger 1999) have described the social power of this information and the cultural and social factors that will likely affect how predictive genetic testing will be used. Evelyn Parsons, in *Culture, Kinship and Genes* (1997), concludes that culture is being overwhelmed by an essentialist view of genetic influences on life. In popular vocabulary, even individual identity has become genetic, and as Marteau (1998) describes, genetic diagnosis not only can determine but also can *reconstruct* identity, in the past as well as the future. That this is a caricature of genetics, which never operates apart from environment, is rarely recognized (see Lewontin 1992).

Incorporation of genetic information into our conception of health and illness is part of the broader context of risk assessment. As Ian Hacking (1990) wrote in *The Taming of Chance*, the rise of probability statistics during the twentieth century provided the tools to recast the way we think about the chances of various events, including the chance of disease. Likewise, changes in the mathematics of epidemiology after the 1940s enabled the construction of a multicausal assessment of factors that put individuals "at risk" for disease (Brandt 1990). Defined in epidemiology it is the probability of an event occurring, combined with the magnitude of the anticipated losses or gains. We are constantly exposed to information about risk, generated mainly by large scale epidemiological surveys, in TV and news media, and in health care settings. Although studies have shown that popular perceptions of risk are influenced by how it is presented (Douglas and Wildavsky 1982), risk data have clearly altered how we understand the relationship between behavior and the occurrence of and responsibility for disease (e.g., Conrad 1999). Risk assessments also have produced the now-familiar concept of "risk groups," whose members have characteristics that place them one or two standard deviations beyond statistical normalcy. Visible or invisible risk group membership often becomes a defining—even stigmatizing—identity for individuals (e.g., adolescent males, people with high cholesterol, women with a family history of breast cancer, etc.).

Empirical research on the meaning of genetic information began in response to the diffusion of prenatal screening technology in the 1970s, and the identification of women whose fetuses were at risk for genetic disease. Initially, the objectives were descriptive. What was taking place? Which women accepted the offer of screening and why? Later researchers began to explore in greater depth the meaning of this new technology, how that might differ across different groups of people, and in so doing, addressed the larger question of how genetic risks are given social meaning. The nature of these questions required that the research methods used be open-ended and qualitative. Charles Bosk, a sociologist who carried out extended observations of genetic counselors in the late 1970s, calls this method of data collection "witnessing." He wrote, "[t]he task of the fieldworker is to witness again and again but not to use the data gathered this way in interaction. . . . This freedom from intervention and from ordinary interaction allows fieldworkers their special purchase on social life" (Bosk 1992, 17).

One of the most powerful studies of this type is Barbara Katz Rothman's 1986 book, *The Tentative Pregnancy: Prenatal Diagnosis and the Future of Motherhood*. Intrigued with how prenatal diagnosis might change the way women experienced pregnancy, Rothman interviewed women who had undergone amniocentesis or refused it. Although her respondents were recruited in a nonrandom manner, through magazine ads, her research powerfully demonstrated the ways in which genetic screening technology—and the choice of having that information—did alter the experience of pregnancy. Drawing on a tradition of qualitative research in sociology, Rothman used a small number of evocative descriptions to characterize the dilemmas caused by genetic information. Communicating their experiences became a mission of sorts for Rothman, who wrote, " . . . I want each person reading this to be able to feel it—I want you to hear the grief, hear the voices of the women who have experienced the new solutions brought by the new technology. Maybe I will sometimes sound morbid, 'wallowing' in grief. I sit at my typewriter with tape recorder, interviewer forms, index cards, stacks of yellow paper, and I cry. There is pain here, and I hear it, and I want you to hear it too" (Rothman 1986, 176).

Rothman's research demonstrated how problematic these new choices were. For her, the issue was as much the *nature* of the information as the impact that the information had on expectant parents. Genetic information is often presented to parents or to individuals before any symptoms are observed or felt. Some prenatal diagnoses, in fact, may never result in observable symptoms. Consequently, what a diagnosis really tells us about the person is often unclear. "Normal" is good news. But normal people vary enormously in physique, abilities, and intelligence. The same variation is also characteristic of different genetic diagnoses, but as Rothman discovered, "[m]ost people are not informed enough to anticipate the range of possible diagnoses or the ambiguity inherent in the diagnostic process" (1986, 160).

It is this ambiguity that presents the most difficult challenges. To illustrate, Rothman featured cases of women who were given ambiguous genetic diagnoses. "Deborah" received the diagnosis of Trisomy X, a female fetus with an extra X chromosome in her cells (three X chromosomes). Deborah and her husband researched the condition, but "got different answers from different sources." She said, "There is very little on that disorder. We have a technology which could tell us what was wrong, but not what its meaning would be in our lives" (1986, 166). They were told their daughter would be sterile, to expect some retardation, and that there was a chance that a Trisomy X female would become schizophrenic. According to Deborah, "I went crazy with it. Hysterical. . . . My emotional rejection of the child came early—embracing her and rejecting her at the same time. Crying for her. Not knowing if I could deal with birthing her knowing what I knew about her. They told me not to tell anyone [so she would not be stigmatized]. What could I tell her?" Hearing this, Rothman concludes, "Deborah was incapacitated by this information; she was made incapable of mothering Amanda. The information was considered damaging enough that she was told not to share it. How could it not damage Deborah?" Deborah terminated the pregnancy, but not, according to Rothman, because she was rejecting an imperfect baby. Rather, she was rendered incapable of proceeding. Deborah said, "It was *knowing* that made continuing intolerable. To have a child be retarded, schizophrenic, that is indeed tragic. To wait for it to happen is torture" (1986, 168).

In Rothman's second case, even a mother who is able to continue the pregnancy has serious reservations about the process. "Roberta" and her husband were told the daughter she was carrying had either full-blown or partial Turner's syndrome, in which the fetus develops as a female with only one X chromosome, or a mosaic variant. Roberta and her husband were thus confronted with both an uncertain diagnosis and an ambiguous one whose prognosis ranged from no outward signs of abnormality to a child with growth problems and failure to develop secondary sex characteristics. Roberta chose to continue the pregnancy, and after producing an apparently healthy child, she observed, "I am not sure if it has been helpful or not to have this unique diagnosis. Certainly it would have been easier to not know and to not have the anxiety, stress, and uncertainty. However, if May does have some of the problems associated with Turner's, we are more prepared by having known. I guess I really feel that unless the outcome is truly knowable and clear it is more humane and ethical to not share this information—but that doesn't feel right either" (1986, 171–72). Rothman concludes that we are caught in a bind—we *cannot not* offer screening; but she cautions, "What does it do to a child to arrive in the world as the embodiment of a diagnosis?" (1986, 173).

Shirley Hill's interviews with mothers of children with sickle-cell anemia investigated the reasons that poor women were not coming in for carrier screening, nor modifying reproductive decisions because of sickle cell disease (Hill 1994). Most articles on the ethics of genetic testing and screening refer to the poorly implemented screening programs for sickle cell carriers and patients in the 1970s. Yet little was done to investigate why this occurred and what screening and testing meant to the population at risk. As Hill notes (as of the early 1990s), "[v]irtually no research has been done on how having the sickle cell trait affects the reproductive decisions of blacks" (1994, 72).[4] She found that low-income, African American women in her study saw themselves and their children as victims of the historic neglect of sickle cell disease. They advocated education as a strategy for controlling the disease, yet they were often unable to persuade their male partners to be tested for the sickle cell trait, and they lacked access to health care that would have offered them such options as prenatal screening. Hill thus concludes, "[s]tructural barriers to health care, gender inequality between these women and their males partners, and the cultural ideology that valued motherhood, all served to undermine the power of education to affect change" (1994, 72). Hill's research follows a theoretical tradition in sociology that posits the importance of social structure in the creation of social meaning. It also adds to the long list of empirical research in medical sociology that demonstrates the importance of race, gender, and social class as critical influences on access to health care and on medical care decision making.

Like Hill and Rothman, Rayna Rapp's interviews with women also focused on prenatal screening. Rapp conducted field-based anthropological research on the social impact and cultural meaning of prenatal diagnosis for poor women in New York City. She found that differences in appraisal of the value of genetic information and possible outcomes contributed significantly to patient-provider misunderstanding. For poor and/or immigrant pregnant women and their families, statistical information on age-related risk rates for chromosome abnormality may appear unimportant in contrast to more pressing vulnerabilities. In addition, for some people, detection of fetal mental retardation is not always viewed as an appropriate reason to test. Finally, Rapp found that variation in individual reproductive histories and social values strongly shape acceptance and rejection of the test (Rapp 1997, abstract). Each of these observations highlights the importance of the social position and social experiences of women involved in prenatal screening decision making, and reinforces the findings of Rothman and Hill.

In addition to these qualitative studies on prenatal screening, the meaning of genetic information is also featured in recent personal narratives. Martha Beck's account of anticipating the birth of her son (1999) is a compelling description of the personal transformation engendered by his prenatal diagnosis of Down's Syndrome. In *Mapping Fate: A Memoir of Family, Risk, and Genetic Research,* Alice Wexler (1995) recounts her family's history with an adult-onset condition, Huntington Disease (HD), from which her mother suffered and eventually died. Each remaining family member became deeply involved in trying to find the gene for HD. Much of the book details how she and her sister, Nancy, a noted HD genetic researcher, and their father dealt with the question of testing for the disease. Reflecting on this issue for *60 Minutes,* Nancy Wexler said, "I've always believed in knowledge for its own sake. And it is ironic that after working for precisely that, I'm now finding it much more complex than I ever thought it would be." When Diane Sawyer asked if she had thought she would take the test when the linkage was discovered, Nancy replied, "Absolutely. Yes. I never doubted it. And now I'm not sure." Nancy Wexler (1995) has also written about the ethical issues involved, and her concern over the powerful and often unanticipated meanings attached to genetic information. She warns that the "harm to people at risk is whether those who agree to a test really understand what they are doing" (1995, 401). She points out that in a pilot study of the linkage test for HD, researchers found that although two-thirds said they wanted the test, only 15 percent actually were tested.

In summary, empirical studies that focus on the meaning of genetic information have, for the most part, used ethnographic and qualitative methods, with open-ended questions that focus on meaning, experience, and identity, and on understanding complex and often ambiguous information. Quantitative surveys are simply not appropriate for these kinds of inquiries. Rather, researchers rely on deeply textured, individual accounts to identify the ways that people experience and make sense of genetic information and risk for genetic disease. The findings of these studies have raised concerns about the difficulties inherent in obtaining truly informed and voluntary consent to genetic screening and testing. We turn now to research that assesses the processes of informed consent.

CONSENT FOR GENETIC DIAGNOSIS: HOW IS IT DONE AND HOW CAN IT BE IMPROVED?

The majority of recent empirical studies related to genetic testing and screening have focused on some aspect of informed consent.[5] This body of research assesses a variety of interrelated aspects of the consent process, including adherence to minimum standards, the adequacy and understandability of the information conveyed, the quality of the patient-provider interaction, and differences in response to the offer of testing. Interestingly, the issue of voluntariness of consent as a separate subject has not been the focus of many studies.

Newborn screening is the most common form of genetic screening in the United States. All newborns, four million per year, are checked for between two to ten genetic and nongenetic conditions. Various studies have shown how screening has been done in the past. Farfel and Holtzman (1984), for example, reported on a 1980 survey of sickle cell screening programs in Maryland. Out of 52,000 people screened in one year, 13,000 were screened without informed consent. Many did not receive education or counseling.

In 1993, a comprehensive review article made recommendations for the development of national policy for the clinical application of genetic diagnostic technologies (Wilfond and Nolan 1993). The authors recommended that "appropriate procedural mechanisms be established at both state and federal levels to prevent the unnecessary confusion, expense, and personal or social harms to result from completely unrestrained application of developing genetic technologies" (1993, 2948). They concluded, "Given the rapidly increasing availability of genetic diagnostic services, occurring at the time of heightened awareness of concerns about equitable access, quality of care, allocation of resources, and cost containment, we believe new genetic diagnostic services must be held to carefully considered and practicable evidentiary standards" (1993, 2953). The authors remind us of the "long-standing consensus among health care professionals, bio-ethicists, and policy analysts . . . that the mere availability of a test is not in itself a sufficient criterion for [its] clinical implementation" (1993, 2948).

Despite this wise caution, the diffusion of screening technology has continued, with inadequate safeguards. In one of the few studies to examine commercial testing, Giardello and colleagues (1997) reported on a nationwide sample of 177 patients in 125 families who underwent colon cancer testing from a commercial laboratory in 1995. They found that patients often received inadequate counseling and incorrectly interpreted results. Based on telephone interviews with physicians and genetic counselors, it appeared that 17 percent of the 177 patients were not at risk and should not have been tested. Of the 177 patients, only 18.6 percent received genetic counseling before test, and only 16.9 percent provided written informed consent. In 31.6 percent of cases, physicians misinterpreted test results, believing that negative means normal, whereas actually 20 percent of the test negatives are false negatives.

Other studies echo these findings. Bernhardt and colleagues (1998) reported on analyses of tape-recorded discussions during first prenatal visits of 169 pregnant women with obstetricians and nurse-midwives. Although the amount of discussion time varied by age (2.5 minutes for women younger than thirty-five, and 6.9 minutes for women older than thirty-five), based on the content of the discussions, the authors concluded that "information about genetic testing is inadequate for ensuring informed autonomous decision making." Durfy and colleagues (1998) surveyed consent forms for BRCA1 and BRCA2 mutation testing (mutations that are associated with increased susceptibility to breast and ovarian cancers), and did a content analysis of ten consent forms from seven of the major testing centers in the United States. All forms described in varying ways the purpose of genetic testing, limitations of the test, implications of both positive and negative results, and confidentiality procedures. However, the authors found substantial variation in content and organization and, importantly, that not all forms discussed potential psychological or insurance risks. Similarly, an assessment of information in cystic fibrosis screening pamphlets, based on a content analysis of twenty-eight pamphlets from commercial and noncommercial organizations in the United States and Britain, also revealed lack of uniformity and mixed messages (Loeben, Marteau, and Wilford 1998).

At the same time that studies such as these demonstrate the failure of procedures to insure minimally consistent transmission of appropriate information, other researchers call attention to the need for more individualized and sophisticated interactions around the consent process. Reflecting the qualitative research described above, Geller et al. (1997) argue that uncertainties in genetic testing "greatly complicate the process of informed consent, creating an excellent opportunity to reconsider exactly how it should be conducted." Based on a series of focus groups to investigate women's reactions to BRCA testing, their results "dramatically underscore that informed consent ought to be highly individualized" (1997, 28).

The clear need for improvement in the consent process continues to be demonstrated by recent research, and has also produced interventions aimed at improving some aspect of the process. Using a variety of qualitative, quantitative, and experimental methods, the research falls into three broad categories: longitudinal survey investigations of screening decision making, surveys of the views of consumers in contrast to providers, and assessment of various attempts to improve the entire screening process. One of the most innovative is a study that tests an experimental consent form for hemophilia screening in a randomized clinical trial.[6]

An example of the longitudinal surveys is a study by Mischler and colleagues (1998), who conducted an evaluation of cystic fibrosis (CF) neonatal screening of more than 650,000 infants in Wisconsin over a nine-year period, from 1985 to1994. Assessment of 135 families with children diagnosed with CF included a questionnaire administered three months after diagnosis that asked about reproductive knowledge, attitudes, and behaviors. Seventy-three of these families were re-interviewed in 1994. By that time, there were forty-three subsequent pregnancies in thirty-one families. Eight of the thirty-one families used prenatal diagnosis and three pregnancies with CF were detected, all of which were carried to term. The study found that nearly all the families retained the information that when both parents are carriers there is a one-in-four chance of having a child with CF with each pregnancy. However, as Hill (1994) found in her study of sickle cell screening, a number of parents went ahead with more pregnancies, understanding the risk of CF. These data contradicted earlier reports that parents with a risk of having a CF child would modify their reproductive behavior after learning their carrier status. In this study, only a minority of individuals changed their reproductive behavior based on genetic information. Mischler and colleagues note that "the psychologic implications of prenatal diagnosis and possibly being faced with a decision about abortion have unique complexities for families with a child who has CF" (1998, 49).

Research protocols involving genetic testing for mutations linked to breast cancer involving families with high-risk members have been a focus of research on how to improve screening for adult-onset diseases. Many say they would be interested in testing, but as noted earlier regarding Huntington's Disease, far fewer accept testing. Lerman and colleagues (1996) carried out a prospective, observational study, in 1994–95, of 279 members of thirteen BRCA1-linked families to evaluate the psychological and functional health status of people who have been tested for the BRCA1 gene. The goals of the study were to assess predictors of the decision to be tested, to evaluate the effects of testing, and to evaluate how testing affects people's medical decisions. The average age of those studied was forty-three; the group was all white, mostly female (67 percent) and married (77 percent).

Ninety percent had completed high school or more, and 93 percent had health insurance. The 279 family members were contacted and interviewed by telephone; an educational session was given, followed by offering the test results and a follow-up session. Sixty-nine percent (192 people) completed the telephone interview, and 60 percent of those who completed the telephone interview (116 people) requested the education and test results. Requesting the results was most strongly associated with having health insurance (odds ratio 3.74), as well as with having first-degree relatives with breast cancer, higher baseline knowledge, and perceived importance of the benefits of testing. Even in this experimental setting, with a select sample of people already in a cancer registry who are offered free and easy testing, half rejected testing and many did not have adequate information. The authors expressed concern about the implications of these findings for commercial testing, where careful provision of information is less likely (as shown in the study by Giardello and colleagues [1997] described above).

Other studies have focused on ethnic differences in response to information, and the decision to be tested. For example, Hughes et al. (1997) examined ethnic differences (black vs. white) in knowledge and attitudes about BRCA1 testing in women at increased risk, defined as women, age 18–75, with at least one first-degree relative with breast and/or ovarian cancer. Compared to white women, black women had lower levels of knowledge and more positive attitudes about the benefits of genetic testing. Richards and colleagues (1997) evaluated screening for BRCA1 among Ashkenazi Jews (an identified risk group) and found that that the great majority (94 percent) requested testing. Their reasons included concern for their own risk, concern for the risk of their children and desire to learn about surveillance options. The most common reason given by those who declined testing was concern about health insurance. Similarly, a recent report (Eng et al. 1997) found that among 2,824 Ashkenazi Jewish individuals referred to screening for Tay-Sachs disease, more than 95 percent were also willing to be tested for Gaucher disease and cystic fibrosis. The study conducted pre- and postcounseling knowledge testing, and found, in this well-educated group, high levels of understanding and retention of genetic concepts and disease-related information. Twenty-one carrier couples were identified, all of whom opted for prenatal diagnosis. In contrast, Sorenson and colleagues (1997) report on a study of home- versus clinic-based CF carrier education and testing, offered free of charge to first-, second-, and third-degree relatives of (mainly white) cystic fibrosis patients in North Carolina. Overall, 58 percent accepted, with more accepting testing in the home (67 percent) compared to a clinic (45 percent).

As noted earlier, African American women in Hill's 1994 small sample of mothers with sickle cell children either did not want to be tested or did not act on the information. This was related to a number of factors, including not being in touch with the father or not being able to convince him to be tested. Wright and colleagues (1994) confirmed Hill's finding that many young black adults do not know their sickle cell status. They interviewed a convenience sample of 147 black patients presenting to the emergency department at a university hospital in Tennessee, and found that while almost all had heard of sickle-cell anemia and three-quarters knew it was a genetic disorder, only 31 percent knew their own sickle cell status. Women were more likely than men to know their status. Another study also confirmed the importance of childbearing to this population. Neal-Cooper and Scott (1988) reported on a cohort of seventy-four sickle trait-carrying couples in

Virginia, identified and provided counseling in 1970. Initial responses to risk information varied widely, and stated intentions regarding childbearing did not accurately predict subsequent events. While the majority of pregnancies occurred in a subgroup who had not borne an affected child, the authors (echoing Hill) observed that concern about the risk is often "offset by a strong desire to have children regardless of risk" (1988, 174). A later account by Rowley et al. (1991) also found a low rate of acceptance of genetic testing by carriers. In their study of women offered screening during a five-year period in Rochester, N.Y., 810 pregnant women (4.3 percent of all screened) were found to have hemoglobinopathy, 60 percent of which was sickle-cell anemia. Eighty-six percent of these said they wanted their partner tested and 55 percent had their partner tested. For those seventy-seven pregnancies found to be at risk, prenatal diagnosis was offered to fifty-three pregnancies, and was accepted by only twenty-five couples.

In addition to differences in patients' views about testing, researchers have looked at providers and have compared the views of patients and providers. Geller and Holzman (1995) reported on a qualitative assessment of primary care physicians' perceptions about the implications of offering genetic testing. Following up a national survey of physicians' knowledge and attitudes regarding genetics, five focus groups were conducted with thirty-nine physicians. They found that these physicians "believed that the goals of full disclosure and non-directiveness in genetic counseling were neither possible to achieve nor desirable in primary care." Female physicians reported deferring to patients in decision making more than male physicians did. Geller and colleagues (1998) surveyed patients and providers to determine what they would want to discuss about breast cancer susceptibility testing and their preferred role in testing decisions. Their findings showed discrepancies between providers and patients. Eighteen percent of physicians underestimated the importance patients placed on informed consent for testing, and 34 percent underestimated the importance of discussing the risk of insurance discrimination. Patients were less likely to say they would undergo prophylactic mastectomy than providers were to recommend it. Providers emphasized the importance of understanding false negative results more than patients; patients wanted providers to make recommendations more than providers did.

In summary, many of the studies cited above could be characterized as fact-finding missions, generated by a familiar concern that technology may be racing ahead of our ability to manage its dissemination ethically. Researchers have focused on the information provided to participants in screening and testing and how much of that is understood. What are they being told? How consistent is the information provided, and how much is remembered? What do potential clients say about their willingness to be tested, and about their fears? What proportion actually get tested? What proportion act on a genetic diagnosis? There is no *a priori* expectation that everyone who is offered a test would or should agree. Rather, the concern is that the process of offering a genetic test is carried out in as clear and thorough a manner as possible. Studies also examined whether there are group differences in understanding genetic information and acceptance of testing. Although many studies are forced to use convenience samples, or small samples based on a select population offered genetic testing at this time, a few are more broadly representative.

It seems that of the many people offered some kind of genetic screening or testing, far fewer accept. This may indicate failure to communicate information effectively, or it may indicate individual voluntariness of choice. The studies were not designed to address this issue. The research does show that among those who accept testing, some testing is inappropriate, some patients do not give written informed consent, and for many, the information included in the consent process varies, sometimes considerably. Perceptions of what motivates people to be tested and what they would want after they have the information also vary, across patients and between patients and providers.

Surprisingly, although the qualitative research reviewed in the first section focuses on the meaning of genetic information, and the studies of informed consent also explore informational aspects of the consent process, these two literatures rarely reference each other. This is unfortunate. When the studies of informed consent are considered in light of the qualitative data, richer interpretations are possible. For example, survey results that identify a percent of patients who reject a prenatal screening test or a diagnosis that may result in symptoms later in life are brought to life by Rothman's cases and the Wexlers's personal accounts. Likewise, the quantitative data provide a context in which such cases can be interpreted. The validity of Hill's interviews with a small group of sickle cell mothers is substantiated by the studies of screening for sickle cell disease cited above. These advantages are seen only in a review such as this, however, and reveal the most obvious gap in the literature on genetic diagnosis—the need for research that addresses the complex nature of informed consent with the strengths of both qualitative and quantitative methods.

ECONOMIC AND SOCIAL OUTCOMES OF GENETIC DIAGNOSIS: DISCRIMINATION AND EUGENICS

Genetic discrimination—in the workplace, in access to health insurance, and in society at large—is a key issue in some of the literature described above, and is seen by some as an inevitable result of the production of genetic information, no matter what kind of safeguards are employed. Because they do not believe that confidentiality can be assured, many authors call for anonymous genetic counseling and testing (e.g., Mehlman et al. 1996).

Many patients and family members also worry that genetic information cannot be kept confidential. In her family memoir, Alice Wexler (1995) reported a disturbing event that resonates with this concern. "April 16, 1986 . . . The other day I got a copy of my medical records from my new gynecologist. 'Patient has a high probability of developing Huntington's disease,' he wrote on the record he submitted to the insurance company. I was furious and called him to protest. 'I'm sorry,' he said. If I'd asked him earlier to delete the disease from the record he would have done so, but now it was too late. 'But it's not true,' I said, 'I don't have a high probability. I'm forty-four years old and my odds are going down.' 'I'm sorry, there's nothing I can do.' Doesn't he know that the risk for Huntington's is one of the conditions, along with sickle-cell anemia, muscular dystrophy, insulin-dependent diabetes, and AIDS, for which insurance companies unconditionally deny medical coverage?" (1995, 231). Many believe that Wexler's experience is just as likely to occur today as in 1986.

An article in *Science* appeared to confirm this, with a study of genetic discrimination as seen from the perspective of people with genetic disorders in the family (Lapham, Kozma, and Weiss 1996). The authors recruited respondents for a forty-minute telephone interview through chapters of the Alliance of Genetic Support Groups. Three hundred thirty-two respondents from across the United States participated; they were mainly female, highly educated, married, and Caucasian—characteristics typical of genetic support groups. The study found that 25 percent believed they or affected family members were refused life insurance; 22 percent believed they were refused health insurance; and 13 percent believed they were denied or let go from a job. Fear of genetic discrimination resulted in 17–18 percent not revealing genetic information to insurers and employers. While not a representative survey, this study and others have identified considerable fear of discrimination and concern over losing health insurance among people with genetic diagnoses.

There have been a number of recent legislative and regulatory responses to this issue, although their ultimate effectiveness has yet to be tested. Several bills whose objectives are to increase the protection of individual privacy and confidentiality of genetic information are currently pending in Congress.[7] Among these, for example, is the Genetic Privacy and Nondiscrimination Act of 1999, whose goal is "to establish limitations on disclosure and use of genetic information in connection with health insurance coverage, hospital care, medical services, and to prevent employment discrimination on the basis of genetic information and testing" (H. R. 2555, 106th Cong. [1999]). The bill also mandates that the National Bioethics Advisory Commission submit recommendations to Congress regarding standards for increased protection for collection, storage, and use of identifiable DNA samples and genetic information obtained from those samples.

The second potential for discrimination results from stigma related to being part of a group with increased risk for a genetic condition. A 1997 *Washington Post* article by Rick Weiss featured this issue. In "Discovery of 'Jewish' Cancer Gene Raises Fears of More than Disease," he reports on the discovery of a genetic alteration that is present in one of six Jews of East European descent, and absent in non-Jews, which doubles the odds of getting colon cancer. Quoting several Jewish leaders, he writes, "Is too much research focusing on the Jewish community and are we at risk of stigmatization? . . . We are still living with some history, a history of discrimination" (Weiss 1997).

Once risk for a particular condition becomes associated with ethnic group membership, it is difficult to change. Sickle-cell anemia, for example, is typically considered a genetic disease of blacks. Yet recent studies have found that the sickle trait is not uncommon in white subjects. Shafer and colleagues (1996) reviewed data from four years of screening two million infants in California and found that targeted screening would have missed fifty-eight nonblack infants with sickle-cell disease and 6,921 nonblack infants with sickle-cell trait. The Agency for Health Care Policy Research (AHCPR) clinical practice guidelines for sickle-cell disease, in fact, recommend universal screening "as the only way to ensure that all infants with sickle-cell disease will be identified early. . . . Screening programs that target specific high-risk racial or ethnic groups will not identify all infants with sickle-cell disease because it is not possible to determine reliably an individual's racial or ethnic background by physical appearance, surname, presumed racial heritage, or self-report" (Clinton 1993, 2158). The lack of diffusion of these recommendations into the general medical community demonstrates the persistence of stigma attached to a risk group even after that risk relationship has been challenged.

The predominance of this disease among African Americans, however, raises an equity question of a different sort, regarding genetic screening in an already disadvantaged and stigmatized population. In the early 1980s, Bowman wrote an article that attempted to place this program in a broader context with regard to the allocation of resources for all health problems. He stated, "A woman should have the right to decide whether or not she wishes to have a child with a genetic disorder, and recent advances in research on prenatal diagnosis, particularly when supported by public funds, should be made available to all, and not just the affluent." However, "[p]resent-day dire poverty and callous health care public policies lead to the inescapable conclusion that a concerted attempt to alleviate poverty and its consequent adverse effects on maternal, neonatal, and infant mortality should take precedence over, or at least coincide with, a national program to prevent sickle-cell disease" (Bowman 1983, abstract).

This equity issue was revisited in 1997, in an extensive review of state policies on newborn screening. Hiller and colleagues conducted a survey of all policies and practices of newborn screening programs, finding that they vary considerably across the states. While all but two states require newborn-screening programs, only thirty-two states require educational programs or materials, and only California requires that a mother be provided information in a language she understands. Parental refusal of newborn screening is allowed in all states except South Dakota, although in many there is no mechanism to inform parents of this right. Only two states require parental signed consent to the testing (Maryland and Wyoming). Georgia requires it only for targeted hemoglobinopathy screening. Thirty-six states have newborn-screening advisory committees. In at least seventeen states, the public played no role in deciding which conditions should be screened, and in the other states, the extent of public participation varied considerably. Even more important, there is substantial variation in follow-up for individuals with metabolic and/or congenital disorders. "Consequently," the authors observe, "an underlying premise of newborn screening, that early diagnosis will lead to effective treatment, is not always valid because of legislative and other gaps in access to treatment" (Hiller, Landenburger, and Natowicz 1997, 1285).

Finally, many commentators on developments in contemporary genetics explicitly link the power of a genetic diagnosis to a caution about the ultimate discrimination, eugenics. Daniel Kevles, editor of *The Code of Codes: Science and Social Issues in the Human Genome Project*, comes to the genome project from his study of the continuity of eugenics with modern genetics (Lewontin 1992, 64). Duster (1990), in *Backdoor to Eugenics*, argues that our present-day eugenics is, in fact, elimination of a defective fetus.

Yet the studies described above should assuage fears about eugenics. They demonstrate that despite expectations to the contrary, a surprising number of high-risk couples do not choose to be tested, to modify their reproductive behavior, or to terminate their pregnancies. In fact, cross-national comparisons reveal that pregnancy termination after genetic diagnosis is higher in several other countries. In a recent study on prenatal diagnosis of cleft palate in Israel, for example, the majority of couples terminated the pregnancies, while similar studies in the United States have reported a much lower percentage of terminations (Blumenfeld, Blumenfeld, and Bronstein 1999). In Cuba, Granda and colleagues (1991) report on a program for prevention of sickle-cell disease where the percentage of carriers of the sickle-cell gene ranges from 3 percent to 7 percent. Between 1983 and 1989, more than 800,000 pregnant women, as well as 67 percent of the fathers, were screened and counseled. Twelve hundred sixty-eight at-risk couples were detected. Five hundred thirty-one (42 percent) elected to have prenatal diagnosis; ninety-eight affected fetuses were found, and in seventy-two cases, the pregnancy was terminated.

On the other hand, research also demonstrates that genetic screening has been applied most poorly to those who are already disadvantaged, while the research needed to examine these issues has been carried out, for the most part, among better educated, more advantaged patient groups. Abortion *is* the main alternative for most conditions identified by screening, yet the implications of selective abortion for populations that might have a heightened sensitivity to ethnic cleansing is relatively unexamined. Calls for control over the rapid diffusion of genetic testing technology, and continued concerns from all parties over lack of confidentiality and anticipation of discrimination based on access to this information, have not elicited strong regulatory responses. In this situation, caution about possible eugenic uses of this technology may well be justified.

CONCLUDING COMMENTS

In the first section of this essay, data on the meaning of genetic information was drawn from qualitative and ethnographic accounts of personal experience. The moral dilemmas that genetic information often pose are most vividly captured in these accounts. In fact, some argue that this kind of information is so different from other types of medical information that it requires more controls than we have applied thus far. For example, Weaver (1997) argues that we must guarantee a right *not* to know our genetic diagnoses. He writes, "While genetic technologies offer great promise for the future of medicine, and the eradication of certain genetically linked diseases, until there are cures for persons with the faulty genes, such knowledge can lead to anxious preoccupation with the ever-present disease potential within, and discrimination by employers, insurers, governmental agencies, and health care providers without. Given these unpleasant results of genetic screening or monitoring, it is important to assert the individual's right not to know." Rothman (1986) draws the same conclusion from her interviews with pregnant women. She writes, " . . . knowledge does not always empower. . . . *Seeing the inevitable end of a life at the threshold of that life cuts us at our essence*" [author's emphasis] (1986, 176).

These are compelling arguments, and many of the studies reviewed in the second section of this essay were generated, at least indirectly, by concerns that the special moral features of genetic information make the goals of informed consent especially difficult to achieve. Yet, much of this research also is based on the assumption that the solution lies in improving the delivery of information to individual patients so that they are able to make informed choices. If the question of individual rights is raised, it is in terms of equity in access to information. The choice *not* to choose is not on the agenda. Researchers aim to promote the autonomy of patients by equipping them with information. However, Bosk's observation that "genetic counselors at times use the goal of patient autonomy as a ground for patient abandonment" (Bosk 1992, 10) raises a troubling concern that also relates to the direction of research on genetic screening and testing.

The literatures reviewed for this chapter suggest that social disadvantage is related to problems in equitable access to genetic testing services, to failure to understand and retain information about the tests, and to miscommunication and misunderstanding between patients and providers. In the current era, 16 percent of the U.S. population lacks medical insurance, and managed care continues to limit medical encounters. It may be that well-documented recommendations for more thoughtful, lengthy, and personal consent interactions to overcome the difficulties of communicating about genetic diagnoses miss the point. It is possible that a different level of analysis is needed to bring the most relevant factors into focus, a level that is not generally included in the research designs of empirical studies of informed consent. Perhaps the critical issue for genetic testing is not revealed in studies of individual level factors, but rather, is found in the social and economic context of increasingly commercialized medical care. Some of the studies reviewed in the last section of this chapter address the presence of stigma and discrimination. However, notable for their absence are system-level studies or experiments designed to test innovative reforms in the organization, financing, and management of genetic diagnostic services.

The literatures that address, in some fashion, the moral features of genetic information are, indeed, fragmented. Yet considered together, they provide a rich portrait of the challenges of the new genetic era. Empirical research documents the nature of these challenges to informed consent, to confidentiality and privacy, and to justice. In our individually oriented culture in the United States, and its market-driven medical care environment, it should come as no surprise that the bulk of the research focuses on an autonomous individual. This review suggests that we would be well served to focus research on the forces in our society that have prevented implementation of the wise cautions (e.g., Wilfond and Nolan 1993) against unregulated and commercially driven genetic testing.

NOTES

1. Grateful acknowledgment is made to Larry Churchill, Arlene Davis, Sue Estroff, Sara Hull, Nancy King, Ron Strauss, and Ben Wilfond for comments on an earlier draft of this chapter.
2. The *Encyclopedia* entry for "Genetic Testing and Screening" is twenty-six pages long and covers the following topics: (1) preimplantation diagnosis; that is, screening an embryo for genetic defects before implantation); (2) prenatal diagnosis, screening a fetus for both genetic and other defects; (3) newborn screening for conditions such as phenylketonuria (PKU), a genetic disease that can lead to severe mental retardation, but that with screening discovered in the 1960s, can be prevented with a special diet; (4) carrier screening, for people with one defective copy and one normal copy of a gene (either autosomal recessive or X-linked recessive disorders), to provide information to potential parents; (5) predictive and workplace screening, for genetic traits that might predispose exposed workers to greater risk; (6) legal issues; and (7) ethical issues. All the sections identify a common set of ethical concerns, including access to testing services, informed consent, confidentiality and privacy of genetic information, group or individual stigmatization, and the interests of third parties, including family members, employers, and insurers (Seashore 1995, 992).
3. As Larry Churchill pointed out to me, much of what I am describing is research on issues that have ethical implications, rather than research on ethics per se.
4. An exception is Hull (1999).
5. That informed consent is a popular research topic is documented in a recent annotated bibliography of close to 400 articles reporting on empirical research on informed consent (Sugarman et al. 1999).

6. This RCT is conducted by James Sorenson at University of North Carolina, under a grant funded by the Program on Ethical, Legal and Social Implications of the Human Genome Project, NIH, NHGRI.
7. See http://thomas.loc.gov.

REFERENCES

Beck, M. 1999. *Expecting Adam: The True Story of Birth, Rebirth, and Everyday Magic.* New York: Random House.

Bernhardt, B. A., G. Geller, T. Doksum, S. M. Larson, D. Roter, and N. A. Holtzman. 1998. "Prenatal Genetic Testing: Content of Discussions between Obstetric Providers and Pregnant Women." *Obstetrics and Gynecology* 91(5): 648–55.

Blumenfeld, Z., I. Blumenfeld, and M. Bronstein. 1999. "The Early Prenatal Diagnosis of Cleft Lip and the Decision Making Process." *Cleft Palate Journal* 36:105–07.

Bosk, C. L. 1992. *All God's Mistakes: Genetic Counseling in a Pediatric Hospital.* Chicago: University of Chicago Press.

Bowman, J. E. 1983. "Is a National Program to Prevent Sickle-Cell Disease Possible?" *American Journal of Pediatric Hematology-Oncology* 5(4): 367–72.

Brandt, A. 1990. "The Cigarette, Risk, and American Culture." *Daedalus* 116(4): 155–76.

Clinton, J. J. 1993. "Sickle-Cell Disease." *Journal of the American Medical Association* 270(18): 2158.

Conrad, P. 1997. "Public Eyes and Private Genes: Historical Frames, New Constructions, and Social Problems." *Social Problems* 44(2): 139–54.

———. 1999. "A Mirage of Genes," *Sociology of Health and Illness* 21(2): 228–41.

Conrad, P., and J. Gabe, eds. 1999. *Sociological Perspectives on the New Genetics.* Oxford: Blackwell Publishers.

Douglas, M., and A. Wildavsky. 1982. *Culture and Risk.* Berkeley: University of California Press.

Durfy, S. J., T. E. Buchanan, and W. Burke. 1998. "Testing for Inherited Susceptibility to Breast Cancer: A Survey of Informed Consent Forms for BRCA1 and BRCA2 Mutation Testing." *American Journal of Medical Genetics* 75(1): 82–87.

Duster, T. 1990. *Backdoor to Eugenics.* New York: Routledge.

Eng, C., C. Schechter, J. Robinowitz, G. Fulop, T. Burgert, B. Levy, R. Zimberg, and R. Desnick. 1997. "Prenatal Genetic Carrier Testing Using Triple Disease Screening." *Journal of the American Medical Association* 278(15): 1268–72.

Farfel, M. R., and N. A. Holtzman. 1984. "Education, Consent, and Counseling in Sickle-Cell Screening Programs: Report of a Survey." *American Journal of Public Health* 74(4): 373–75.

Geller, G., B. A. Bernhardt, T. Doksum, K. Helzlsouer, P. Wilcox, and N. Holtzman. 1998. "Decision Making about Breast Cancer Susceptibility Testing: How Similar Are the Attitudes of Physicians, Nurse Practitioners, and At-Risk Women?" *Journal of Clinical Oncology* 16(8): 2868–76.

Geller, G., and N. A. Holtzman. 1995. "A Qualitative Assessment of Primary Care Physicians' Perceptions about the Ethical and Social Implications of Offering Genetic Testing." *Qualitative Health Research* 5(1): 97–116.

Geller, G., M. Strauss, B. A. Bernhardt, and N. A. Holtzman. 1997. "'Decoding' Informed Consent: Insights from Women Regarding Breast Cancer Susceptibility Testing." *Hastings Center Report* 27(2): 28–33.

Giardello, F. M., J. D. Brensinger, G. M. Petersen, M. C. Luce, L. M. Hylind, J. A. Bacon, S. V. Booker, R. D. Parker, and S. R. Hamilton. 1997. "The Use and Interpretation of Commercial APC Gene Testing for Familial Adenomatous Polyposis." *New England Journal of Medicine* 336(12): 823–27.

Granda, H., S. Gispert, A. Dorticos, M. Martin, Y. Cuadras, M. Calvo, G. Martinez, M. Zayas, J. Oliva, and L. Heredero. 1991. "Cuban Programme for Prevention of Sickle-Cell Disease." *Lancet* 337:152–53.

Hacking, I. 1990. *The Taming of Chance.* Cambridge: Cambridge University Press.

Henderson, L., and J. Kitzinger. 1999. "The Human Drama of Genetics: 'Hard' and 'Soft' Media Representations of Inherited Breast Cancer." In *Sociological Perspectives on the New Genetics*, ed. P. Conrad and J. Gabe. Oxford: Blackwell Publishers, pp. 59–76.

Hill, S. A. 1994. *Managing Sickle-Cell Disease in Low-Income Families.* Philadelphia: Temple University Press.

Hiller, E., G. Landenburger, and M. Natowicz. 1997. "Public Participation in Medical Policy-Making and the Status of Consumer Autonomy: The Example of Newborn-Screening Programs in the United States." *American Journal of Public Health* 87(8): 1280–88.

Hughes, C., A. Gomez-Caminero, J. Benkendorf, J. Kerner, C. Isaacs, J. Barter, and C. Lerman. 1997. "Ethnic Differences in Knowledge and Attitudes about BRCA1 Testing in Women at Increased Risk." *Patient Education and Counseling* 32(1–2): 51–62.

Hull, S. 1999. Sickle-Cell Disease, Cystic Fibrosis, and Reproduction: A Qualitative Study of Affected Adult and Health Care Provider Perspectives. Unpublished dissertation manuscript. Baltimore, MD: Johns Hopkins University.

Lapham, V. E., C. Kozma, and J. O. Weiss. 1996. "Genetic Discrimination: Perspectives of Consumers." *Science* 274:621–24.

Lerman, C., S. Narod, K. Schulman, C. Hughes, A. Gomez-Caminero, G. Bonney, K. Gold, B. Trock, D. Main, J. Lynch, C. Fulmore, C. Snyder, S. Lemon, T. Conway, P. Tonin, C. Lenoir, and H. Lynch. 1996. "BRCA Testing in Families with Hereditary Breast-Ovarian Cancer: A Prospective Study of Patient Decision Making and Outcomes." *Journal of the American Medical Association* 275(24): 1885–92.

Lewontin, R. C. 1992. *Biology as Ideology: The Doctrine of DNA.* New York: Harper Collins.

Loeben, G. L., T. M. Marteau, and B. S. Wilfond. 1998. "Mixed Messages: Presentation of Information in Cystic Fibrosis-Screening Pamphlets." *American Journal of Human Genetics* 63(4): 1181–89.

Marteau, T. 1998. "Revealed Identity: A Study of the Process of Genetic Counseling." *Social Science and Medicine* 47(1): 1653–58.

McEwen, J., and P. Reilly. 1995. "Genetic Testing and Screening: Legal Issues." In *Encyclopedia of Bioethics*, ed. W. T. Reich. New York: Simon and Schuster Macmillan, pp. 1000–1004.

Mehlman, M. J., E. D. Kodish, P. Whitehouse, A. Zinn, S. Sollitto, J. Berger, E. Chiao, M. Dosick, and S. Cassidy. 1996. "The Need for Anonymous Genetic Counseling and Testing." *American Journal of Human Genetics* 58(2): 393–97.

Mischler, E. H., B. S. Wilfond, N. Frost, A. Laxova, C. Reiser, C. Sauer, L. Makholm, G. Shen, L. Feenan, C. McCarthy, and P. Farrell. 1998. "Cystric Fibrosis Newborn Screening: Impact on Reproductive Behavior and Implications for Genetic Screening." *Pediatrics* 102(1): 44–52.

Murray, T. H., and J. R. Botkin. 1995. "Genetic Testing and Screening: Ethical Issues." In *Encyclopedia of Bioethics*, ed. W. T. Reich. Rev. ed. New York: Simon and Schuster Macmillan, pp. 1005–11.

Neal-Cooper, F., and R. B. Scott. 1988. "Genetic Counseling in Sickle-Cell Anemia: Experiences with Couples at Risk." *Public Health Reports* 103(2): 174–78.

Nelkin, D. 1990. "Genetics and Social Policy" *Bulletin of the New York Academy of Medicine* 68(1): 135–43.

Nelkin, D., and M. S. Lindee. 1995. *The DNA Mystique: The Gene as a Cultural Icon.* New York: Freeman and Company.

Parsons, E. 1997. "Culture and Genetics: Is Genetics in Society or Society in Genetics?" In *Culture, Kinship and Genes: Toward Cross-Cultural Genetics*, ed. A. Clarke and E Parsons. New York: St. Martin's Press, Inc., pp. 245–60.

Rapp, R. 1997. "Communicating about Chromosomes: Patients, Providers, and Cultural Assumptions." *Journal of the American Medical Women's Association* 52(1): 28–29, 32.

Richards, C. S., P. A. Ward, B. B. Roa, L. Friedman, A. Boyd, G. Kuenzli, J. Dunn, and S. Plon. 1997. "Screening for 185delAG in the Ashkenazim." *American Journal of Human Genetics* 60(5): 1085–98.

Rothman, B. K. 1986. *The Tentative Pregnancy: Prenatal Diagnosis and the Future of Motherhood.* New York: Viking.

Rowley, P. T., S. Loader, C. J. Sutera, M. Walden, and A. Kozyra. 1991. "Prenatal Screening for Hemoglobinopathies: I. A Prospective Regional Trial." *American Journal of Human Genetics* 48(3): 439–46.

Seashore, M. R. 1995. "Genetic Testing and Screening: Newborn Screening." In *Encyclopedia of Bioethics*, ed. W. T. Reich. Rev. ed. New York: Simon and Schuster Macmillan, pp. 991–93.

Shafer, F. E., F. Lorey, G. C. Cunningham, C. Klumpp, E. Vichinsky, and B. Lubin. 1996. "Newborn Screening for Sickle-Cell Disease: 4 years of Experience from California's Newborn Screening Program." *Journal of Pediatric Hematology/Oncology* 18(1): 36–41.

Sorenson, J. R., B. Cheuvront, B. DeVillis, N. Callahan, L. Silverman, G. Koch, T. Sharp, and G. Fernald. 1997. "Acceptance of Home and Clinic-Based CF Carrier Education and Testing." *American Journal of Medical Genetics* 70(2): 121–29.

Sugarman, J., D. McCrory, D. Powell, Al. Krasny, B. Adams, E. Ball, and C. Cassell. 1999. "Empirical Research on Informed Consent: An Annotated Bibliography." *Hastings Center Report* Special Supplement (Jan.–Feb.): S1–42.

Weaver, K. D. 1997. "Genetic Screening and the Right Not to Know." *Issues in Law and Medicine* 13(3): 243–81.

Weiss, Rick. 1997. "Discovery of 'Jewish' Cancer Gene Raises Fears of More than Disease," *Washington Post*, 3 September, sec. A03.

Wexler, A. 1995. *Mapping Fate: A Memoir of Family, Risk, and Genetic Research.* New York: Random House.

Wexler, N. 1995. "Presymptomatic Testing for Genetic Disease." In *Classic Cases in Medical Ethics*, ed. G. E. Pence. 2nd ed. New York: McGraw-Hill, pp. 384–412.

Wilfond, B. S., and K. Nolan. 1993. "National Policy Development for the Clinical Application of Genetic Diagnostic Technologies: Lessons from Cystic Fibrosis." *Journal of the American Medical Association* 270(24): 2948–54.

Wright, S. W., M. H. Zeldin, K. Wrenn, and O. Miller. 1994. "Screening for Sickle-Cell Trait in the Emergency Department." *Journal of General Internal Medicine* 9(8): 421–24.

16

Reading the Medical Ethics Literature: A Discourse on Method

Daniel P. Sulmasy

What constitutes a good paper or book in medical ethics? This important question cannot be decided merely by whether or not one agrees with the conclusion of a paper or a book! As the previous chapters should make clear, there are many fine works in medical ethics, written by talented authors employing a wide variety of methods. The best of these works genuinely expand knowledge, expose hidden assumptions, challenge prevailing convictions, make rigorous arguments, enrich understanding, or illuminate contentious issues in fresh ways. However, frankly speaking, the medical ethics literature is also filled with chaff—often sincere chaff, but chaff nonetheless. The aim of this chapter is to provide an overview on how to read the medical ethics literature critically, separating the golden grains of wheat from the inconsequential chaff.

The many methods of medical ethics make this a very challenging task. Many readers of the literature of medical ethics do not have a background in particular research disciplines. Clinicians, for example, are often keenly interested in medical ethics, yet their training rarely equips them to read studies about ethics sensibly and critically. Many scholars in the field of medical ethics read research studies conducted by scholars in other disciplines, often examining the same questions they themselves are examining. However, they may be unfamiliar with the methods and disciplinary assumptions of these, and unsure how to apply this work to their own inquiry. The editors of medical journals are often scientists for whom any paper that does not present empirical data in numerical form is considered "opinion." They might have little experiential basis for distinguishing an editorial from a philosophical essay or a qualitative empirical study, let alone judging whether these are good or bad pieces of scholarship. In such cases, editors generally rely upon the judgments of peer reviewers. However, without sufficient background, they might even have difficulty determining who should play the role of "peer." Finally, many persons who are neither clinicians nor scholars are interested in the writings of medical ethicists. Since the issues of medical ethics affect the lives of almost everyone, all readers of the medical ethics literature have an interest in distinguishing sound bites from sound scholarship.

This chapter provides suggestions about aspects of medical ethics research that readers might want to look for in assessing the quality of scholarship in the field. If there is to be a genuinely interdisciplinary exchange in medical ethics research, readers must know at least the rudiments of how to read the work of colleagues in other disciplines critically. Otherwise, discourse about medical ethics will remain fragmented and much less helpful than it might be otherwise.

At the risk of creating a false dichotomy, the discussion is divided into two categories: humanities research and descriptive research.[1] Each category is discussed in turn.

JUDGING GOOD HUMANITIES RESEARCH IN MEDICAL ETHICS

The authors of chapters 3 though 8 all have offered some insights into what counts as good quality scholarship in their respective disciplines. Some of these are widely applicable to all the other humanities. For example, DeGrazia and Beauchamp (chapter 3) outline some of the features they believe are evidence of excellent work in philosophical medical ethics, such as (1) the importance of the topic, (2) the clarity of the writing, (3) the strength of the arguments, and (4) the novelty of the ideas presented. Other authors have delineated features of good scholarship particular to their own disciplines. For example, Amundsen (chapter 8) posits that good historical work in medical ethics should be "descriptive," not "prescriptive," and should avoid the twin fallacies of "presentism" and "essentialism."

However, it would seem that there are some features that are common to excellent humanities research in medical ethics that have not been addressed specifically in any of the previous chapters of this book. Some of these may seem obvious, but precisely because they are so obvious they may be overlooked. Others concern the ways in which scholarship in medical ethics crosses disciplinary boundaries and must therefore be addressed not in individual chapters about particular methods, but only in a chapter that surveys work in medical ethics as a whole. This first section of this chapter proposes standards by which one can be a critical reader of the humanities literature in medical ethics. This section draws upon well-established standards for essay composition (e.g., Strunk and White 1959; Crews 1974), as well as recent works on philosophical writing (Martinich 1996; Watson 1992). Even if everything proposed in this chapter is not endorsed wholeheartedly by all scholars, this chapter will provide at least a point of departure for future discussion and refinement of these standards.

Structure

The contribution of the humanities to medical ethics generally will be to make normative arguments, and normative arguments have a generally expected structure. Good normative writing usually requires a beginning, a middle, and an end; that is, an introduction stating the thesis, an argument to prove it, and a conclusion. This more or less has been the structure of a good argument since the time of Aristotle (1941). Of course, the very best writers manage to do this in such an effortless way that the underlying structure is not so apparent. But this structure will be expected by most serious readers of a normative argument, just as a clinician expects a chief complaint at the beginning of a case presentation, or a scientist expects that a description of the methods will follow the introduction to a scientific paper. Readers who fail to find such a structure will be either confused or forced to conclude that the author either is trying to hide something, or is himself confused.

Assumptions

Second, since investigations in the humanities in medical ethics are generally concerned with arguments, good writing in this field will move from premises to conclusions. Yet it is important to recognize that all of these arguments are based upon assumptions. Arguments cannot start from scratch. There is no spontaneous generation of arguments. Therefore, a well-written paper in medical ethics using the methods of the humanities will include an explicit discussion of the underlying assumptions. If the assumptions are not given directly, the critical reader will need to arrive at them inferentially after having read the whole paper. For example, philosophers often have definite theoretical orientations. They therefore should acknowledge explicitly that their analysis is utilitarian, or Rawlsian, or libertarian, or based upon some other theoretical orientation. It is difficult to evaluate a nonempirical paper critically without knowledge of the underlying assumptions and the author's theoretical orientation.

Further, as Brody (1990) has pointed out, the work is better if it also acknowledges that the assumptions of the author may not be shared by all readers, and attempts to show how other theoretical orientations might lead to similar conclusions. Quality scholarship in medical ethics is aware of and in dialogue with moral traditions other than those of the author.

Definitions

Third, medical ethics research by scholars in the humanities often makes use of technical terms, or employs ordinary words in technical ways. Good research in the humanities defines the terms used in the book or paper. This may be done up front, early in the work. Alternatively, terms may be defined as they are introduced. Critical readers will look for such definitions.

Sometimes entire arguments turn upon how the terms are defined. The informal logical fallacy of *petitio principii* ("begging the question") means that the conclusion of the argument is already contained in the premises (Copi 1982). For example, if one defines killing as morally unjustified, then defines euthanasia as killing, and then concludes that euthanasia is morally unjustified, one has "begged the question." This is a very common error in the medical ethics literature. It often goes unnoticed because the terms have not been clearly defined. The definitions are simply assumed, or are obliquely acknowledged, or are separated by long strings of additional but unnecessary premises. When the terms are defined clearly, however, the logical error becomes obvious.

The term "begging the question" itself is often misconstrued and misused. It does not mean, "this question cries out for an answer." Definitions count. This rule also applies to words or phrases like "begging the question" that proscribe the improper use of definitions.

Internal Consistency

Fourth, arguments must be internally consistent. One can disagree with an author's premises, but this does not mean that the argument is wrong, unless one can prove that the premises are wrong. Regardless of whether one agrees with the premises or the conclusion, to show that one part of an argument contradicts another is to show that the argument is invalid. Good arguments (sound arguments) are at least internally consistent.

Factual Correctness

Fifth, work in the humanities in medical ethics must not employ any factual misconceptions. It is sometimes the case that a philosophical or theological or legal argument in medical ethics is based upon misconceptions about the medical facts. This provides an easy way to refute the argument. Such a refutation can be a genuine embarrassment to the author.

In pointing to the importance of correct medical facts, however, it must be acknowledged that some medical "facts" are in dispute and open to interpretation. When this is the case, authors should be careful to consider alternative interpretations of the scientific or medical data and the ways in which this might affect the arguments, even in a work employing methods from the humanities to address issues in medical ethics.

Firm Grasp of the Literature

Sixth, what DeGrazia and Beauchamp (chapter 3) say about philosophical medical ethics is true of all the humanities research in medical ethics: the author should demonstrate a firm grasp of the relevant literature. This often is demonstrated by citation of these other works, but citation alone does not suffice to establish either that the author has truly grasped this literature, or that the author has been able to situate his or her work within this wider discourse. Sometimes, particularly in medical journals, authors seem to feel that since they have no "data," they must prove that they have read dozens, even hundreds of books and papers in preparing their own essay by citing all of these works. One should be cautious about such essays. Citing 150 books and papers can be a poor substitute for demonstrating the type of genuine grasp of the relevant literature that is necessary to make a good nonempirical argument. Sometimes, for example, whole books are cited in support of very specific points, yet the relevant page number may not be included in the citation. Quite often, authors engage in what has been dubbed "proof-texting," plucking isolated quotes out of the context of the larger body of works of a classical or renowned scholar in order to claim an authority in support of the author's own thesis. Sometimes, it seems as if the author has only read the online abstract of a work, yet has cited the entire paper or book. While this practice is almost always inappropriate, in looking for *medical facts* one sometimes can "cut corners" this way without serious damage to one's work. However, this is not the case in the humanities. The arguments made in the humanities are usually too complex and too subtle, and need to be read and understood before they can be cited properly. The point is that a good essay in casuistry or history or theology or law, for example, must demonstrate either a grasp of the subtleties of the extant literature or a profound, sweeping, "for-est-for-the-trees" interpretation of this literature as an integrated body of work. Otherwise, it is not very good scholarship.

Counterarguments

Seventh, it is important to be sure that the authors of a humanities work in medical ethics have considered counterarguments. Good investigators know that others may dis-agree with them, or have differing arguments. These arguments must be weighed carefully, and major objections to the author's own position ought to be considered and addressed in a nonempirical paper. Works that do this well are stronger works. One should be wary, however, of counterarguments that unfairly represent the position of those who hold the opposite view, or present only the weakest sort of counterarguments that no serious oppo-nent would endorse. These weak counterarguments are called "straw man" arguments. One should be vigilant for these arguments as a critical reader of humanities studies in medical ethics.

JUDGING GOOD DESCRIPTIVE RESEARCH IN MEDICAL ETHICS

Chapters 9 through 13 describe many of the empirical methods used in descriptive medical ethics. Obviously, some studies in descriptive medical ethics are better than others. The authors of these chapters on empirical methods have described in detail how to con-duct excellent studies in descriptive ethics. But what should a reader of the medical ethics literature look for in attempting to separate the wheat from the chaff in these fields?

As the chapters in this volume make clear, descriptive medical ethics is remarkably multidisciplinary. Each of a multitude of disciplines contributes a set of methods and crite-ria for scholarly excellence. These methods are applied to the investigation of moral ques-tions and are to be judged according to the criteria for scholarly excellence proper to the dis-cipline. The methods may be quantitative or qualitative. They may be unique to a particular discipline or shared by several. They may be high tech or low tech. But the work that results is to be judged according to how well it meets the criteria for scholarly excellence established for studies in its discipline. Thus, one judges an anthropological study in medi-cal ethics according to the standards of the discipline of anthropology and an economic study according to the standards of the discipline of economics.

One factor complicates this situation tremendously. What draws all these scholars together is a common interest in the study of moral questions in medical practice. Medical ethics is a single field of inquiry, studied by many empirical disciplines, using a variety of methods. Yet, no single scholar is capable of mastering all of these various disciplines, each with its own proper methods, technical vocabulary, and standards. Thus, it is critical that these scholars be able to communicate their research in a way that emphasizes the rigors that are proper to their own disciplines, but in a manner that is accessible to a very diverse audi-ence. Since such communication skills are difficult to cultivate, this can be extremely challenging. Scholars in medical ethics should make an effort to understand the rudiments of the methods of the numerous other disciplines that contribute to this field. But no one can be the master of all of these various trades. The onus really falls upon each scholar to communicate research results in jargon-free language without sacrificing the scholarly rigors of the field. This makes the multidisciplinary character of descriptive medical ethics research very challenging.

Qualitative Research

Many topics in medical ethics are not readily amenable to quantitative research using surveys that consist of closed-ended questions with multiple choice answers. Such a survey is appropriate when the researchers have a sufficient level of understanding of the research population that they can create a range of responses that will capture the opinions of the respondents. However, making such an assumption in the case of medical ethics could be presumptuous. This is one of the main reasons that researchers in descriptive ethics have begun increasingly to turn to qualitative methods.

Qualitative research does not simply consist of a group of well-intentioned researchers devising a few open-ended questions and then presenting their interpretation of the responses. Careful readers will want to be sure that the research has been conducted according to the standards of excellence delineated by Hull, Taylor, and Kass in chapter 9, and Marshall and Koenig in chapter 10. Such readers will look for evidence that the authors have used appropriate methods, such as observational studies, ethnographic interviews, focus groups, and delphi panels.

Observational Studies

The authors of qualitative studies in medical ethics that are based on observation should clarify whether they have used direct observation, or participant-observer techniques, as distinguished by Hull, Taylor, and Kass (chapter 9). They should specify their methods of data collection (e.g., whether they have used field notes, tape recordings, or both). They should comment on the degree of engagement by participant-observer, as described by Marshall and Koenig (chapter 10). The length of time devoted to this type of study should be specified in the report. In good studies, this time period is rather extended. For example, a report based on a weekend spent interviewing refugees in a border camp should be viewed with skepticism. Participant observation is very labor intensive. Studies that report having utilized this technique are preferred to studies that simply report anecdotal experiences or episodic observations.

Ethnographic Interviews

Ethnographic interviews are another important type of qualitative research method in medicine (Ventres and Frankel 1996). A research report of a study that used this technique and was well conducted will report whether interviews were structured or semistructured, and whether the subjects were chosen randomly, by convenience-sampling, or by key-informant methods, as Marshall and Koenig point out (chapter 10).

Good ethnographic interviews will clearly define the research question. The report of a well-conducted study will describe how the data were analyzed, using specific techniques such as saturation, triangulation, and "thick description" (chapter 9). Reports of these studies will also include frank acknowledgment of sources of bias in interpretation of the observations. Studies that include such methodological rigor can give excellent information about the actual behavior of health care professionals in settings of interest to medical ethics, or about medical ethics decision making in certain familial or cultural contexts.

Focus Groups

Focus groups are a systematic method for gathering qualitative information in a setting in which individuals are able to generate ideas by discussing a defined topic in a group setting and to respond to the remarks of others in the group (Morgan 1997). There are many opportunities to make use of such techniques in descriptive medical ethics. However, critical readers will be wary of whether such studies have conformed to the methodologic rigor described by Hull, Taylor, and Kass (chapter 9) and by Marshall and Koenig (chapter 10). Good reports should describe the focus group technique employed, and this method should be appropriate to the goals of the study. For example, the Nominal Group Technique is designed to avoid dominance by any particular member and to generate a wide variety of ideas arranged in a hierarchy of importance (Delbecq, van de Ven, and Gustafson 1975). Other kinds of focus groups can be run using techniques to achieve consensus. Like reports of good ethnographic analyses, reports of focus group research should describe the composition of the groups, who ran them, how the data were collected, and what method was used to generate themes from the data, and frankly acknowledge potential sources of bias in interpretation and steps taken to minimize this bias. Without such information, the reader should be skeptical of whether the research was well conducted.

Delphi Panels

An important semiquantitative technique not discussed in either chapter 9 or 10 is the use of delphi panels. A delphi panel is a formal method for achieving a consensus opinion among a group of experts regarding a particular topic (Delbecq, van de Ven, and Gustafson 1975). This technique is particularly useful when it is not feasible to bring the members of the group together in a single, face-to-face session. Experts are asked to respond to a question, rank their answers, and explain their answers in a written fashion. The responses are collated, kept anonymous, and circulated among the group through a series of iterations until consensus is reached. Sometimes, this technique is used to provide information that is fed into formal decision analyses (see chapter 13).

Quantitative Methods

Survey Research

In chapter 11, Pearlman and Starks describe how excellent survey research should be conducted in medical ethics. Since survey research is probably the most common type of research technique in descriptive medical ethics (see chapter 2), anyone interested in medical ethics should know the rudiments of how to read a report of a medical ethics survey in a careful, critical fashion. Surveys serve good purposes, pointing out both areas of disagreement and interesting associations between particular opinions and certain characteristics of the population under study. More sophisticated survey instruments try to elicit more basic underlying attitudes, psychological tendencies, cultural norms, or stages of moral development.

Careful readers ought to remember that while simple opinion surveys can be very important in identifying ethical controversies, the best studies do more than simply ask a few questions and count up the answers. In assessing the quality of descriptive ethics research using surveys, critical readers should expect that the authors will state clearly that they have designed the study according to the sorts of standards outlined by Pearlman and Starks (chapter 11). The authors of a research study should indicate the hypotheses that led them to design the survey. Questions should avoid framing bias (i.e., phrasing a question in such a way as to influence the response). Ideally, the exact wording of the most important question in the study should be reported in the paper, so that readers can judge for themselves whether the question was properly constructed. There should be some evidence that the questions validly reflect the information being sought. Better studies will report having done this by actual testing for face validity, criterion validity, and/or construct validity, as described in chapter 11. There should also be some mention that the questions were pilot tested before the actual survey was completed.

The main outcome variable in a survey tends to be more valid if it is a scale based on several questions than if it is a single item on a survey (Neuman 1994). This is especially important if the researchers are trying to examine deep underlying attitudes, cultural norms, psychological tendencies, or stages of moral reasoning. As Pearlman and Starks discuss, these scales need to be checked for internal consistency. Research reports should indicate this using appropriate statistical tests such as Cronbach's α.

Certain factors that are often of interest in descriptive ethics research have been studied extensively by multiple other investigators who have developed valid and reliable instruments. Thus, there is generally no need for researchers to create new instruments to measure anxiety, depression, dementia, confusion, functional status, severity of illness, or quality of life. There are plenty of scales available to measure such factors. One should be wary of studies that include idiosyncratic measures of well-studied factors such as dementia, and even more wary of studies that report on such complex phenomena on the basis of single questions rather than scales.

Of course, there may be valid reasons for descriptive ethics researchers to develop their own scales for such factors in particular circumstances, but the justification for doing so should be stated clearly. For example, there could be *a priori* reasons to suspect that severity-of-illness scales developed for unselected patients might differ from severity-of-illness scales for patients suffering from chronic, terminal conditions, leading researchers to develop and validate their own instruments particular to a group of patients who generate considerable ethical interest (Knaus et al. 1995).

Basic demographic characteristics of the respondents also should be presented in a good survey report. Response rates should be adequate (generally about 70 percent or more for patients, nurses, house officers, or students, and about 50 percent or more for practicing physicians). Some reporting on the characteristics of nonrespondents should be given to help to support the contention that there has been little response bias.

Survey research in descriptive ethics can be very helpful and very interesting, but there must be clear evidence in the research reports that the survey has been carefully constructed, administered, analyzed, and interpreted.

Experimental Methods

The ability to introduce the experimental method into medical ethics could, as Thomasma (1985) has put it, only enhance the field. Critical readers will want to be sure they know when experimental methods are appropriate in medical ethics. As described in detail by Danis, Hanson, and Garrett (chapter 12), experimental methods are best employed when ethical or legal theory has proposed a normative standard and one wishes to test whether or not that standard can be met in actual clinical practice. A program designed to promote a particular clinical behavior deemed morally praiseworthy (e.g., better informed-consent practices) or designed to educate clinicians about a new law or about ethics in general can be tested by a controlled trial. As pointed out in chapter 12, all of the rigorous standards appropriate to the conduct of excellent randomized clinical trials in any field of medicine should be applied to the assessment of the quality of randomized clinical trials in medical ethics (Meinert 1986).

The Analysis of Quantitative Data

Analysis of data in reports of research in descriptive ethics should follow standard procedures for statistical testing, as detailed in chapter 12. Readers who are unfamiliar with statistics, but skeptical about a finding, can ask colleagues who are skilled in this area to review the research report.

Readers should be particularly careful in evaluating studies that present correlations. Correlations between outcome variables and sociodemographic, clinical, or other respondent characteristics should be reported in a manner that takes into account multiple associations, using, for example, multivariable regression models (Concato, Feinstein, and Holford 1993). There should be adequate numbers of events so that any regression model reported is neither underfitted (too few events to detect important associations) nor overfitted (too many subjects with too few events). Correlations are not sufficient to infer causation, and authors should be very careful not to imply that this is so.

An additional issue is the difference between statistical significance and clinical or moral importance. For example, if one has 10,000 study subjects and wants to investigate factors associated with responses to a single question—e.g., Do you want to be resuscitated?—even the patient's shoe size might randomly show a statistically significant association. In these cases, researchers bear important responsibility for justifying the sample size and for sorting out the important variables.

Subgroup analyses should reflect genuine preconceived hypotheses or be acknowledged explicitly as an exercise in hypothesis generation. "Data dredging" for statistically significant results is all too common and should be avoided. If the study was not designed to compare subgroups, such analysis may be misleading.

Interpretation of the data should scrupulously avoid normative conclusions. It may be interesting, for example, if one were to discover that 75 percent of physicians do not believe they are bound by the precepts of the Hippocratic Oath. It would be inappropriate, however, to suggest that this means that the Hippocratic Oath should no longer be considered normative for medical practice. That may or may not be the case, depending upon the strength of various normative arguments.

Theoretical Framework

Empirical research in sociology, anthropology, and psychology is often judged on the basis of whether or not it specifies a particular theoretical framework. This will be true as well of empirical research in medical ethics that is approached from any of these disciplines. But while this is a necessary ingredient for the highest-quality research in descriptive ethics, it is not sufficient. Excellent descriptive research in medical ethics will not only specify the theoretical framework particular to the empirical discipline, it will also explicitly designate the ethical theory that undergirds the research. So, for example, a study on end-of-life decision making that employs a willingness-to-pay utility analysis and also acknowledges specifically that the moral theory undergirding the study is preference-based utilitarianism is superior to a study in which the authors do not appear to understand whether or not they are operating within the framework of any particular theory of ethics (see chapter 13).

As Brody (1993) has pointed out, even in the absence of a specifically acknowledged theoretical orientation, the investigators must be able to conceptualize the question from an ethical perspective in order to conduct solid projects in descriptive ethics. Failure to conceptualize the research adequately from an ethical point of view will make the study less ethically illuminating.

Detached Disinterest

These concerns about the quality of descriptive studies in medical ethics are important for all readers of the medical ethics literature, not just ethicists. Some studies will be published because they appear to support a particular point of view, regardless of their quality. Especially in ethics, a more detached and disinterested spirit would ideally be expected, but this does not always obtain in reality. Whether reviewers, editors, or readers agree with the position that appears to be supported by the study should not influence the decision to publish. If an editor or reviewer has a particular viewpoint regarding an issue, it should not be necessary that a paper persuade the editor or reviewer to change his or her mind on the issue in order for the paper to be deemed publishable. It pays to recall that no descriptive study ever answers a normative question. One should be more concerned about whether the results are of intrinsic interest, whether the study answers an empirical question relevant to a normative argument, or whether the study adequately tests the implementation of a normative standard. These studies should make no claims to answer any normative questions. Regardless of one's normative position on the issue under study, one should support quality in descriptive research.

CONCLUDING COMMENTS

In this chapter, I have tried to outline some of the indicators of quality scholarship in medical ethics, emphasizing that these quality indicators are largely those of the methods and disciplines that are being employed. Nonetheless, there are also some indicators of quality that are common to many methods and disciplines within the broad categories of the "humanities" and "descriptive research." Where possible, these factors have been delineated in the hope that this chapter will help ethicists, clinicians, journal editors, students, and lay readers to become more careful, critical readers of the vast literature of medical ethics.

NOTE

1. The term "humanities" is used despite its awkwardness. The methods employed by the disciplines represented in chapters 3 through 8 all seem to fit together and to be distinguishable from the empirical methods and disciplines presented in chapters 9 through 13. However, labeling these methods is not easy. On the one hand, it is not quite proper to call law or history or a casuistic discussion of actual case studies either "nonempirical" or "nondescriptive." On the other hand, it would not be proper to call such studies "theoretical," either. Historical studies also should not be labeled "normative," even though law and casuistry, as well as philosophy and theology, might make normative arguments. So, it seems that the term "humanities" best covers these methods and disciplines, and distinguishes them from those in chapters 9 through 13. Admittedly, "humanities" may be too inclusive, implying the inclusion of literature, the arts, and architecture—fields that might enhance discussions of medical ethics but might not properly be said to constitute research in medical ethics. But the word at least includes what we want it to include, and excludes the chapters we want it to exclude. In a multidisciplinary field like medical ethics, achieving even this much clarity seems sufficient.

REFERENCES

Aristotle. 1941. "Rhetoric." In *The Basic Works of Aristotle,* Richard McKeon, ed. New York: Random House, pp. 1325–1454.

Brody, B. A. 1990. "The Quality of Scholarship in Bioethics." *The Journal of Medicine and Philosophy* 15:161–78.

———. 1993."Assessing Empirical Research in Bioethics." *Theoretical Medicine* 14: 211–19.

Concato, J., A. R. Feinstein, and T. R. Holford. 1993. "The Risk of Determining Risk with Multivariable Models." *Annals of Internal Medicine* 118:201–10.

Copi, I. M. 1982. *Introduction to Logic.* 6th ed. New York: Macmillan, pp. 107–08.

Crews, F. 1974. *The Random House Handbook.* New York: Random House.

Delbecq, A. L., A. H. van de Ven, and D. H. Gustafson. 1975. *Group Techniques for Program Planning: A Guide to Nominal Group and Delphi Processes.* Middleton, WI: Green Briar Press.

Knaus, W. A., F. E. Harrell, J. Lynn, L. Goldman, R. S. Phillips, A. F. Connors, N. V. Dawson, W. J. Fulkerson, R. M. Califf, and N. Desbiens. 1995. "The SUPPORT Prognostic Model: Objective Estimates of Survival for Seriously Ill Hospitalized Adults." *Annals of Internal Medicine* 122:191–203.

Martinich, A. P. 1996. *Philosophical Writing: An Introduction.* 2nd ed. Oxford: Blackwell Publishing.

Meinert, C. L. 1986. *Clinical Trials.* New York: Oxford University Press.

Morgan, D .L. 1997. *Focus Groups as Qualitative Research.* 2nd ed. Thousand Oaks, CA: Sage Publications.

Neuman, W. L. 1994. *Social Science Methods: Qualitative and Quantitative Methods.* 2nd ed. Boston: Allyn and Bacon, pp. 227–69.

Strunk, W., and E. B. White. 1959. *The Elements of Style.* New York: Macmillan, 1959.

Thomasma, D. C. 1985. "Empirical Methodology in Medical Ethics." *Journal of the American Geriatric Society* 33:313–14.

Ventres, W. B., and R. M. Frankel. 1996. "Ethnography: A Stepwise Approach for Primary Care Researchers." *Family Medicine* 28:52–56.

Watson, R. A. 1992. *Writing Philosophy: A Guide to Professional Writing and Publishing.* Carbondale, IL: University of Illinois Press.

Index